MW00835252

TRACE ELEMENTS AND IRON IN HUMAN METABOLISM

TOPICS IN HEMATOLOGY

Series Editor: Maxwell M. Wintrobe, M.D.
University of Utah, Salt Lake City

THE RESPIRATORY FUNCTIONS OF BLOOD
Lars Garby, M.D. and Jerry Meldon, M.D.

HEMOLYTIC ANEMIA IN DISORDERS OF RED CELL METABOLISM
Ernest Beutler, M.D.

TRACE ELEMENTS AND IRON IN HUMAN METABOLISM
Ananda S. Prasad, M.D., Ph.D.

TRACE ELEMENTS AND IRON IN HUMAN METABOLISM

Ananda S. Prasad, M.D., Ph.D.

Wayne State University School of Medicine
and Department of Medicine, Harper-Grace Hospital
Detroit, Michigan

and

Veterans Administration Hospital
Allen Park, Michigan

PLENUM MEDICAL BOOK COMPANY · New York and London

Library of Congress Cataloging in Publication Data

Prasad, Ananda Shiva.
Trace elements and iron in human metabolism.

(Topics in hematology)
Includes bibliographies and index.
1. Trace element metabolism. 2. Iron metabolism. I. Title. II. Series. [DNLM: 1. Trace Elements – Metabolism. 2. Iron – Metabolism. QU130.3 P911t]
QP534.P7 612′.3924 78-13446
ISBN 0-306-31142-9

227 West 17th Street, New York, N.Y. 10011

Plenum Medical Book Company is an imprint of Plenum Publishing Corporation

Printed in the United States of America

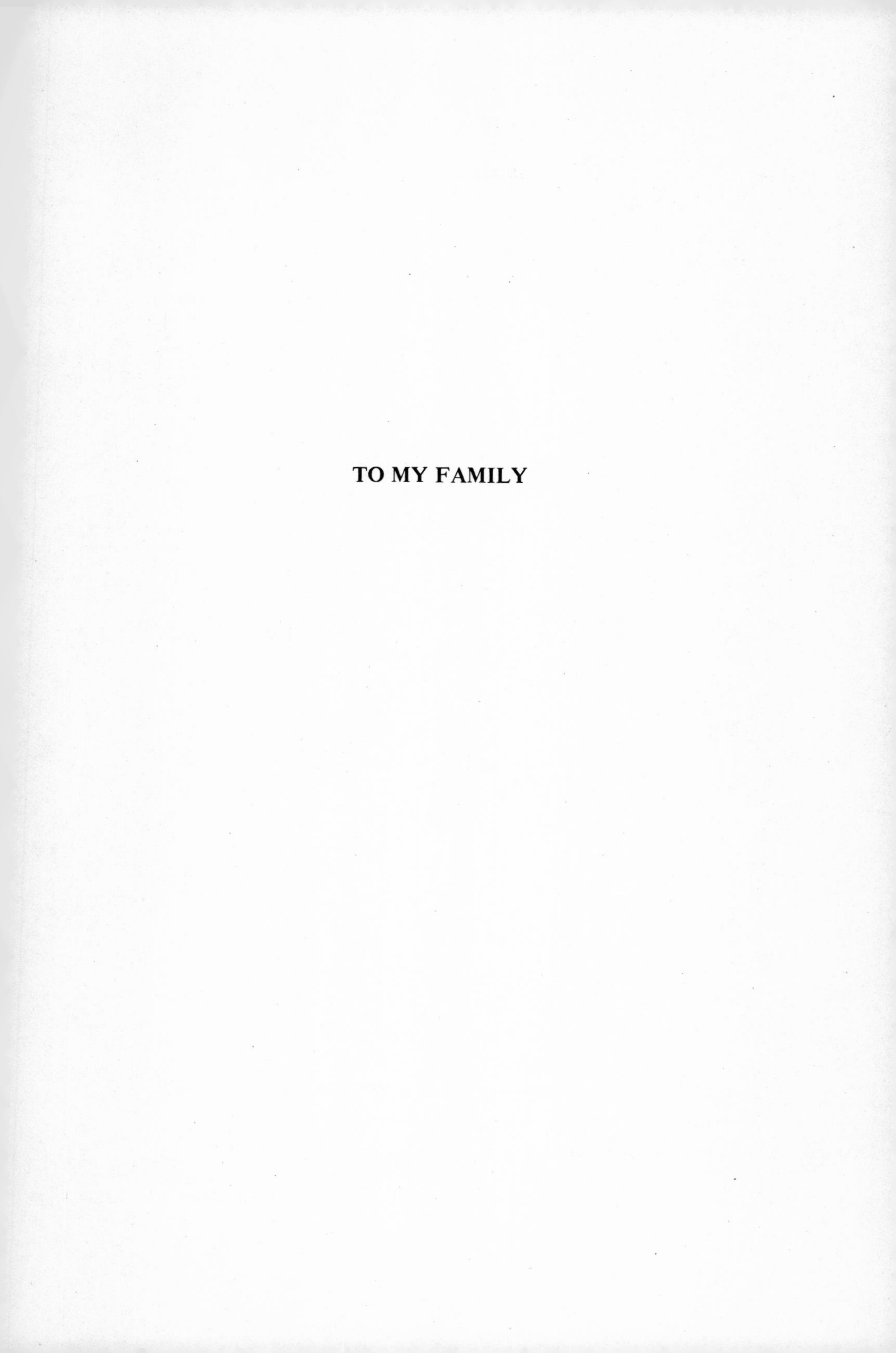

TO MY FAMILY

FOREWORD

Each year, it becomes more apparent that trace elements play an important role in human metabolism. The concept is no longer new. The literature on the subject is voluminous.

Dr. Prasad, who has been interested in this field for many years, has undertaken the enormous task of bringing our knowledge together in a comprehensive fashion. This monograph should prove very informative and extremely useful to everyone who is concerned with human disease and with the maintenance of good health. His coverage of the subject is broad. Because of the importance of iron, in addition to ''trace'' elements, in human metabolism and nutrition, a chapter dealing with iron has been included.

Maxwell M. Wintrobe, M.D.

PREFACE

It has been known for several decades that many elements are present in living tissues, but it was not possible to measure their precise concentrations until recently. They were therefore referred to as occurring in "trace" amounts, and this practice led to the use of the term "trace elements." Although techniques now available are such that virtually all trace elements can be determined with reasonable accuracy, the designation "trace elements" remains in popular usage.

During the past two decades, remarkable advances have taken place in the field of trace-element research. Although deficiencies of iron and iodine in man have been known for many years, it is only recently that the essentiality of zinc and copper in human metabolism and nutrition has been recognized. Thirty-five years ago, carbonic anhydrase was recognized to be the only enzyme requiring zinc, but now there are approximately seventy related metalloenzymes known for which zinc is needed. The essential role of zinc in growth and development and its basic role in deoxyribonucleic acid (DNA) synthesis have been established only in the past decade.

Recent developments demonstrate that zinc therapy may have a widespread role in various disease processes associated with conditioned deficiency of zinc. Indeed, zinc therapy for patients with acrodermatitis enteropathica has now become a lifesaving measure. It is also becoming clear that besides nutritional deficiency of zinc, conditioned deficiency of this element due to several disease states is probably not uncommon. Awareness of this possibility is likely to uncover many other clinical conditions in which zinc therapy may prove to be beneficial.

Zinc appears to have a fundamental anticalcium action at the cell-membrane level. This mechanism could account for the inhibitory action of zinc on a number of cells, including inflammatory cells and platelets. If this is true, zinc may have potential as an antiinflammatory agent in a variety of diseases, one of which would be rheumatoid arthritis.

The essential role of copper in collagen synthesis, the role of chromium in glucose tolerance factor, the presence of selenium as an integral part of the enzyme glutathione peroxidase of human red cells, and the important role of manganese in the metabolism of cartilage clearly suggest that these elements have vital functions to perform in human metabolism. A proper understanding of their biochemical roles and the application of such knowledge to human diseases could predictably have a great impact on the future practice of medicine.

In this book, all elements known to be essential for man, such as iron, iodine, zinc, copper, manganese, selenium, chromium, and fluoride, with the exception of cobalt, have been included. The only known function of cobalt in man appears to be related to its presence in the vitamin B_{12} molecule. For this reason, this element is not discussed. A short discussion on the role of newer trace elements has been included, inasmuch as future research may implicate these elements in human health and disease. Although magnesium is usually not considered to be a trace element, its biochemical role in enzymatic functions is similar to that of other trace elements. For this reason, it has been included here.

A considerable number of essential trace elements occupy positions in the periodic table between atomic numbers 23 and 34. This atomic-number interval includes two elements, gallium and germanium, for which no vital roles have been described so far. Future studies may uncover essential functions for these two elements.

Toxic elements important for man, such as cadmium, lead, and mercury, are also covered in this book. Recent studies indicate that the toxicity of cadmium and lead may be due to their adverse effects on zinc metalloenzymes. The toxicity of mercury may be diminished by supplementation with selenium in experimental animals. These observations emphasize the interactions of various elements and suggest possible means by which the toxicity of certain metals may be ameliorated. Competition for similar binding sites between zinc and copper, iron and copper, and iron and manganese is a well-known phenomenon. A thorough knowledge of these interactions may provide yet another means by which storage disorders such as Wilson's disease and hemochromatosis may be managed in the future. It is important, however, that one look at these leads very critically and not be indiscriminate in the medical usage of various trace elements in disease conditions.

Physicians, biochemists, nutritionists, and medical researchers should find this book useful, inasmuch as standard textbooks, generally speaking, have thus far not focused on these newer developments in the field of trace elements. It is hoped that an awareness of the metabolic functions of trace elements may lead to better management of some of the diseases associated with their abnormalities.

I wish to thank Dr. Maxwell M. Wintrobe for his helpful suggestions. Ms. Karen Harrington, Clare Giska, Emily Quigley, and Maha Fakhouri provided secretarial help for which I am very grateful. I also wish to thank Doug Door, who checked many references in the library.

CONTENTS

ESSENTIAL ELEMENTS

1. CHROMIUM

2. COPPER

3. FLUORIDE

4. IODINE

5. IRON

6. MAGNESIUM

7. MANGANESE

8. NEWER TRACE ELEMENTS

9. SELENIUM

10. ZINC

TOXIC ELEMENTS

11. CADMIUM

12. LEAD

13. MERCURY

ESSENTIAL ELEMENTS

CHAPTER 1

CHROMIUM

INTRODUCTION

In 1957, Schwarz and Mertz (1957) observed impaired glucose tolerance in rats fed certain diets and postulated that the condition was due to a deficiency of a new dietary agent, designated the glucose tolerance factor (GTF). Later, it was shown that chromium is an integral and active part of GTF, the exact structure of which is not well understood, but is believed to contain two nicotinic acid molecules per chromium atom and possibly contains cysteine, glycine, and even glutamic acid residues.

Deficiency of chromium in experimental animals has been induced and shown to impair glucose tolerance. Recent evidence indicates that deficiency of chromium does occur in some human subjects, presumably due to inadequate intake or poor availability, or both, of this element.

In some foods, refining processes may reduce the content of chromium. Examples of this reduction may be sugar and flour (Czerniejewski *et al.*, 1964; Schroeder, 1968, 1971; Schroeder *et al.*, 1970). In sugar refining, the chromium is concentrated in the molasses fraction, with refined sugar containing less than one tenth the concentration of chromium in molasses (i.e., refined sugar 0.08 μg/g vs. molasses 1.2 μg/g). The geograaphical source of the sugar cane influences the concentration of chromium (i.e., Virgin Islands 0.07 μg/g vs.Colombia, South America, 0.35 μg/g). In the milling of wheat, whole wheat contained 1.75 μg/g of chromium, while white bread contained only 0.14 μg/g. More current analytical data (Schroeder, 1971) suggest that the levels reported earlier may be too high. It must be understood that the determination of chromium in foodstuffs and biological samples presents formidable problems. Differing analytical techniques, sample preparation, and possible contamination, as well as the low levels present, frequently lead to a divergence in reported values (Doisy *et al.*, 1976).

The average American diet contains only a small quantity of chromium (5–115 μg/day), which is poorly absorbed (Levine *et al.*, 1968). A high carbohydrate intake could predispose to chromium deficiency caused by an increased urinary excretion of chromium following carbohydrate loading (Doisy *et al.*, 1976; Schroeder, 1968).

BIOCHEMISTRY

There is no known role for chromium other than in the form of GTF. Various studies have shown some responses to chromium in certain enzyme systems and pathways (Mertz, 1967, 1969). A high concentration of chromium in isolated nucleic acids was noted by Wacker and Vallee (1959).

Trivalent chromium as an integral part of GTF was reported by Schwarz and Mertz (1959). Oral administration of GTF restored impaired glucose tolerance in chromium-deficient animals to normal. Studies *in vitro* suggest that GTF is required for a maximal response to insulin in insulin-sensitive tissues (Mertz, 1969). GTF was concentrated from brewer's yeast, and liver and kidney were recognized to be other rich sources. GTF is an organic, heat-stable, low-molecular-weight complex that contains trivalent chromium.

More recently, Mertz (1974) has prepared biologically active chromium complexes that appear similar to but not identical with the naturally occurring GTF complex. The exact structure(s) remains unknown. Apparently the complex contains two nicotinic acid molecules per chromium atom and might contain cysteine, glycine, and possibly glutamic acid residues. The amino acids may be needed only to convert the complex to a more water-soluble derivative, and the biological activity could be due to the chromium and nicotinic acid in a unique coordination complex (Doisy *et al.*, 1976).

It is believed that GTF and insulin interact to form a complex, and it has been postulated that GTF is required to bind insulin to the cell surface through exposed sulfhydryl groups. The site and synthetic pathway for GTF remain unknown at present.

METABOLISM

CHROMIUM CONTENT OF THE DIET

Results of analyses of various foodstuffs have been reported by many researchers (Schroeder *et al.*, 1962; Gormican, 1970; Maxia *et al.*, 1972; Toepfer *et al.*, 1973), and there are few foodstuffs with appreciable amounts of chromium. In general, spices have the highest concentrations, with lesser amounts in meats, vegetables, and fruits (exceptions are liver and kidney). Usually, the use of spices is based primarily on personal preference and nationality. Determination of the chromium content of foodstuffs gives only limited information regarding dietary adequacy. Availability of the chromium for absorption, and the amount in the form of GTF, are important considerations (Doisy *et al.*, 1976).

In an exhaustive study, Toepfer *et al.* (1973) attempted to correlate the chromium content and GTF avtivity of different foodstuffs. Concerning relative biological values for GTF activity, the following data were obtained: brewer's yeast, 44.88; black pepper, 10.21; calf's liver, 4.52; chicken leg muscle, 1.89; haddock, 1.86; patent flour, 1.86; and skim milk, 1.59. Obviously, a marked variability occurs in the biologically active chromium in natural foodstuffs. Additional work is needed in this area before one can recommend a diet that would supply adequate chromium or GTF. Mertz (1971) tentatively suggested a daily intake of 10–30 μg of GTF-chromium per day to be adequate to meet the daily requirement of man.

It must be considered that stainless steel cooking ware may contribute chromium to the diet if acidic foodstuffs are prepared. Stainless steel is high in chromium content, and this chromium has been found to leach out during the cooking process (Doisy *et al.*, 1976; Schroeder *et al.*, 1962).

CHROMIUM IN DRINKING WATER

Analyses of drinking water in the United States by Durfor and Becker (1964) revealed that water supplies provide only small quantities of chromium. The mean chromium content in 100 selected cities was 0.43 ng/ml, with the range being from nondetectable to 35 ng/ml. The city of Milwaukee, Wisconsin, had water with the highest observed chromium level, although it has since been retested and is no longer high. Water treatment and purification methods can add or remove chromium, depending on the purification processes (Doisy *et al.*, 1976).

ABSORPTION, TRANSPORT, AND EXCRETION OF CHROMIUM

At this time, little work has been done concerning intestinal absorption of chromium in man. Animal studies have suggested that chromium is absorbed in the upper small intestines (Doisy *et al.*, 1976; Donaldson and Barreras, 1966).

Absorption of Chromium

In man and animals, inorganic trivalent chromium salts are poorly absorbed. Chromates are better absorbed, although the preferred valence state for chromium is 3+, and it is likely that any chromates present in the diet are reduced from 6+ to 3+ valence in the gastrointestinal tract (Doisy *et al.*, 1976).

Using labeled ^{51}Cr as chromic chloride, it was reported that only 0.69% of an orally administered dose was absorbed by human subjects (Doisy *et al.*, 1968). This finding is in agreement with the value of 0.5% reported by Donaldson and Barreras (1966). Absorption in elderly subjects did not differ significantly from that in young normal adults (Doisy *et al.*, 1971). Decreased ability to absorb chromium with age therefore does not appear to be the reason for the decreased tissue chromium concentrations with age (Doisy *et al.*, 1976).

The only group of people studied to date who display an abnormal rate of chromium absorption are insulin-requiring diabetics (Doisy *et al.*, 1976). Within the first 24 hr following a single oral dose of chromium, insulin-requiring diabetics (in contrast to maturity-onset diabetics) absorb 2–4 times more chromium than do normal subjects. Paralleling the increased rate of absorption is an increased urinary excretion of chromium. It is tentatively theorized that insulin-requiring diabetics are chromium-deficient and develop an adaptive increase in absorption to help offset the deficiency. Moreover, if insulin-requiring diabetics are given $^{51}CrCl_3$ intravenously, they show an increased urinary excretion in comparison with normal subjects. Therefore, diabetics may not be able to utilize chromium in a normal manner. Morgan (1972) reported that the hepatic chromium content in diabetic autopsy material was 8 μg/g of ash in comparison with 12 μg/g for control subjects. These values are higher than those reported by Schroeder *et al.* (1962); however, Morgan states that background corrections were not made. Hambidge *et al.* (1968) observed that insulin-requiring diabetic children have lower levels of hair chromium than normal children. The average values for the former and latter were, respectively, 0.56 and 0.85 μg/g. It is interesting to note that both diabetic liver and hair concentrations of chromium are proportionately decreased, i.e., by 33% (Doisy *et al.*, 1976).

Transport of Chromium

On the basis of studies by Hopkins and Schwarz (1964), it appears that at least two forms of chromium circulate in the plasma compartment. Some chromium is bound to transferrin (siderophilin) in the β-globulin fraction and is thought to be trivalent chromium. The other form is presumed to be GTF-bound chromium, although definite studies on this point have not been done.

Previous reports by Glinsmann *et al.* (1966) and Levine *et al.* (1968) suggested an increase in serum chromium levels following glucose or insulin administration. With recent advances in atomic absorption techniques, it now seems that the serum chromium values in those earlier reports were too high by a factor of 20- to 40-fold (Doisy *et al.*, 1976).

Current analytical techniques used by a number of investigators suggest that serum or plasma chromium levels in normal subjects in the United States are in the range of 1–5 ng/ml. It appears that a rise in serum chromium levels following oral glucose loading is not a prerequisite to normal glucose tolerance. Pekarek *et al.* (1973a,b) showed that during an induced infectious disease, serum chromium levels declined and glucose tolerance became impaired. On the other hand, intravenous administration of glucose or insulin seems to produce a rapid decline in serum chromium concentration in normal subjects (Davidson and Burt, 1973; Burt and Davidson, 1973).

Placental Transport

Reports by Mertz and Roginski (1971) suggest that inorganic chromium does not cross the placenta to any significant extent, whereas chromium in the form of GTF is readily transported. The ^{51}Cr-labeled GTF seems to be concentrated primarily in the fetal liver. Schroeder *et al.* (1962) observed that postpartum female rats may have nondetectable tissue chromium levels.

Impaired glucose tolerance is a common finding in pregnancy, but whether this impairment is due to GTF deficiency or not is unclear. Davidson and Burt (1973) demonstrated that pregnant women have a circulating plasma chromium level lower than the level in nonpregnant subjects of the same age (2.9 vs. 4.7 ng/ml, respectively). Hambidge (1971, 1974) observed that hair chromium concentrations of the newborn exceeded corresponding maternal hair levels (average values 974 vs. 382 ng/g), which suggested that the fetus extracts chromium from the maternal stores.

Urinary Excretion of Chromium

It appears that orally absorbed chromium is excreted mainly by the kidneys. The daily urinary excretion of chromium is 3–5 μg/24 hr (Hambidge, 1971; Davidson and Secrest, 1972; Wolf *et al.* 1974). Of this amount, it is unknown how much is inorganic chromium or GTF-chromium or both. Schroeder (1968) demonstrated that glucose loading produced an increased chromium excretion in the urine during the first 2-hr following loading. Recent data from Wolf *et al.* (1974) suggest that there is a volatile form of chromium in urine that can be lost, depending on the method of sample preparation (Doisy *et al.*, 1976). Further studies are needed to establish urinary excretion of chromium as a reliable index of chromium status in man.

CLINICAL EFFECTS OF CHROMIUM DEFICIENCY

Chromium deficiency has been induced in animals both accidentally and deliberately by feeding rations that are low in available chromium (Mertz and Schwarz, 1959; Doisy, 1963; Schroeder *et al.*, 1965; Davidson *et al.*, 1967). The hallmark of chromium deficiency is impaired glucose tolerance. In rats and squirrel monkeys maintained on chromium-deficient diets, restoration of a normal glucose tolerance was accomplished by oral administration of Cr^{3+} or GTF (Schwarz and Mertz, 1959; Davidson and Blackwell, 1968). In genetically diabetic mice in which hyperglycemia and hyperinsulinemia coexist, GTF administration, both acutely and chronically, reduced the elevated blood glucose levels to the normal range, while inorganic Cr^{3+} was ineffective. The possibility that the diabetic mice were unable to convert chromium to GTF was considered (Doisy *et al.*, 1973, 1976).

At this time, there is only indirect evidence in the literature to support the theory that chromium deficiency occurs in man. It has been reported that tissue chromium levels decline with increasing age, particularly in the United States (Schroeder *et al.*, 1962; Hambidge and Baum, 1972). Newborn and young children have tissue chromium levels higher than those in adults. Hepatic chromium concentration in children 0–10 years of age was 17.2 μg/g of ash, whereas subjects over 30 years of age had a concentration of 1–2 μg/g of ash. Cause and effect have not been demonstrated; it is possible, however, that the type and quantity of foods ingested in the United States might predispose to the observed low tissue concentrations. Decreased chromium tissue levels are compatible with, but not proof of, deficiency (Doisy *et al.*, 1976).

Maturity-onset diabetics (Glinsmann and Mertz, 1966) and middle-aged (Hopkins and Price, 1968) and elderly subjects (Levine *et al.*, 1968), all from the United States, showed improvement of impaired glucose tolerance by simple addition of 150 μg of inorganic chromium (as Cr^{3+}) to their daily diets (Doisy *et al.*, 1976).

Children in Jordan (Hopkins *et al.*, 1968) suffering from kwashiorkor, and children in Turkey suffering from protein–calorie malnutrition (Gürson and Saner, 1971, 1973), received a chromium supplement (250 μg/day) in their formula. This was followed by restoration of their intravenous glucose tolerance tests to normal (Doisy *et al.*, 1976).

Malnourished children in Egypt (Carter *et al.*, 1968) showed no beneficial response to chromium supplementation of their diets. Chemical analysis of the diets indicated that the dietary intake of chromium in Egypt was higher than elsewhere. Analysis of Egyptian hospital diets showed a mean daily intake of chromium of 129 μg/day, with a range of 76–1057 μg/day (Maxia *et al.*, 1972), in contrast to the estimated United States intake of 52 μg/day (Levine *et al.*, 1968). It must be noted that obviously there are many causes for impaired glucose tolerance, e.g., intercurrent infection, emotional stress, and antecedent diet, but that only in chromium-deficient subjects would one expect to observe a beneficial response with chromium supplementation (unless the response is a pharmacological one). An increasing body of evidence, based primarily on improved glucose tolerance tests after chromium supplementation, suggests that chromium deficiency does occur in man, most likely due to inadequate intake (Doisy *et al.*, 1976).

Jeejeebhoy *et al.* (1977) recently reported the occurrence of severe chromium deficiency in a female patient on total parenteral nutrition for more than 5 years. The infusion, although adequate in other essential nutrients, contained only 8 μg/day of chromium. The patient exhibited weight loss, impaired glucose tolerance, decreased respiratory quotient, peripheral neuropathy, negative nitrogen balance, low blood and hair chromium levels, and negative chromium balance. All these abnormalities were corrected by intravenous administration of 250 μg of chromium per day for 2 weeks.

BIOLOGICAL EFFECTS OF GTF SUPPLEMENTATION OF THE DIET

Normal and Elderly Subjects

Serum Insulin Response. In mammalian systems, the function of GTF is slowly starting to unfold. As reported earlier, chromium, in the form of GTF, seems to act in concert with insulin and thereby help dispose of ingested carbohydrate. GTF seems to be active only in the presence of insulin. Subjects with impaired glucose tolerance tests (GTTs), caused by inadequate GTF or chromium, respond to diet supplementation with a return to normal tolerance and a reduction in the amount of endogenous insulin released (Doisy *et al.*, 1976).

Young subjects (20–25 years of age) having GTTs within normal limits show a reduction in endogenous insulin output during the GTTs following GTF supplementation. Plasma glucose levels during the tests are unchanged, but while the subjects are on the GTF-containing supplement, decreased insulin levels are needed to maintain normal glucose tolerance. This finding might be interpreted to mean that even in "normal" subjects, the dietary intake of chromium (or GTF) is marginal (Doisy *et al.*, 1976).

If insulin determinations from various laboratories may be compared directly, then the following conclusions might be reached. Following oral glucose loading, the peak insulin response is lowest and appears most rapidly (30 min) in childhood. Young adults show intermediate responses, whereas middle-aged and elderly subjects have higher and the most delayed peaks. The magnitude of the insulin response seems to be inversely correlated with tissue chromium levels (Doisy *et al.*, 1976). The older the subjects tested, the lower the chromium content of their tissues and the greater their insulin response to a glucose load. It may be that the body stores of chromium influence the magnitude of the insulin response during GTTs (Doisy *et al.*, 1976).

Serum Lipid Levels. In addition to the reduction in insulin levels, some subjects with impaired GTTs also demonstrate a reduction in the fasting serum cholesterol and triglyceride levels while on the GTF supplement (Doisy *et al.*, 1976). Fasting serum cholesterol levels in the young normal subjects reveal a mean decrease of 36 mg/dl after 1 month of supplementation of the diet with brewer's yeast. One subject revealed an increase of 5 mg/dl, while the other 15 showed decreases ranging from 3 to 107 mg/dl. It was also noted that if the fasting serum cholesterol level was above 240 mg/dl, the decrement was likely to be greater than if the fasting level was 240 mg/dl or below (54 vs. 17 mg/dl). These results are in agreement with those of Schroeder (1968), who reported that trivalent chromium administration in humans caused a mean reduction of 14% in the serum cholesterol levels (Doisy *et al.*, 1976).

Triglyceride levels remained normal and unchanged while the subjects were on the supplement. Some subjects having elevated triglycerides do show reduced triglyceride levels while on the supplement (Doisy *et al.*, 1976).

It is possible that the observed decline in serum cholesterol was due to the nicotinic acid content of brewer's yeast. It seems more likely, however, that the decline was due to the chromium content of the yeast. The usual dosage of nicotinic acid for reduction of elevated cholesterol levels is 1–2 g three times daily. Nicotinic acid may be effective by conversion to GTF, providing adequate tissue stores of chromium are available. It is also possible that the cholesterol-lowering effect resulting from brewer's yeast supplementation is unrelated to the chromium content of the yeast (Doisy *et al.*, 1976).

Curran (1954) implicated chromium in fatty acid and cholesterol synthesis, whereas Schroeder and Balassa (1965) and Staub *et al.* (1969) observed in rats that chromium supplementation of certain diets resulted in a reduction in serum cholesterol levels. Schroeder and Balassa (1965) also noted a decreased incidence of aortic plaques in animals on a chromium supplement.

Insulin-Requiring Diabetics

Earlier evidence indicated that insulin-requiring diabetics have an abnormal pattern in their absorption and excretion of chromium. To date, only a few insulin-requiring diabetics have been studied in terms of their response to brewer's yeast (GTF) supplementation of the diet (Doisy *et al.*, 1976). A reduction in the daily insulin requirement was noted. In 5 diabetics whose daily insulin requirement ranged from 60 to 130 U/day, preliminary results revealed reductions of 20–45 U in their daily requirements over a 1- to 2-month period. This observation confirms a report by McCay (1952), who recommended daily brewer's yeast supplementation for elderly people. McCay also suggested that supplementation could lessen the insulin requirement in elderly diabetics. The elimination of the daily insulin requirement has not been achieved, and would not be expected in these subjects, because in all likelihood they have little endogenous insulin production based on the magnitude of their daily insulin requirement. Yalow and Berson (1960) estimated that a normal adult produces approximately 40 U of insulin per day. It is possible that elimination of the exogenous insulin requirement could occur in subjects who are still capable of making insulin and need only modest amounts, i.e., 5–20 U/day. An attendant risk of hypoglycemia while the supplement is being initiated must be emphasized. The insulin requirement is usually decreased within 24 hr and declines progressively by 1–2 U every 48–72 hr (Doisy *et al.*, 1976).

Siblings or Offspring of Known Diabetics

The incidence of impaired glucose tolerance is higher in the siblings of diabetics than in the general population. In genetically diabetic mice, inorganic chromium was without effect on the elevated blood glucose levels that accompany the genetic diabetic state. GTF preparations produced a reduction in glucose levels to within normal limits in these mice, in which an inability to convert chromium to GTF was considered (Doisy *et al.*, 1973). Similar experience in human studies was reported by Doisy *et al.* (1976). It is suggested that a deficiency of chromium in the United States could occur because of inadequate intake due to chromium loss during the processing of foodstuffs, e.g., flour and sugar (Doisy *et al.*, 1976).

At some point, public health measures to ensure adequate chromium intake might become desirable, although implementation of any such measure would demand careful thought regarding the safety of the procedure, the toxicity of excessive levels, and appropriate safeguards against undesirable excesses (Doisy *et al.*, 1976).

CLINICAL EFFECTS OF CHROMIUM EXCESS

Chromium, particularly trivalent chromium, has a low order of toxicity. A wide margin of safety exists between the amounts usually ingested and those likely to induce adverse effects. Acute toxicity studies in rats with intravenously injected chromium (III) established the lethal dose for 50% of the animals at about 1 mg of the element per 100 g body weight (Mertz *et al.*, 1965). This amount is several times greater than the 0.05–0.10 μg Cr/100 g required to correct the impairment of glucose metabolism *in vivo*. Hexavalent chromium is much more toxic than trivalent. Chronic exposure to chromate dust has been correlated with an increased incidence of lung cancer (Brinton *et al.*, 1952), and oral administration of excessive levels (50 ppm) has been associated with growth depression and liver and kidney damage in experimental animals (Mackenzie *et al.*, 1958).

TREATMENT OF CHROMIUM POISONING

Chromic acid and its salts, the chromates and bichromates, are used in electroplating, steel-making, leather-tanning, photography, dyeing, and chemical synthesis. Due to liberation of O_2 and H_2 at electrodes, a fine spray of chromic acid arises over the bath, and toxic chromium trioxide escapes into the air that is inhaled. The lethal dose of potassium chromate is 5 g. Contact with chromate salts may cause eczematous dermatitis, edema, and ulcer (punched-out). Allergic reaction, conjunctivitis, and ulceration of nasal septum have also been reported. Prolonged exposure to chromate salts may produce gastrointestinal symptoms, hepatitis, and carcinoma of the lung (Arenas, 1970).

In case of ingestion, gastric lavage, followed by administration of demulcents to alleviate gastritis, should be carried out. If oliguria is present, fluid and electrolyte balance should be carefully monitored (Arenas, 1970).

For dermatitis, 1% aluminum acetate wet dressing may be useful; 10% ethylenediamine tetraacitate (EDTA) ointment is also beneficial. If chronic systemic poisoning is present, British anti-lewisite (BAL) may be used (Arenas, 1970).

REFERENCES

Arenas, J. M. 1970. *Poisoning: Toxicology—Symptoms—Treatments,* 2nd ed. Charles C. Thomas, Springfield, Illinois, p. 198.

Brinton, H. P., Fraiser, E.S., and Koven, A.L. 1952. Morbidity and mortality experiences among chromate workers; respiratory cancer and other causes. *Public Health Rep.* **67,** 835–847.

Burt, R. L., and Davidson, I.W.F. 1973. Carbohydrate metabolism in pregnancy: A possible role of chromium. *Acta Diabetol. Lat.* **10,** 770–778.

Carter, J. P., Kattob, A., Abd-El-Hodi, Davis, J.T., El Cholmy, A., and Patwardhan, V.N. 1968. Chromium III in hypoglycemia and in impaired glucose utilization in kwashiorkor. *Amer. J. Clin. Nutr.* **21,** 195–202.

Curran, G. L. 1954. Effect of certain transition group elements on hepatic synthesis of cholesterol in the rat. *J. Biol. Chem.* **210,** 765–770.

Czerniejewski, C. P., Shank, C.W., Bechtel, W.G., and Bradley, W.B. 1964. The minerals of wheat, flour, and bread. *Cereal Chem.* **41,** 65–72.

Davidson, I. W. F., and Blackwell, W. L. 1968. Changes in carbohydrate metabolism of squirrel monkeys with chromium dietary supplementation. *Proc. Soc. Exp. Biol. Med.* **127,** 66–72.

Davidson, I. W. F., and Burt, R. L. 1973. Physiologic changes in plasma chromium of normal and pregnant women: Effect of glucose load. *Amer. J. Obstet. Gynecol.* **116,** 601–608.

Davidson, I. W. F., and Secrest, W. L. 1972. Determination of chromium in biological materials by atomic absorption spectrometry using a graphite furnace atomizer. *Anal. Chem.* **44,** 1808–1813.

Davidson, I. W. F., Lang, C. M., and Blackwell, W. L. 1967. Impairment of carbohydrate metabolism of the squirrel monkey. *Diabetes* **16,** 395–401.

Doisy, R. J. 1963. Plasma insulin assay and adipose tissue metabolism. *Endocrinology* **72,** 273–278.

Doisy, R. J., Streeten, D. H. P., Levine, R. A., and Chodos, R. B. 1968. Effects and metabolism of chromium in normals, elderly subjects, and diabetics. In: *Trace Substances in Environmental Health,* Vol. II (D.D. Hemphill, ed.). University of Missouri Press, Columbia, pp. 75–82.

Doisy, R. J., Streeten, D. H. P., Souma, M. L., Kalafer, M. E., Rekant, S. I., and Dalakos, T. G. 1971. Metabolism of ^{51}chromium in human subjects—normal, elderly, and diabetic subjects. In: *Newer Trace Elements in Nutrition* (W. Mertz and W. E. Cornatzer, eds.). Dekker, New York, pp. 155–168.

Doisy, R. J., Jastremski, M. S., and Greenstein, F. L. 1973. Metabolic effects of glucose tolerance factor and trivalent chromium in normal and genetically diabetic mice. *Excerpta Med. Found. Int. Congr. Ser.* **280,** 155 (abstract).

Doisy, R. J., Streeten, D. H. P., Freiberg, J. M., and Schneider, A. J. 1976. Chromium metabolism in man and biochemical effects. In: *Trace Elements in Human Health and Disease,* Vol. II (A.S. Prasad, ed.). Academic Press, New York, pp. 79–104.

Donaldson, R. M., and Barreras, R. F. 1966. Intestinal absorption of trace quantities of chromium. *J. Lab. Clin. Med.* **68,** 484–493.

Durfor, C. N., and Becker, E. 1964. Public water supplies of the 100 largest cities in the United States, 1962. U.S. Government Printing Office, Washington, D.C. Geological Survey Water Supply Paper 1812.

Glinsmann, W. H., and Mertz, W. 1966. Effect of trivalent chromium on glucose tolerance. *Metab. Clin Exp.* **15,** 510–520.

Glinsmann, W. H., Feldman, F. J., and Mertz, W. 1966. Plasma chromium after glucose administration. *Science* **152,** 1243–1245.

Gormican, A. 1970. Inorganic elements in foods used in hospital menus. *J. Amer. Diet. Assoc.* **56,** 397–403.

Gürson, C. T., and Saner, G. 1971. Effect of chromium on glucose utilization in marasmic protein–calorie malnutrition. *Amer. J. Clin. Nutr.* **24,** 1313–1319.

Gürson, C. T., and Saner, G. 1973. Effect of chromium supplementation on growth in marasmic protein–calorie malnutrition. *Amer. J. Clin. Nutr.* **26,** 988–991.

Hambidge, K. M. 1971. Chromium nutrition in the mother and the growing child. In: *Newer Trace Elements in Nutrition,* Proceedings of an International Symposium (W. Mertz and W. E. Cornatzer, eds.). Dekker, New York, Chapt. 9, pp. 169–194.

Hambidge, K. M. 1974. Chromium nutrition in man. *Amer. J. Clin. Nutr.* **27,** 505–514.

Hambidge, K. M., and Baum, J. D. 1972. Hair chromium concentrations of human newborn and changes during infancy. *Amer. J. Clin. Nutr.* **25,** 376–379.

Hambidge, K. M., Rodgerson, D. O., and O'Brien, D. 1968. The concentration of chromium in the hair of normal and children with juvenile diabetes mellitus. *Diabetes* **17,** 517–519.

Hopkins, L. L., Jr., and Price, M. G. 1968. Effectiveness of Chromium III in improving the impaired glucose tolerance of middle-aged Americans. In: *Proceedings of the 2nd Western Hemisphere Nutrition Congress, 1968,* Vol. 2, pp. 40–41 (abstract).

Hopkins, L. L., Jr., and Schwarz, K. 1964. Chromium binding to serum proteins, specifically siderophilin. *Biochim. Biophys. Acta* **90,** 484–491.

Hopkins, L. L., Jr., Ransome-Kuti, O., and Majaj, A. S. 1968. Improvement of impaired carbohydrate metabolism by Chromium III in malnourished infants. *Amer. J. Clin. Nutr.* **21,** 203–211.

Jeejeebhoy, K. N., Chu, R. C., Marliss, E. B., Greenberg, G. R., and Robertson, A. B. 1977. Chromium deficiency, glucose intolerance, and neuropathy reversed by chromium supplementation, in a patient receiving long-term total parenteral nutrition. *Amer. J. Clin. Nutr.* **30,** 531–538.

Levine, R. A., Streeten, D. H..P., and Doisy, R. J. 1968. Effects of oral chromium supplementation on the glucose tolerance of elderly human subjects. *Metab. Clin. Exp.* **17,** 114–125.

MacKenzie, R. D., Byerrum, R. U., Decker, C. F., Hoppert, C. A., and Langham, R. F. 1958. Chronic toxicity studies. II. Hexavalent and trivalent chromium administered in drinking water to rats. *AMA Arch. Ind. Health* **18,** 232–234.

Maxia, V., Melini, S., Rollier, M. A., Brandone, A., Patwardhan, V. N., Waslien, C. I., and Said-El-Shami. 1972. Selenium and chromium assay in Egyptian foods and blood of Egyptian children by activation analysis. In: *Nuclear Activation Techniques in the Life Sciences.* IAEA-SM 157/67, IAEA, Vienna, pp. 527–550.

McCay, C. M. 1952. Chemical aspects of aging and the effect of diet upon aging. In: *Cowdry's Problems of Aging,* 3rd ed. (A.J. Lansing, ed.). Williams & Wilkins, Baltimore, Chapt. 6, pp. 139–202.

Mertz, W. 1967. Biological role of chromium. *Fed. Proc. Fed. Am. Soc. Exp. Biol.* **26,** 186–193.

Mertz, W. 1969. Chromium occurrence and function in biological systems. *Physiol. Rev.* **49,** 169–239.

Mertz, W. 1971. Human requirements: Basic and optimal. *Ann. N. Y. Acad. Sci.* **199,** 191–199.

Mertz, W. 1974. Biological function of chromium–nicotinic acid complexes. *Fed. Proc. Fed. Am. Soc. Exp. Biol.* **33,** 659 (abstract).

Mertz, W., and Roginski, E. E. 1971. Chromium metabolism: Glucose tolerance factor. In: *Newer Trace Elements in Nutrition,* Proceedings of an International Symposium (W. Mertz and W. E. Cornatzer, eds.). Dekker, New York, Chapt. 7, pp. 123–153.

Mertz, W., and Schwarz, K. 1959. Relation of glucose tolerance factor to impaired glucose tolerance in rats on stock diets. *Amer. J. Physiol.* **196,** 614–618.

Mertz, W., Roginski, E. E., and Reba, R. 1965. Biological activities and fate of trace quantities of intravenous chromium (3) in the rat. *Amer. J. Physiol.* **209,** 489–494.

Morgan, J. M. 1972. Hepatic chromium content in diabetic subjects. *Metab. Clin. Exp.* **21,** 313–316.

Pekarek, R. S., Hauer, E. C., Wannemacher, R. W., Jr., and Beisel, W. R. 1973a. Serum chromium concentrations and glucose utilization in healthy and infected subjects. *Fed. Proc. Fed. Am. Soc. Exp. Biol.* **32,** 930 (abstract).

Pekarek, R. S., Hauer, E. C., Wannemacher, R. W., Jr., and Beisel, W. R. 1973b. The direct determination of serum chromium by an atomic absorption spectrophotometer with heated graphite atomizer. *Anal. Biochem.* **59,** 283–292.

Schroeder, H. A. 1968. The role of chromium in mammalian nutrition. *Amer. J. Clin. Nutr.* **21,** 230–244.

Schroeder, H. A. 1971. Losses of vitamin and trace minerals resulting from processing and preservation of foods. *Amer. J. Clin. Nutr.* **24,** 562–573.

Schroeder, H. A., and Balassa, J. J. 1965. Influence of chromium, cadmium, and lead on rat aortic lipids and circulating cholesterol. *Amer. J. Physiol.* **209,** 433–437.

Schroeder, H. A., Balassa, J. J., and Tipton, I. H. 1962. Abnormal trace metal in man: Chromium . *J. Chronic Dis.* **15,** 941–964.

Schroeder, H. A., Balassa, J. J., and Vinton, W. H., Jr. 1965. Chromium, cadmium and lead in rats: Effects on life span, tumors, and tissue levels. *J. Nutr.* **86,** 51–66.

Schroeder, H. A., Nason, A. P., and Tipton, I. H. 1970. Chromium deficiency as a factor in atherosclerosis. *J. Chronic Dis.* **23,** 123–142.

Schwarz, K., and Mertz, W. 1957. A glucose tolerance factor and its differentiation from factor 3. *Arch. Biochem. Biophys.* **72,** 515–518.

Schwarz, K., and Mertz, W. 1959. Chromium III and the glucose tolerance factor. *Arch. Biochem. Biophys.* **85,** 292–295.

Staub, H. W., Reussner, G., and Thiessen, R. T., Jr. 1969. Serum cholesterol reduction by chromium in hypercholesterolemic rats. *Science* **166,** 746–747.

Toepfer, E. W., Mertz, W., Roginski, E. E., and Polansky, M. M. 1973. Chromium in foods in relation to biological activity. *J. Agric. Food Chem.* **21,** 69–73.

Wacker, W. E. C., and Vallee, B. L. 1959. Nucleic acids and metals. I. Chromium, manganese, nickel, iron, and other metals in ribonucleic acid from diverse biological sources. *J. Biol. Chem.* **234,** 3257–3262.

Wolf, W., Greene, F. E., and Mitman, F. W. 1974. Determination of urinary chromium by low temperature ashing–flameless atomic absorption. *Fed. Proc. Fed. Am. Soc. Exp. Biol.* **33,** 659 (abstract).

Yalow, R. S., and Berson, S. A. 1960. Immunoassay of endogenous plasma insulin in man. *J. Clin. Invest.* **39,** 1157–1175.

CHAPTER 2

COPPER

INTRODUCTION

The presence of copper in plant and animal tissues was first recognized almost 150 years ago (Bucholz, 1818; Boutigny, 1833). In 1847, copper was shown to be present in the blood proteins of snails (Harless, 1847), and 30 years later, copper-containing pigment (hemocyanin) was recognized to function as a respiratory compound (Fredericq, 1878). In addition, the red pigment turacin (found in the feathers of turaco, a South African bird) was found to be a copper compound (Church, 1869, 1892). Subsequently, turacin was found to be a derivative of the porphyrin pigments normally present in plants and animals (Rimington, 1939).

Suggestive evidence of the dietary importance of copper in rats was first reported by McHargue in 1925 (McHargue, 1925, 1926). In 1928, Hart *et al.* (1928) showed that copper, in addition to iron, was necessary for blood formation in rats. Natural copper deficiency in livestock was recognized in 1931 as an outcome of the report of Neal *et al.* (1931) of "salt-sick" cattle in Florida. Two years later (Sjollema, 1933, 1937), copper deficiency was related to a disease in sheep and cattle occurring in Holland and known locally as lechsucht. Later, enzootic neonatal ataxia in lambs occurring in Western Australia was shown to be due to inadequate intakes of copper from grazing (Bennetts and Chapman, 1937). Defects in the processes of pigmentation, keratinization of wool, bone formation, reproduction, myelination of the spinal cord, cardiac function, and connective tissue formation, in addition to those of growth and hematopoiesis, were found to be manifestations of copper deficiency.

Although anemia as a common expression of copper deficiency was recognized earlier (Beck, 1941), it was much later that Lahey *et al.* (1952) showed that addition of copper to the diet of pigs suffering from a combined iron and copper deficiency anemia elicits a marked and persistent reticulocyte response, whereas iron had little effect. Gubler *et al.* (1952) documented that copper-deficient pigs have an impaired ability to absorb iron, mobilize it from the tissues, and utilize it in hemoglobin synthesis. More recently, four defects in iron metabolism were delineated in copper-deficient pigs: (1) impaired synthesis of heme from Fe(III) and protoporphyrin; (2) impaired mobilization of iron from reticuloendothelial cells to transferrin; (3) impaired mobilization of iron from hepatic parenchymal cells to transferrin; and (4) impaired absorption of iron from the gastrointestinal tract (Lee *et al.,* 1968b).

The role of copper in the cross-linking and maturation process has been clarified since the simultaneous discovery that pigs (Shields *et al.,* 1962) and chicks (O'Dell *et al.,* 1961) fed copper-deficient diets frequently die suddenly from massive internal hemorrhage caused by structural defects in major arteries. Many copper-protein compounds have been isolated from tissues, several of which are enzymes with oxidative functions. Copper enzymes are unique in catalyzing the reduction of molecular oxygen to water. Tyrosinase, lysl oxidase, laccase, ascorbic acid oxidase, cytochrome oxidase, uricase, monoamine oxidase, and dopamine-β-hydroxylase have been identified as copper enzymes. Several manifestations of copper deficiency in the animals have been related to altered tissue activities of some of these enzymes, thus providing basic biochemical mechanisms of the effects of copper deficiency.

Copper deficiency has now been implicated in the etiology of three distinct clinical syndromes in the human infant. In the first of these, anemia, hypoproteinemia, hypoferremia, and hypocupremia are present, and combined therapy with iron and copper is necessary to promote complete recovery (Sturgeon and Brubaker, 1956; Zipursky *et al.,* 1958; Schubert and Lahey, 1959). The second syndrome is known to affect malnourished infants being rehabilitated on high-caloric and low-copper-containing diets who exhibit anemia, neutropenia, diarrhea, "scurvylike" bone changes, and hypocupremia (Cordano *et al.,* 1964). The third clinical condition in infants is Menke's kinky hair syndrome, which is caused by a genetically determined defect in copper absorption from the intestinal tract (Danks *et al.,* 1972a,b). In addition to these syndromes, copper deficiency resulting from prolonged administration of total parenteral nutrition (TPN) without copper supplementation has been reported (Karpel and Peden, 1972). More recently, copper deficiency due to TPN (Vilter *et al.,* 1974; Dunlap *et al.,* 1974) and secondary to prolonged zinc administration in adults has been observed (Prasad *et al.,* 1978). The observations described above thus clearly demonstrate the important role of copper in clinical medicine.

BIOCHEMISTRY AND PHYSIOLOGY

The first evidence that copper plays an important role in vertebrates was provided by Hart *et al.* (1928), who showed that it is required for prevention of anemia. Soon thereafter, Cohen and Elvehjem (1934) showed that copper is essential for the synthesis of heme A, a component of cytochrome oxidase, and thus copper was established as a biochemically significant catalyst. An important cuproprotein was first isolated from bovine erythrocytes (Mann and Keilin, 1938), although its function as an enzyme was not known until much later (McCord and Fridovich, 1969; O'Dell, 1976).

Since the isolation of hemocuprein, several copper-containing enzymes have been isolated and characterized (O'Dell, 1976). A list of copper metalloenzymes found in tissues of higher animals is shown in Table I. Although most of the proteins listed are cuproenzymes, there is lack of firm evidence in some cases and controversy in others (O'Dell, 1976).

Brady *et al.* (1972) reported that tryptophan-2,3-dioxygenase purified from both rat liver and *Pseudomonas acidovorans* contains 2 g atoms copper and 2 mol heme per mole of tetrameric enzyme. Ishimura and Hayaishi (1973), however, purified the oxygenase from *Pseudomonas fluorescens* and did not find a stoichiometric quantity of copper (O'Dell, 1976).

Most of the cuproenzymes listed in Table I catalyze physiologically important reactions. However, the physiological functions of some, including ceruloplasmin and the amine oxidases, are not well understood. Aside from its enzymatic oxidase activity, ceruloplasmin contains essentially all

Table I. Cuproenzymes Found in Vertebrate Tissues[a]

Enzyme	Source
Cytochrome *c* oxidase	Mitochondria
Superoxide dismutase (hemocuprein)	Erythrocytes and heart
Ceruloplasmin	Plasma
Tyrosinase	Melanomas and skin
Uricase	Liver and kidney
Dopamine-β-hydroxylase	Adrenal gland
Lysyl oxidase	Aorta and cartilage
Spermine oxidase	Bovine plasma
Benzylamine oxidase	Pig plasma
Diamine oxidase (histaminase)	Kidney
(Tryptophan-2,3-dioxygenase)	Liver

[a]From O'Dell (1976).

the plasma copper, and it probably plays a role in copper transport from the liver to extrahepatic organs (O'Dell, 1976).

MELANIN FORMATION AND TYROSINASE

Failure of pigmentation of hair and wool due to copper deficiency has been observed in numerous mammalian species (Underwood, 1977). In black-wooled sheep, bands of pigmented and unpigmentated wool can be correlated with copper supplementation. It seems probable that depressed tyrosinase activity may be responsible for the lack of melanin formation. Tyrosinase (EC 1.10.3.1) catalyzes two reactions, the hydroxylation of tyrosine to 3,4-dihydroxyphenylalanine (dopa) and the oxidation of dopa to the quinone, leading ultimately to the formation of melanin (Pomerantz, 1963), as shown below:

Tyrosine → dopa → dopaquinone → 2,3-dihydro-5,6-dihydroxyindole-2-carboxylate → dopachrome →→→ melanin (O'Dell, 1976)

CROSS-LINKING OF THE CONNECTIVE TISSUE PROTEINS, COLLAGEN AND ELASTIN

Skeletal Defects due to Copper Deficiency

Spontaneous fractures of bones occur in sheep and cattle grazing in copper-deficient pastures. Bone abnormalities have also been observed experimentally in rabbits, pigs, chicks, and dogs (Underwood, 1977). In the dog, the bone cortices are abnormally thin, and the trabeculae are lacking or deficient. The ash as well as the calcium and phosphorus content remains unaltered in the copper-deficient dog and chick. The defect seems to reside in the organic matrix. The copper-deficient chick bones contain a higher proportion of soluble collagen than normal bone, and the soluble collagen from deficient bone has a lower aldehyde content (Rucker *et al.*, 1969). The cross-linking of bone collagen is impaired in copper deficiency, and this defect is probably the basis for the commonly observed bone abnormalities (O'Dell, 1976).

Cardiac Defects due to Copper Deficiency

Bennetts described "falling disease" in cattle (Underwood, 1977) and reported that cardiac lesions occur as a result of copper deficiency. The sudden death was believed to be due to heart failure, and the lesion consisted of atrophy of the myocardium with replacement fibrosis. Kelley *et al.* (1974) also reported the occurrence of heart failure among young rats the dams of which were fed a copper-deficient diet. In contrast to the lesion in cattle, the hearts in rats were grossly enlarged, and some displayed aneurysms at the apex. Variable areas of necrosis in both the ventricular and atrial musculature were noted, and hemopericardium occurred frequently. These lesions implicate a direct myocardial defect resulting from copper deficiency (O'Dell, 1976).

Vascular Defects due to Copper Deficiency

Integrity of the cardiovascular system, particularly of the major arteries, is largely dependent on the quality and quantity of collagen and elastin. The role of copper in the maturation of these connective-tissue proteins has been known since 1961. O'Dell *et al.* (1961) and Shields *et al.* (1962) showed that chicks and pigs fed copper-deficient diets die suddenly from massive internal hemorrhage due to dissecting aneurysms in the walls of intact aortas (O'Dell, 1976).

The biochemical defect leading to angiorrhexis is a failure to form the normal cross-linking compounds in elastin and collagen. The concentration of elastin in the aortas of copper-deficient chicks is reduced to less than one half that of the supplemented controls. There is no defect in elastin polypeptide synthesis, but rather a failure of cross-linking and the inability of immature elastin to resist the solubilizing effect of hot 0.1 N NaOH or formic acid used to determine elastin. The concentration of total collagen in the aortas is unchanged, but the proportion soluble in cold saline solution is increased fivefold. Solubility of collagen in cold 1 M NaCl is a measure of intermolecular cross-linking, and the results show that copper deficiency interferes with this process (O'Dell, 1976).

Intramolecular cross-linking is also impaired as a result of copper deficiency. The collagen molecule is made up of three polypeptide chains, commonly two α_1 chains and one α_2 chain. Part of the α chains are covalently linked to form β_{11} and β_{12} chains. Soluble collagen from copper-deficient chick tendon contained a much higher proportion of α_1 chains and no detectable β_{11} chains. The ratio of α to β chains was greater than 3 compared with a normal ratio of less than 1 (O'Dell, 1976).

Tropoelastin and Cross-Link Biosynthesis

A soluble, elastin like protein, tropoelastin, has been isolated from aortas of copper-deficient pigs (Smith, D. W., *et al.*, 1968; Sandberg *et al.*, 1969) and chicks (Roensch *et al.*, 1972). A soluble elastin from normal tissue has not been isolated, although it has been found in lathyritic chick aortas (Sykes and Partridge, 1972). The soluble elastins isolated from both pig and chick aorta have amino acid compositions similar to that of mature

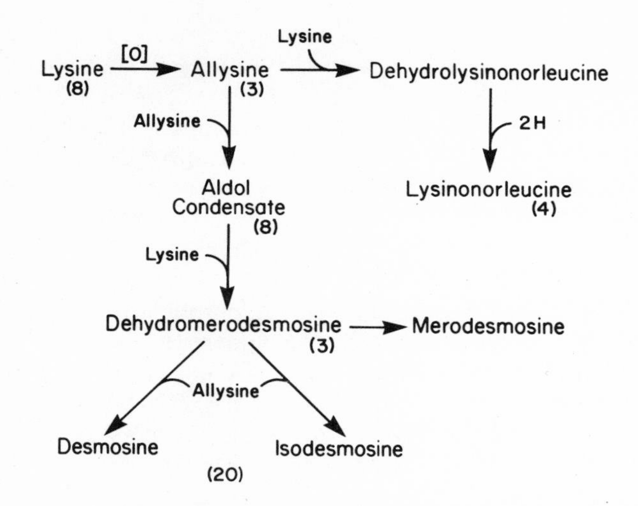

Fig. 1. Scheme for biosynthesis of the cross-linking compounds in elastin. All proposed reactions involve lysine residues in peptide linkage. The numbers in parentheses indicate the distribution of lysine and lysine-derived residues per 1000 residues in mature mammalian elastin (Gallop *et al.,* 1972). From O'Dell (1976).

elastin. The cross-linking compounds desmosine and isodesmosine are lacking in the soluble elastins. Also, the concentration of lysine is much higher in the soluble elastin as compared with its concentration in the insoluble elastin (O'Dell, 1976).

The differences in lysine content of the soluble and insoluble elastins are accounted for by the lysine-derived cross-linking compounds found in elastin (Fig. 1). Desmosine and isodesmosine, the first cross-links isolated from elastin (Partridge, 1969), account for 8 residues in chick aorta elastin (4 lysines per desmosine). According to Gallop *et al.* (1972), the desmosines, including the dihydro and tetrahydro forms, account for 20 lysine residues in mammalian elastin. The remaining lysine residues are present as intermediates involved in the biosynthesis of the desmosines (O'Dell, 1976).

The formation of the cross-linking compounds of collagen and elastin is dependent on the oxidative deamination of the epsilon carbon of specific lysyl residues in polypeptide chains to form an aldehyde. Such reactions, involving molecular oxygen, are commonly catalyzed by amine oxidases. These enzymes catalyze the following type of reaction:

$$R{-}CH_2{-}NH_2 + O_2 \rightarrow R{-}\overset{H}{C} = O + H_2O_2 + NH_3 \text{ (O'Dell, 1976)}$$

Lysyl Oxidase

In 1968, Pinnell and Martin (1968) identified an enzyme, lysyl oxidase, in embryonic chick bone that catalyzes the conversion of peptidyllysine to the corresponding aldehyde residue. Although the complete stoichiometry of the reaction has not been determined, it is clear that the reaction requires oxygen and produces the allysine residue (O'Dell, 1976).

Siegel *et al.* (1970) were able to extract lysyl oxidase from cartilaginous bone with phosphate-buffered saline, but were not entirely successful in purifying this enzyme. Nevertheless, the crude enzyme was inactivated by α,α-dipyridyl, and the activity was restored by copper, iron, and cobalt. Although copper was the most effective cation, the lack of specificity suggests that part of the reversal was related to reaction of the ions with bound α,α-dipyridyl. Cartilage extracts from chicks fed a copper-deficient diet showed no lysyl oxidase activity, whereas control extracts were active, thus providing further evidence that this enzyme was copper-dependent. Later studies have confirmed that aortic lysyl oxidase is a copper metalloenzyme (O'Dell, 1976).

There appear to be at least two proteins in chick aorta that possess lysyl oxidase activity. Narayanan *et al.* (1974) presented evidence for only one enzyme in the chick cartilage. Since aorta contains both collagen and elastin, the two forms may possess different specificities for collagen and elastin, or they may be isozymes (O'Dell, 1976).

Lysyl oxidase is believed to play the key role in the cross-linking of connective tissue proteins. Whether or not other enzymes are involved in this process is not known (O'Dell, 1976).

CENTRAL NERVOUS SYSTEM DISORDERS DUE TO COPPER DEFICIENCY

Neonatal Ataxia and Hypomyelination

Copper deficiency leads to nervous disorders in the neonates of various species, including lambs, goats, pigs, guinea pigs, and rats (Underwood, 1977). The most frequently observed nervous disorder among lambs due to copper deficiency is neonatal ataxia, or swayback. In Australia, the ataxia is associated with subnormal levels of copper in the forage and in the tissues of the affected animals. In other areas of the world, the incidence of ataxia is not so well correlated with copper status, but can be prevented by copper supplementation. The latter observation suggests a conditioned copper deficiency induced by other environmental factors, such as high levels of molybdenum and sulfate (O'Dell, 1976).

Incoordination of movement, particularly of the hindquarters, is associated with lack of myelination in the brainstem and spinal cord. Whether the nerve lesion is the result of demyelination or simply failure of myelin formation is not clear. Recent studies suggest that it is the result of myelin aplasia. In animals severely affected at birth, there may be cavitation of the cerebrum, but more generally there is cell necrosis and fiber degeneration in the brainstem and spinal cord. Everson *et al.* (1968) studied the brain and spinal cord of ataxic neonatal guinea pigs born to dams fed a low-copper diet during gestation. The cerebellum was damaged, and histologically, lack of myelin development throughout the brain was demonstrated. There was no cellular change in the cerebrum, brainstem, or spinal cord (O'Dell, 1976).

Carlton and Kelly (1969) described neurological changes in the offspring of female rats fed a copper-deficient diet. Histological changes consisting of rarefaction and edema were observed in the cerebral cortex and corpus striatum, but not in the brainstem or spinal cord. Demyelination was not reported. In rats, DiPaolo *et al.* (1974) observed behavioral disturbances due to copper deficiency. Histologically, the deficient brains contained less myelin. The deficient brains showed a decrease in cholesterol, galactocerebroside, and sulfatide, but the total phospholipid concentration was normal. At present, it is not possible to define clearly the primary metabolic defect in the central nervous system of copper-deficient animals. Hypomyelination appears to be the most common lesion, but whether it is the primary cause of ataxia or the result of a more fundamental neuron damage is unclear (O'Dell, 1976).

Cytochrome oxidase activity in many tissues, including liver, heart, and brain, is depressed in copper-deficient animals. It is possible that the basic biochemical defect in neonatal ataxia is a lack of cytochrome oxidase in the motor neurons (Underwood, 1977). A reduction of cytochrome oxidase activity in various regions of the brains of swayback lambs, including the red nucleus of the brainstem, was reported by Howell and Davison (1959) and Mills and Williams (1962). Both cytochrome a and a_3 and cytochrome oxidase activities in cerebral cortex mitochondria of copper-deficient, ataxic lambs were reduced to approximately one half control levels, but the other cytochromes were unaffected (O'Dell, 1976). Whether or not these biochemical changes account for clinical and pathological nervous lesions cannot be settled at present.

Copper and Catecholamines

Similarity of the ataxic signs in the lamb to those of the extrapyramidal motor diseases, such as Parkinson's disease, suggests that the dopaminergic system may be defective. O'Dell (1976) measured the catecholamine and serotonin concentrations in the brainstem of ataxic lambs with and without copper supplementation. Copper supplementation significantly increased the dopamine levels in the ataxic brains, but did not cure the locomotor disorder. Serotonin concentrations were unchanged. Norepinephrine concentrations were lower in both the anterior and posterior (medulla and pons) portions of the untreated animals, but because of the sample size, the differences were not statistically significant. Prohaska and Wells (1974) observed lower levels of norepinephrine in the whole brain (minus cerebellum) of perinatal rats as a result of copper deficiency (O'Dell, 1976).

Sourkes (1972) showed that the conversion of dopamine to cardiac norepinephrine in copper-deficient rats is reduced. Inasmuch as dopamine-β-hydroxylase is a copper-dependent enzyme, a decreased concentration of norepinephrine in the brains of copper-deficient animals may be expected. An explanation for the low dopamine concentration, however, is not obvious. It is conceivable that copper status affects the activity of tyrosine hydroxylase directly or indirectly. It is also possible that because of low superoxide dismutase activity, the superoxide anion accumulates in brain tissue and destroys catecholamines by a mechanism similar to the one proposed by Misra and Fridovich (1972) for the conversion of epinephrine to adrenochrome (O'Dell, 1976).

Whether or not the hypomyelination observed in copper-deficient brains is directly related to the decreased concentrations of catecholamines remains unsettled. It is also not known whether the lower catecholamine levels are responsible for neonatal ataxia. Copper supplementation of an affected animal increases the dopamine concentration, but it neither cures the ataxia nor eliminates the myelin defect. Although it is possible that these defects are related during the development of the disease, they certainly do not appear to be related in the later stages (O'Dell, 1976).

STEELY WOOL AND HAIR IN COPPER DEFICIENCY

Copper deficiency in adult sheep is characterized by a change in the physical characteristics of the wool (Underwood, 1977). The fibers lose their normal crimp, and have a decreased concentration of disulfide bonds with concomitant increase in sulfhydryl groups. A similar biochemical defect has been found in the hair of children who suffer from Menke's syndrome, which is a genetic disorder caused by a failure to absorb copper. The hair of these infants has a tortuous appearance when magnified (Danks *et al.*, 1972a,b; O'Dell, 1976).

Failure of hair and wool to form disulfide bonds in copper deficiency suggests that the process is normally catalyzed by a copper-dependent enzyme; however, such an enzyme has not yet been identified (O'Dell, 1976).

CUPROENZYMES UNASSOCIATED WITH SPECIFIC PATHOLOGY

Cytochrome *c* Oxidase

Cytochrome *c* oxidase (EC 1.9.3.1) is composed of cytochrome *a* and a_3, and it contains 1 g atom of copper per mole of heme A (O'Dell, 1976). Cytochrome oxidase is the terminal oxidase in the mitochondrial electron-transport system, catalyzing the transfer of electrons from cytochrome *c* to oxygen. This is a key reaction in energy metabolism, but it is difficult to associate this enzyme with a specific pathology. Although low brain cytochrome oxidase levels have been associated with neonatal ataxia, a causal relationship has not been established. Copper deficiency usually has a greater effect on cytochrome oxidase levels in liver than in brain, and hepatic mitochondria become progressively enlarged and grossly misshapen with advancing copper deficiency (Gallagher *et al.*, 1973; O'Dell, 1976).

Superoxide Dismutase

Superoxide dismutase catalyzes the dismutation of the superoxide anion free radical according to the following reaction:

$$O_2^- + O_2^- + 2H^+ \rightarrow O_2 + H_2O_2$$

The enzyme was isolated from bovine erythrocytes (McCord and Fridovich, 1969) and shown to be identical with the protein variously designated as hemocuprein, erythrocuprein, and cerebrocuprein. Carrico and Deutsch (1970) showed that this enzyme contains 2 g atoms of zinc as well as 2 of copper per mole of the protein. This type of superoxide dismutase is located in the cell cytosol, and has been isolated from a wide range of eukaryotic species. Another type of superoxide dismutase has been isolated from prokaryotes and shown to contain manganese instead of copper and zinc. Chicken liver has been shown to contain both types of enzyme, the manganoprotein being localized in mitochondria and the copper–zinc enzyme in the cytosol (Weisiger and Fridovich, 1973; O'Dell, 1976).

No pathology in higher animals has been attributed to a lack of superoxide dismutase activity. If one extrapolates from microorganisms, superoxide dismutase may be an extremely important protective catalyst. Oxidation of some substrates by O_2, e.g., xanthine catalyzed by xanthine oxidase, proceeds by univalent reduction of O_2 and produces O_2^-.Thus, aerobic organisms may need superoxide dismutase to degrade this highly reactive free radical. A survey of several species of microorganisms showed that obligate anaerobes, those that cannot survive in oxygen, contained no superoxide dismutase (Fridovich, 1972). All aerobes surveyed contained relatively high levels of the enzyme, while oxygen-tolerant anaerobes contained low levels. Prohaska and Wells (1974) reported lower levels of superoxide dismutase in the brains of copper-deficient neonatal rats than in those of controls, thus indicating that this enzyme is copper-dependent (O'Dell, 1976).

Uricase

Uricase (EC 1.7.3.3) catalyzes the oxidation of uric acid by molecular oxygen:

$$\text{Uric acid} + O_2 + 3\ H_2O \rightarrow \text{allantoin} + H_2O_2 + HCO_3^-$$

There is no evidence that the activity of this enzyme is decreased in copper deficiency (O'Dell, 1976).

Dopamine-β-hydroxylase

Dopamine-β-hydroxylase (EC 1.14.2.1) is a monooxygenase that catalyzes the oxidation of the β-carbon of dopamine to form norepinephrine:

$$\text{3,4-Dihydroxyphenylethylamine (dopamine)} + O_2 + \text{ascorbate} \rightarrow \text{norepinephrine} + \text{dehydroascorbate} + H_2O$$

The activity is stimulated by fumarate, and catechol can serve as a poor substitute for ascorbate. This enzyme is relatively nonspecific inasmuch as many phenylethylamine derivatives serve as substrates. The bovine adrenal enzyme has a molecular weight of 290,000 and contains 2 g atoms of copper per mole. The copper in the enzyme undergoes reversible reduction during the enzymatic reaction. The adrenal enzyme consists of four subunits, two pairs of which are linked by disulfide bonds (Craine *et al.*, 1973; O'Dell, 1976).

Dopamine-β-hydroxylase plays a key role in the biosynthesis of norepinephrine in the adrenal gland, but there is no evidence that its activity becomes limiting during copper deficiency. Although this enzyme has not been isolated from brain, it is presumed that a similar enzyme catalyzes the formation of norepinephrine in brain. Although the brain norepinephrine level is reduced in copper-deficient animals, it is not known whether this reduction plays any role in pathogenesis (O'Dell, 1976).

Amine Oxidases

There are many different amine oxidases found in vertebrate tissues. They all catalyze the oxidative deamination of amines by molecular oxygen to give an aldehyde and hydrogen peroxide. They can be divided into two major types based on the cofactors involved. Mitochondrial membrane-bound monoamine oxidase is a flavoprotein that does not contain copper. The other general class of amine oxidases contains copper and pyridoxal phosphate or a closely related compound (O'Dell, 1976).

Among the copper-containing amine oxidases are benzylamine oxidase isolated from pig plasma (Buffoni and Blaschko, 1964), spermine oxidase isolated from bovine plasma (Yamada and Yasunobu, 1962), diamine oxidase isolated from pig kidney (Mondovi *et al.,* 1967), and lysyl oxidase isolated from connective tissues (Siegel *et al.,* 1970; Harris *et al.,* 1974). Lysyl oxidase has an important function in collagen and elastin metabolism. Connective tissues also contain amine oxidases the properties of which are highly similar to those of amine oxidases found in the plasma of the same species (Rucker and O'Dell, 1971; Rucker and Goettlich-Rieman, 1972). Polyamines are the best substrates for the enzyme purified from bovine aorta, and it might be considered a spermine oxidase. Benzylamine is a good substrate for the rabbit aorta enzyme, whereas the polyamines are inactive. Thus, it might be classed as a benzylamine oxidase. It has been suggested that the plasma enzymes arise from connective tissues. Although the connective-tissue amine oxidases have not been purified to homogeneity, there is circumstantial evidence that they are copper-dependent enzymes (Bird *et al.*, 1966; Chou *et al.,* 1968). The benzylamine oxidase activities in chick aorta, heart, kidney, skin, cartilage, and tendon are depressed by copper deficiency. Addition of Cu^{2+} *in vitro* partially restores the activity in copper-deficient aortas (O'Dell, 1976).

ROLE OF COPPER IN IRON METABOLISM

DEFECTIVE GASTROINTESTINAL ABSORPTION OF IRON

Iron absorption is impaired in copper-deficient pigs (Lee *et al.,* 1976). Two observations are pertinent in this respect: First, despite oral iron supplements given to copper-deficient swine, the total body iron became considerably less than that of control animals (Gubler *et al.,* 1952). Second, when radioactive iron was fed to a control and two deficient pigs, the control animal absorbed 6.1% of the iron, whereas both copper-deficient pigs absorbed less than 2% (Lee *et al.,* 1976).

Copper-deficient pigs receiving oral iron supplements deposited iron granules in the proximal duodenum within macrophages of the lamina propria as coarse, large granules, and within the columnar epithelial cells as fine, dustlike granules (Lee *et al.,* 1968b, 1976). No such granules were seen in intramuscularly iron-supplemented pigs, indicating that the stainable iron was of dietary origin. Such deposits of iron were not seen in the mucosa of the control animals. These observations suggest that the defect in iron absorption represents impaired transfer from mucosa to plasma, rather than from duodenal lumen to mucosa (Lee *et al.,* 1976).

Whereas in the liver of the control swine, all stainable iron was confined to macrophages (Kupffer cells), easily visible excessive deposits of iron were present in parenchymal cells of the deficient pigs (Lee *et al.,* 1968b, 1976).

Nearly all copper-deficient animals developed transient hypoferremia of several days' to several weeks' duration, even though they received intramuscular iron injections and their body iron stores were maintained at normal levels (Lee *et al.,* 1968a,b, 1976; Roeser *et al.,* 1970). Hypoferremia occurred after an average of 9.5 weeks (range 7–12 weeks) of copper deficiency (Roeser *et al.,* 1970) and concided with the occurrence of hypoceruloplasminemia (Lee *et al.,* 1976).

Administration of ceruloplasmin to copper-deficient animals induced a prompt increase in plasma iron (Ragan *et al.,* 1969). This increase was not observed when inorganic copper in the amount contained in the ceruloplasmin was administered, nor was there an observable response following administration of ceruloplasmin-deficient plasma (Lee *et al.,* 1976).

Although there was lack of response to small doses of inorganic copper, an increase in plasma iron was observed when larger doses of copper were administered. There was a lag of about 30 min before any appreciable response was measurable. During this time, plasma ceruloplasmin levels steadily increased to 1% normal level by the time an increase in plasma iron was observed. Thus, it appears reasonable to attribute the effect of inorganic copper to its influence on ceruloplasmin levels, rather than to a direct effect of copper (Lee *et al.,* 1976).

These studies indicate that ceruloplasmin plays an important role in the normal flow of iron from cells to plasma. Although ceruloplasmin is known to catalyze the oxidation of a number of substrates *in vitro,* including purified protein derivative and ascorbate, an *in vivo* oxidative function essential to normal metabolism could not be established (Lee *et al.,* 1976). Curzon and O'Reilly (1960) and Osaki and co-workers (Osaki, 1966; Osaki *et al.*, 1966) first reported that the oxidation of ferrous iron was catalyzed by ceruloplasmin. Osaki and co-workers pointed out that the oxidase activity of ceruloplasmin was greater for iron than any other substrate. They proposed that ceruloplasmin be renamed "ferroxidase." They also suggested that the ceruloplasmin-catalyzed oxidation of iron was an essential step in normal iron metabolism. According to this hypothesis, iron is presented to the cell surface in the form of ferrous iron and must be oxidized to the ferric form in order to be bound by transferrin (Gaber and Aisen, 1970). Although spontaneous oxidation is to be expected, Osaki (1966) calculated that the spontaneous rate would be inadequate for physiologic needs (Lee *et al.*, 1976).

Certain facts, however, do not directly support the hypothesis that ceruloplasmin is essential for iron oxidation *in vivo*. In patients with Wilson's disease, despite low ceruloplasmin level, there is no evidence that defective iron mobilization exists. Anemia in particular is not a feature of Wilson's disease except when liver failure is severe or during transient episodes of hemolysis (Lee *et al.*, 1976).

In copper-deficient swine, hypoferremia was not observed until the ceruloplasmin levels fell below 1% of normal. Hypoceruloplasminemia of this degree is uncommon in untreated Wilson's disease. By an immunological method, ceruloplasmin values of 2–22 mg/100 ml (normal 27–38) were found in 28 patients (Cartwright *et al.*, 1962). Similarly, plasma ceruloplasmin exceeded 5 mg/100 ml in 84 of 111 patients in another investigation (Sternlieb and Scheinberg, 1965; Lee *et al.*, 1976). Thus, the absence of defects in iron metabolism in Wilson's disease may be partly explained by a lack of a severe degree of hypoceruloplasminemia in this disorder.

Another explanation for the lack of abnormalities of iron metabolism in Wilson's disease is the possibility that alternate pathways of iron flow, not dependent on ceruloplasmin, are utilized. At least two other nonceruloplasmin ferroxidases have been found to exist in plasma (Lee *et al.*, 1969, 1976; Williams *et al.*, 1974). The physiological significance of these substances remains to be determined (Lee *et al.*, 1976).

It appears that ceruloplasmin plays an important role in the transfer of iron from reticuloendothelial cells to plasma. A similar mechanism may be required for optimal release of iron from duodenal mucosal cells and from hepatic parenchymal cells, which may account for the defective intestinal iron absorption and the excessive iron in duodenal mucosa and hepatic cells in the copper-deficient animals (Lee *et al.*, 1976).

The mechanism whereby ceruloplasmin exerts its effect on iron metabolism is by no means completely settled. It may be that the Osaki hypothesis accounts for the observed effect on iron flow (Osaki, 1966; Osaki and Walaas, 1967; Osaki *et al.*, 1966). However, the relatively low ferroxidase activity of the rat protein and the observation that ceruloplasmin ferroxidase activity at physiologic pH has only about one seventh the activity it has at pH 6.7 may be cited as evidence against this hypothesis (Williams *et al.*, 1974; Lee *et al.*, 1976).

Another mechanism of action of ceruloplasmin may be that it interacts with specific sites occupied by ferrous iron on the reticuloendothelial cell surface, and thus remove iron and transfer it to transferrin (Lee *et al.*,

1976). One other possibility is that ceruloplasmin may be responsible for regeneration of cytochrome oxidase (Broman, 1967), a copper protein known to be depleted in the copper-deficient animal. It is conceivable that cytochrome oxidase is required for the intracellular reduction of iron and that this reaction enhances the formation of a membrane iron pool available to transferrin (Lee *et al.,* 1976).

EFFECT OF COPPER DEFICIENCY ON NORMOBLASTS

The anemia of copper deficiency has many characteristics of bone marrow failure with ineffective erythropoiesis. Associated with the high plasma iron level are the low values for reticulocytes. Kinetic studies indicate that plasma iron turnover is normal. but erythrocyte iron incorporation is reduced. The bone marrow is cellular, and sideroblasts are increased. These findings are compatible with an intracellular defect in iron utilization (Lee *et al.,* 1976).

Screening procedures failed to detect deficiencies of the heme biosynthetic enzymes in copper deficiency (Lee *et al.,* 1968a, 1976). Nevertheless, intracellular defect in iron utilization was observed by means of *in vitro* studies of the transfer of [^{59}Fe]transferrin to reticulocytes and its incorporation into heme. Early in the course of copper deficiency, reticulocyte iron uptake was normal, but heme synthesis was impaired. Later, reticulocyte iron uptake was also impaired as the heme biosynthetic defect worsened (Lee *et al.,* 1976).

Goodman and Dallman (1969) concluded that a copper protein was required for normal mitochondrial iron uptake, a step that presumably must precede heme biosynthesis, inasmuch as the heme synthetase reaction takes place on the inner surface of the inner mitochondrial membrane (Jones and Jones, 1969). It is possible that the defect in heme synthesis in copper-deficient mitochondria is a consequence of the deficiency of cytochrome oxidase. Cytochrome oxidase, by donating electrons to ferric iron, could provide a steady supply of ferrous iron to serve as a substrate for heme synthesis (Lee *et al.,* 1976).

METABOLISM OF COPPER

Copper is absorbed mainly from the duodenum in man (Sacks *et al.,* 1943). Up to 32% of orally administered copper is absorbed in normal human subjects (Cartwright and Wintrobe, 1964a,b). Copper absorption and retention depend on the chemical forms in which the metal is ingested, the dietary levels of several other minerals and organic substances, and the acidity of the intestinal contents in the absorptive area. The mechanism of copper absorption is not known (Underwood, 1977).

High dietary intakes of calcium carbonate and ferrous sulfide depress copper absorption in sheep (Dick, 1954). The former presumably reduces absorption by raising the intestinal pH; the latter, by the formation of insoluble copper sulfide.

Copper absorption is inhibited by phytate (Davis *et al.,* 1962), and ascorbic acid increases the severity of copper deficiency in chicks (Carlton and Henderson, 1965; Hill and Starcher, 1965). Zinc, molybdenum, and cadmium also affect copper availability adversely. These observations suggest competition among various cations for similar binding sites at the intestinal level (Underwood, 1977).

Copper in the plasma is reversibly bound to serum albumin and forms the small, direct-reacting pool of plasma copper that is distributed widely to the tissues (Bush *et al.,* 1956a,b). The copper-albumin serum pool also receives copper from the tissues. The copper in ceruloplasmin does not appear to be so readily available for exchange or for transfer. A small fraction of serum copper is ultrafiltrable, and consists of copper that is free and another small fraction that is liganded to the amino acids (Sass-Kortsak, 1965).

The copper reaching the liver is incorporated into the mitochondria, microsomes, nuclei, and soluble fraction of the parenchymal cells in proportions that vary with the age, the strain, and the copper status of the animal (Gregoriadis and Sourkes, 1967; Herman and Kun, 1961; Milne and Weswig, 1968; Porter, 1970; Porter *et al.,* 1961; Thiers and Vallee, 1957). The copper is either stored in these sites or released for incorporation into erythrocuprein and ceruloplasmin and the various copper-containing enzymes of the cells. Ceruloplasmin is synthesized in the liver and secreted into the serum. Erythrocuprein is probably synthesized in normoblasts in the bone marrow. The hepatic copper is also secreted into the bile.

A high proportion of ingested copper appears in the feces. Most of this normally consists of unabsorbed copper, but active excretion via the bile occurs in all species. The biliary system is the major pathway of excretion in humans (van Ravesteyn, 1944). It has been estimated that of the 2–5 mg copper ingested daily by adult man, 0.6–1.6mg (32%) is absorbed, 0.5–1.3mg is excreted in the bile, 0.1–0.3 mg passes directly into the bowel, and 0.01–0.06 mg appears in the urine (Cartwright and Wintrobe, 1964a,b) (Fig. 2). Intravenous injection of copper is followed by a greater excretion of copper in the bile, and hence in the feces, but does not normally raise urinary copper output. Increased urinary excretion of copper occurs in patients with liver cirrhosis if associated with biliary obstruction (Bearn and Kunkel, 1954). Only a small amount of copper (10–60 μg) is excreted in urine daily in human subjects (Schroeder *et al.,* 1966).

In Wilson's disease, urinary copper excretion may be as high as 1500 μg/day. Amino acid excretion is also high in this disease, and some copper may be excreted in the urine as copper–amino acid complexes. In

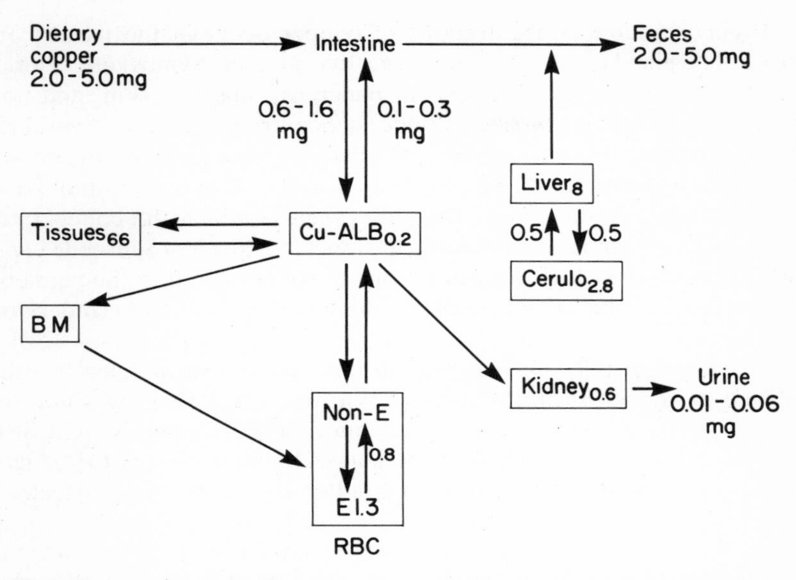

Fig. 2. Schematic representation of some metabolic pathways of copper in man. The numbers in the boxes refer to milligrams of copper in the pool. The numbers next to the arrows refer to milligrams of copper transversing the pathway each day. (Cu-ALB) direct-reacting fraction; (Cerulo) ceruloplasmin; (Non-E) nonerythrocuprein; (BM) bone marrow; (RBC) red blood cell. From Wintrobe (1974).

nephrosis, increased urinary copper may be correlated with proteinuria and excreted as copper–protein complexes.

Negligible amounts of copper are lost in the sweat (Mitchell and Hamilton, 1949). An average of 0.5 mg copper may be lost per menstrual cycle. This loss may account for less than 0.02 mg/day negative balance in females who are in their reproductive phase of life. Although the loss of copper in the milk at the height of human lactation is much higher (approximately 0.4 mg/day), there is no evidence that this loss imposes any nutritional hazard.

COPPER IN BODY TISSUES AND FLUIDS

The adult human body contains approximately 80 mg of copper (Cartwright and Wintrobe, 1964a,b). Newborn and very young subjects contain more copper per unit of body weight than adults (newborn 4.7 ppm vs. adults 1.7 ppm).

Cartwright and Wintrobe (1964a,b) reported a total of 23 mg in the liver, heart, spleen, kidneys, brain, and blood of normal subjects. Of this total, 8 mg was present in the liver and, surprisingly, 8 mg in the brain.

Highly variable concentrations of copper occur in the tissues of all species. The glands (prostate, pituitary, thyroid, and thymus) are examples of tissues low in copper; the spleen, pancreas, muscles, skin, and bones represent organs of intermediate copper concentration; and the liver, brain, kidneys, heart, and hair are tissues of relatively high copper concentration (Cunningham, 1931; Smith, H., 1967). In a study of the variation of copper levels with age, the brain was the only organ in which the concentration increased from birth to about double the level at maturity (Schroeder *et al.*, 1966). Exceptionally high concentrations of copper occur in the pigmented parts of the eye. The role of copper in these sites is not clear (Underwood, 1977).

Lea and Luttrell (1965) found, in contrast to the findings of others (Gopalan *et al.*, 1963; McDonald and Warren, 1961), that kwashiorkor is not necessarily accompanied by a reduction in the copper content of the hair. The copper concentration in the hair of humans does not rise significantly with age as it does in rats (Reinhold *et al.*, 1966, 1967; Underwood, 1977).

In the liver of the rat, at birth, over 80% of the total copper is present in the mitochondrial and nuclear fractions and less than 20% in the microsomes and soluble (supernatant) fractions (Gregoriadis and Sourkes, 1967). In the adult rat, the supernatant fraction contains about one half the total copper of the liver, with the copper content of nuclei, mitochondria, and microsomes following in that order. Porter (1970) showed that the copper in newborn liver is chiefly accounted for by mitochondrocuprein, a protein compound extraordinarily high in copper (more than 3%), localized in the mitochondrial fraction and specific to the neonatal period. Determination of liver copper may be a useful aid in the diagnosis of copper deficiency. The concentration of copper in the liver is influenced by several dietary factors other than copper. An increase in dietary molybdenum reduces the storage of copper in the livers of sheep and cattle (Dick and Bull, 1945). Copper retention in the liver and other tissues is also influenced by the levels of zinc and iron and of calcium carbonate in the diet. High intake of zinc depresses both copper and iron absorption (Cox and Harris, 1960; Grant-Frost and Underwood, 1958; Magee and Matrone, 1960; Van Campen, 1966). A marked zinc–copper antagonism is evident both when copper is limiting (Hill and Matrone, 1962) and in copper toxicity (Suttle and Mills, 1966a,b). A highly significant inverse correlation between hepatic iron and copper concentrations has also been demonstrated in rats.

Liver Copper in Disease States

Abnormally high liver copper concentrations are characteristic of a number of diseases of man. These diseases include thalassemia, hemochromatosis, cirrhosis and yellow atrophy of the liver, tuberculosis, carcinoma, severe chronic diseases accompanied by anemia, and Wilson's disease (hepatolenticular degeneration) (Cartwright, 1950).

Copper in Blood

A colorless copper protein, called erythrocuprein, has been isolated from human erythrocytes (Kimmel *et al.*, 1959; Markowitz *et al.*, 1959; Shields *et al.*, 1961). This compound is distinct from ceruloplasmin and from the human hepatocuprein isolated by Shapiro *et al.* (1961). Erythrocuprein has a molecular weight of 31,000, contains 3.4 μg Cu/mg protein, and comprises 60% or more of the total red cell copper (Shields *et al.*, 1961). It remains fairly constant under different conditions in man (Cartwright and Wintrobe, 1964a,b). The remainder of the erythrocyte copper is more loosely bound to unidentified proteins and is much more labile than erythrocuprein.

The copper in plasma also occurs in two main forms—one firmly bound to ceruloplasmin and the other reversibly bound to albumin. Ceruloplasmin is an α_2-globulin with a molecular weight of 151,000 containing 8 atoms of copper per molecule and accounts for roughly 80% of plasma copper in man (Butler, 1963; Cartwright, 1950; Holmberg and Laurell, 1947, 1948, 1951; Milne and Weswig, 1968; Starcher and Hill, 1965; Wintrobe *et al.*, 1953). Ceruloplasmin is an oxidase that catalyzes the oxidation of a variety of substrates including various polyphenols and biological compounds such as serotonin and epinephrine (Holmberg and Laurell, 1947, 1948, 1951; Martin *et al.*, 1964; Underwood, 1977).

"Direct-reacting" copper reacts directly with dithizone, is nondialyzable, and is reversibly bound to serum albumin (Bowland *et al.*, 1961; Bush *et al.*, 1956a,b; Moustgaard and Hojgaard-Olsen, 1951; Wintrobe *et al.*, 1953). This albumin-bound plasma copper is believed to constitute transport copper. In addition, the plasma contains copper enzymes, such as cytochrome oxidase and monoamine oxidase, in concentrations that vary with the copper status of the animal. A small amount of copper also exists in the serum in an ultrafiltrable form, as free copper and copper bound to amino acids. Although the exact physiological role of the amino-acid-bound copper fraction is not established, its role may be important for absorption of copper and cellular metabolism (Sass-Kortsak, 1965).

In human subjects, plasma copper does not increase following meals or decrease during fasting (Cartwright, 1950). The small diurnal variation in plasma copper observed in some studies is of doubtful statistical significance (Cartwright, 1950; Heilmeyer *et al.*, 1941; Vallee, 1954). Physical exertion in man produces no change in plasma copper. Plasma copper is higher in females than in males (105.5 $\pm$ 5.03 μg Cu/100 ml for men vs. 114.0 $\pm$ 4.67 μg Cu/100 ml for women) (Cartwright, 1950). Plasma copper can be significantly increased by the administration of estradiol in humans

(Johnson *et al.,* 1959; Russ and Raymunt, 1956). Serum copper levels are increased in women taking oral contraceptives (Halsted *et al.*, 1968; Clemetson, 1966; Prasad *et al.,* 1975).

Nielsen (1944a,b), in a study of 31 pregnant women, found serum copper to increase from the third month to an average of 2.7 μg/ml, compared with a normal level of 1.2 μg/ml in nonpregnant women. Similar results were reported by Krebs (1928), Röttger (1950), Fay *et al.* (1949), and Halsted *et al.* (1968). In these studies, the red cell copper remained at normal levels throughout pregnancy. The high serum copper levels of pregnancy return to normal in the first few weeks postpartum. The serum copper of the newborn infant is much lower than that of the mother, but rises to adult level by the second week of life (Fay *et al.,* 1949; Underwood, 1977).

The copper content of human erythrocytes is 1.2 ± 0.2 μg/ml (Prasad *et al.,* 1976). The amount of copper in the individual leukocyte and platelet is approximately one quarter of the red cell content. Plasma copper is a more sensitive indicator of the copper status of an animal than whole blood copper (Dreosti and Quicke, 1968; Underwood, 1977).

Influence of Disease on Serum Copper

In man, hypocupremia is associated with nephrosis and Wilson's disease, both of which are accompanied by increased urinary copper excretion. Hypocupremia also occurs in kwashiorkor and cystic fibrosis associated with a low dietary intake of protein. In one study, the mean plasma copper of nephrotics was found to be 0.6 ± 0.2 μg/ml, compared with 1.2 μg/ml in normal subjects (Cartwright *et al.,* 1954). The mean total serum copper of 36 patients with Wilson's disease was 0.61 ± 0.21 μg/ml, and that of 205 normal subjects, 1.14 ± 0.17 μg/ml. In this disease, serum copper levels are positively correlated with ceruloplasmin concentrations (Cartwright *et al.,* 1960). Almost all patients with Wilson's disease have less than 23 mg ceruloplasmin per 100 ml serum, which can be taken as the lower limit of normal.

Hypercupremia is present in most chronic and acute infections in man. In leukemia, Hodgkin's disease, various anemias, "collagen" disorders, hemochromatosis, and myocardial infarction, serum copper is increased (Vallee, 1954; Wintrobe *et al.,* 1953). In hyperthyroidism, an increase in plasma copper is accompanied by a decrease in erythrocyte copper (Underwood, 1977).

Copper in Milk

The copper content of milk during lactation ranges from 0.62 to 0.89 μg/ml (Underwood, 1977). Cavell and Widdowson (1964) also obtained a mean value of 0.62 μg Cu/ml (range 0.51–0.77) for the milk of 10 women sampled at the end of the first week of lactation.

COPPER DEFICIENCY IN HUMANS

Copper deficiency has been implicated in a syndrome affecting infants that is characterized by anemia, hypocupremia, and low serum iron and serum copper levels (Sturgeon and Brubaker, 1956; Zipursky *et al.,* 1958; Schubert and Lahey, 1959). Combined iron and copper administration is necessary for complete recovery. The hypocupremia is believed to result from an inability of the infants to obtain sufficient copper from a low-copper milk diet to prevent copper depletion from the increased loss of copper-protein into the bowel.

Until recently, the concept of uncomplicated copper deficiency in man was not widely accepted (Graham and Cordano, 1976). Despite evidence dating back to Josephs (1931), it was stated that copper deficiency could not exist in man (Wintrobe, 1961). Its development in severely malnourished infants rehabilitated on milk-based, low-copper diets (Cordano *et al.,* 1964), and its presence in untreated malnourished infants (Holtzman *et al.,* 1970), have been reported. During the past few years, copper deficiency has been reported in small premature infants (Al-Rashid and Spangler, 1971), in malnourished infants alimented exclusively by the intravenous route (Karpel and Peden, 1972), and in adults receiving TPN (Dunlap *et al.,* 1974).

A full-term infant, or a premature of more than 1500 g at birth, does not become copper-deficient on a low-copper diet without first experiencing prolonged and significant body losses of the element. These infants have normal concentrations of copper in the liver, which are adequate for many months after birth (Morrison and Nash, 1930). On the other hand, the livers of smaller premature infants contain less copper, and are thus unable to meet the demands for rapid growth on a diet based on unmodified cow's milk, which has a significantly lower concentration of copper than human milk (Fomon, 1974). With this single exception, no instance of copper deficiency has been reported that has not resulted from repeated and prolonged diarrhea and poor dietary copper intake. The principal route of excretion of copper is the bile (Underwood, 1977), and the main cause of deficiency is, presumably, failure to reabsorb this copper. Urinary loss is usually insignificant (Graham and Cordano, 1976).

In Peru, prior to 1964, malnourished infants were routinely treated with modified cow's-milk formula. This formula used to be given for 2–8 weeks before other feedings were substituted. Occasionally, and for special reasons, it was continued for a number of months. Because of relative lactose intolerance, the modified milk used to be diluted with sucrose and cottonseed oil. The water used to prepare the formula came from galvanized iron plumbing and was deionized to control electrolyte imbalance. These conditions undoubtedly served to accentuate the inadequacy of copper in the diet.

Cordano and Graham (1966) noted that four infants on this formula, despite rapid growth and normal serum proteins (albumin and globulins), developed neutropenia and anemia. The response to copper administration was dramatic (Graham and Cordano, 1976).

The earliest evidence of copper deficiency was persistent neutropenia, although the ability of the deficient patients to respond to infection with a significant neutrophil response was unimpaired. In some of the more severe and prolonged cases, a maturation arrest of the granulocyte series in the bone marrow was detected (Cordano *et al.*, 1964). A fall in serum copper and ceruloplasmin level was also found early in the depletion phase (Graham and Cordano, 1976).

Late in the course of copper deficiency, scurvylike bone lesions (by X ray) and occasional pathological fractures without any hemorrhage were observed (Cordano *et al.*, 1964; Cordano and Graham, 1966). The existence of similar bone lesions, without anemia and neutropenia, in Menkes' syndrome (Menkes *et al.*, 1962), which is believed to be a congenital defect in copper absorption (Danks *et al.*, 1972a,b), has not been explained. It is suggested that copper was available *in utero* for marrow development but not for calcified bone, central nervous system, or elastic tissue of the arterial vessels (Graham and Cordano, 1976).

Following the administration of oral copper sulfate to deficient infants, an initial fall in serum copper was observed in the first few hours, followed by a steep rise that preceded the increases in serum ceruloplasmin (Holtzman *et al.*, 1970, 1973; Graham and Cordano, 1976).

The peak incidence of copper deficiency in infants was under 1 year of age. This finding suggested that beyond that age, the infant or child was more likely to have consumed foods sufficiently rich in copper that the incidence of clinical deficiency was less detectable (Graham and Cordano, 1969, 1976).

Cordano and Graham (1966) reported two effects of copper deficiency on iron metabolism. The first, occurring early, was an adverse effect of copper deficiency on iron absorption (or mobilization). Untreated hypochromic iron deficiency that predated or developed simultaneously with copper deficiency persisted despite treatment with copper alone. It was suggested that the impairment of iron metabolism may be due to the loss of ferroxidase activity due to a lack of copper. The second and later effect of copper deficiency on iron metabolism was inadequate erythropoiesis, even in the presence of abundant iron stores. The neutropenia responded better to free copper than to ceruloplasmin (Graham and Cordano, 1976).

Another clinical condition in infants, Menke's kinky hair syndrome, is an X-linked genetic disorder in which copper absorption from intestine to blood is defective. The disease is characterized by hypocupremia, a decreased level of copper in the liver and hair, progressive mental deterioration, hypothermia, defective keratinization of hair, metaphyseal lesions, and degenerative changes in the aortic elastin (Danks *et al.,* 1972a,b).

Deficiency of copper has now been reported to occur in adults who received TPN for several weeks without copper supplementation (Vilter *et al.,* 1974; Dunlap *et al.,* 1974). Recently, copper deficiency characterized by hypochromic microcytic anemia and neutropenia was observed in adult patients with sickle cell disease who received 150 mg zinc daily in divided doses orally for nearly 2 years (Prasad *et al.,* 1978). Zinc was primarily given for the healing of leg ulcer and control of pain crisis. Once recognized, the hematological changes were promptly corrected by administration of 1 mg copper orally daily.

COPPER EXCESS

Acute copper poisoning occurs in man when grams of copper sulfate are ingested accidentally (Chuttani *et al.,* 1965; Wahal *et al.,* 1965). Acidic food or drink—vinegar, carbonated beverages, citrus juices—in prolonged contact with the metal has been known to produce copper toxicity (Hopper and Adams, 1958; Semple *et al.,* 1960; Bohre *et al.,* 1965; Paine, 1968; McMullen, 1971). Symptoms include metallic taste, ptyalism, nausea, vomiting, epigastric burning, and diarrhea (Hopper and Adams, 1958). Systemic toxic effects of copper poisoning include hemolysis, hepatic necrosis, gastrointestinal bleeding, oliguria, azotemia, hemoglobinuria, hematuria, proteinuria, hypotension, tachycardia, convulsions, coma, and death (Chuttani *et al.,* 1965; Davenport, 1953). Hemolysis has been reported following the application of solutions of copper salts to large areas of burned skin (Holtzman *et al.,* 1966), or following the introduction of copper from copper-containing semipermeable membranes or copper tubing into the circulation during hemodialysis (Blomfield *et al.,* 1969, 1971; Manzler and Schreiner, 1970; Barbour *et al.*, 1971; Klein *et al.,* 1972). Drinking water with an unusually high copper concentration (800 μg/liter) may have caused acrodynia (pink disease in a 15-month-old infant (Salmon and Wright, 1971; Scheinberg and Sternlieb, 1976).

Pulmonary copper deposition and fibrosis occur in the lungs of some vineyard workers after years of spraying fungicidal copper sulfate solutions (Pimentel and Marques, 1969). Yet, in copper miners, hepatic and serum concentrations of copper are normal despite years of exposure to an environment containing about 1% copper (Scheinberg and Sternlieb, 1969).

Gingivitis (Trachtenberg, 1972), lichen planus (Frykholm *et al.*, 1969), and eczematous dermatitis (Barranco, 1972) have been attributed to the copper alloys used in some dental or other prostheses. Penetration of a fragment of metallic copper into the eye can cause its loss, sunflower cataracts, or merely the visible corneal deposits of copper known as Kayser–Fleisher rings (Rosen, 1949; Hanna and Fraunfelder, 1973).

Human copper toxicity may occur in the following situations: (1) Wilson's disease; (2) the use of copper-containing intrauterine contraceptive devices; (3) the addition of copper salts to animal feeds; and (4) the use of copper sulfate as a fungicide, algicide, or molluscacide (Scheinberg and Sternlieb, 1976).

WILSON'S DISEASE (HEPATOLENTICULAR OR HEPATOCEREBRAL DEGENERATION)

This disease is inherited as an autosomal recessive trait with a general prevalence of about 1 in 200,000 and affects all races. The heterozygous state is found in about 1 in 200 people. The heterozygotes remain free of pathological manifestations of Wilson's disease (Scheinberg and Sternlieb, 1976).

Patients with Wilson's disease exhibit a deficiency of the plasma copper-protein ceruloplasmin (Scheinberg and Gitlin, 1952) and an excess of hepatic copper (Goldfischer and Sternlieb, 1968; Scheinberg and Sternlieb, 1965; Sternlieb and Scheinberg, 1968, 1974; Sternlieb, 1972). The latter finding is probably due in part to impairment of hepatic lysosomal excretion of copper into bile (Sternlieb *et al.,* 1973; Osborn and Walshe, 1967; Strickland *et al.,* 1969; O'Reilly *et al.,* 1971; Frommer, 1972) and in part to diminished or absent hepatic synthesis of ceruloplasmin (Sternlieb *et al.,* 1961; Scheinberg and Sternlieb, 1976).

The capacity of the liver to bind 50 times or more the normal hepatic concentration of copper is ultimately exceeded in patients with Wilson's disease. Copper may then suddently be released into the bloodstream, or it may diffuse into the circulation slowly (Sternlieb, 1972; Sternlieb and Scheinberg, 1974; Scheinberg and Sternlieb, 1976). The release of large amounts of copper from degenerating hepatocytes into the plasma may induce severe or fatal hemolysis characterized by jaundice that is both hemolytic and hepatocellular in origin (Roche-Sicot *et al.,* 1973; Scheinberg and Sternlieb, 1976).

If the copper in the liver is released slowly, the plasma concentration of free copper may rise to about 25–50 μg/100 ml (5–10 times normal). Free copper may diffuse out of the vascular compartment into both extracellular and intracellular fluids. The presence of excessive deposits of copper may be unsuspected for years, despite the progression of pathological changes in several organs, primarily in the liver. Characteristic changes in the liver include fatty degeneration of hepatocytes eventuating in necrosis, collapse of parenchyma, and postnecrotic cirrhosis (Sternlieb, 1972; Sternlieb and Scheinberg, 1974).

Unless the patient with Wilson's disease succumbs to his liver disease, the toxic effects of copper ultimately become manifest in the central nervous system, in the kidneys, and in the corneas (Sternlieb, 1966; Sussman and Scheinberg, 1969; Scheinberg and Sternlieb, 1976). Pathological changes in the brain are widespread (Konovalov, 1960; Wilson, 1912; Cumings, 1959; Schulman, 1968). In the kidney, glomerular and tubular changes, seen in biopsy and autopsy specimens of patients, are nonspecific (Wolff, 1964; Gilsanz *et al.,* 1960; Reynolds *et al.,* 1966). A number of renal functional abnormalities, including the Fanconi syndrome (aminoaciduria, phosphaturia, and glycosuria), proteinuria, uricosuria, hematuria, and tubular acidosis (Strickland and Leu, 1975), are generally reversible effects of copper toxicity in many patients (Bearn, 1972; Scheinberg and Sternlieb, 1976).

When copper is deposited in the corneas, it is visible as the Kayser–Fleischer ring, or crescent, which is seen best with the slit lamp as a golden or greenish-brown ring in Descemet's membrane (Sternlieb, 1966; Sussman and Scheinberg, 1969) at the outer circumference of the cornea. In some patients, copper is also deposited on the capsular surfaces of the lens in the form of a sunflower cataract (Cairns *et al.,* 1969). Neither of these phenomena interferes with vision (Scheinberg and Sternlieb, 1976).

Diagnosis. In about half of all symptomatic patients, the first clinical evidence of disease is dysfunction of the liver. There may be ascites, esophageal variceal hemorrhage (Sternlieb *et al.,* 1970), a syndrome mimicking toxic or infectious hepatitis, hemolysis caused by sudden release of sequestered copper (Deiss *et al.,* 1970), deficiency of clotting components, hypersplenism, or gonadal dysfunction (Sass-Kortsak, 1965; Scheinberg and Sternlieb, 1959, 1965, 1976; Sternlieb and Scheinberg, 1974).

In almost all other patients, neurological or psychiatric disorders are the initial clinical manifestations. The neurological picture may resemble parkinsonism, multiple sclerosis, chorea, dystonia or any combination of these conditions (Scheinberg and Sternlieb, 1965; Konovalov, 1960; Bearn, 1972; Walshe, 1966; Denny-Brown, 1964). The usual onset is insidious. Dysarthria is a frequent sign in children. Incoordination (often subtle), tremors, resting or intention, athetoid movements, rigidity, or dystonic posturing and distortion can occur at all ages. Excessive salivation and drooling are often present. Epileptiform seizures have been reported, but are unusual (Smith and Mattson, 1967; Passouant *et al.,* 1969). Specific disturbances in reflexes, sensation, or muscular strength are rare in Wilson's disease (Scheinberg and Sternlieb, 1976).

Psychiatric disorders may accompany the neurological, or may precede any other evidence of disease (Goldstein *et al.*, 1968; Beard, 1959; Kunath, 1969). The spectrum seen ranges from mild behavioral disturbance to manic–depressive or schizophrenialike psychosis. The emotional disturbance may be partly a reaction to the somatic dysfunction. The possibility that the cerebral deposits of copper may also exert a direct toxic effect on higher brain centers should be considered (Scheinberg and Sternlieb, 1976).

In at least five patients, hematuria was the first evidence of the toxic effects of copper (Fell *et al.*, 1968). In a few patients, Kayser–Fleischer rings are seen in the course of an ophthalmological examination that leads to the proper diagnosis of Wilson's disease (Scheinberg and Sternlieb, 1976).

Because of its autosomal recessive transmission, relatives (particularly siblings) of patients with Wilson's disease must be examined even if they appear perfectly healthy (Sternlieb and Scheinberg, 1968). Less than 20 mg ceruloplasmin/100 ml serum and more than 250 μg copper/gram dry liver and helpful diagnostic biochemical criteria. The liver biopsy samples from the great majority of patients will exhibit hepatocellular steatosis, inflammatory changes, excessive lipofuscin deposits, fibrosis, and/or mitochondrial abnormalities (Sternlieb, 1972; Scheinberg and Sternlieb, 1976).

Treatment of Copper Excess

One gram of penicillamine daily markedly increases the urinary output of copper and is an optimal dose in most patients. Periodic clinical examination of the patient and appropriate analyses of his urine and blood are necessary to detect any of several allergic or toxic side effects of penicillamine (Sternlieb and Scheinberg, 1964; Scheinberg and Sternlieb, 1976). Pyridoxine, 25 mg daily, is sufficient to compensate for any antipyridoxine effect of D-penicillamine (Scheinberg and Sternlieb, 1976).

In Wilson's disease and in chronic copper toxicity of sheep, massive or submassive necrosis of liver can sometimes free large enough amounts of copper over a sufficiently short time to cause considerable hemolysis (Roche-Sicot *et al.*, 1973; Deiss *et al.*, 1970; McIntyre *et al.*, 1967; Passwell *et al.*, 1970; Tönz *et al.*, 1971; Willms *et al.*, 1972). Since copper analyses are rarely performed in blood at the height of the hemolytic process, it is difficult to know the maximal concentration of free plasma copper that is attained. In one report, the value of free plasma copper given during the hemolytic crisis was 0.7 μg/ml (Deiss *et al.*, 1970), or about 10 times the normal free copper concentration. In another patient, 1.8 μg/ml was present temporarily in the plasma at the peak of hemolysis (Scheinberg and Sternlieb, 1976). In five patients not receiving penicillamine, the highest 24-hr urinary copper excretion measured during the hemolysis was 1.2 (Tönz *et al.*, 1971), 3.0 (Deiss *et al.*, 1970), 2.4, 2.5, and 4.7 mg (McIntyre *et al.*, 1967), respectively. These values are much greater than the normal daily copper excretion of 0.5 mg. The cause of hemolysis in Wilson's disease remains unknown (Scheinberg and Sternlieb, 1976).

COPPER-CONTAINING INTRAUTERINE CONTRACEPTIVE DEVICES

Winding several hundred square millimeters of copper wire around a plastic intrauterine device, (IUD) improves its contraceptive efficiency to less than 1.0 pregnancy/100 woman-years of experience (Zipper *et al.*, 1969); Tatum, 1973; Lippes *et al.*, 1973; Hagenfeldt, 1972). The intrauterine presence of copper may be associated with polymorphonuclear leukocytic infiltration of the endometrium (Cuadros and Hirsch, 1972). Analyses of copper IUDs, after their presence *in utero* for varying durations, show that about 20–50 mg of copper can be dissolved in a year. Some of the dissolved copper is lost through menstrual secretions, but experiments in rats show that at least some copper is absorbed within hours and is found in many extrauterine organs and tissues, principally liver and serum (Okereke *et al.*, 1972; Scheinberg and Sternlieb, 1976).

Further studies may determine whether or not the use of copper IUDs will lead to chronic copper toxicity. Such information is not available at present (Scheinberg and Sternlieb, 1976).

COPPER ADDITIVES TO ANIMAL FEEDS

Pigs fed rations containing 250 ppm copper for the purpose of accelerating increases in carcass weight have significant elevations in their hepatic copper concentrations from the normal mean of 24 to a mean of 220 μg/gram dry tissue (Braude *et al.*, 1973; Scheinberg and Sternlieb, 1976). Porcine liver is a principal constituent of many prepared meats, and much is eaten fresh. One quarter pound of liver from pigs fed rations with 250 ppm copper contains about 10 mg copper, which is 2–3 times the average daily supply of the metal in the Western diet. There are no data on the effects of eating this amount of copper for long periods. It would seem probable that except for persons with Wilson's disease, the normal homeostatic mechanisms could maintain zero copper balance in the face of an oral intake of this magnitude two or three times weekly (Scheinberg and Sternlieb, 1976).

COPPER AS A FUNGICIDE

A 1–2% solution of copper sulfate, neutralized with hydrated lime and known as Bordeaux mixture, is widely used as a fungicidal spray to prevent mildew on grape vines, principally in France, Portugal, and southern Italy (Pimentel and Marques, 1969). The copper in this spray has been incriminated in the pathogenesis of interstitial pulmonary lesions in the lungs of some vineyard workers. Their lungs were blue, suggesting the presence of excess copper, though analyses for copper were not reported. Similar lesions have also been observed in the lungs of guinea pigs exposed experimentally to the same sprays (Pimentel and Marques, 1969; Scheinberg and Sternlieb, 1976).

REFERENCES

Al-Rashid, R. A., and Spangler, J. 1971. Neonatal copper deficiency. *N. Eng. J. Med.* **285,** 841–843.

Barbour, B. H., Bishel, M., and Abrams, D. E. 1971. Copper accumulation in patients undergoing chronic hemodialysis: The role of cuprophan. *Nephron* **8,** 455–562.

Barranco, V. P. 1972. Eczematous dermatitis caused by internal exposure to copper. *Arch Dermatol.* **106,** 386–387.

Bearn, A. G. 1972. Wilson's disease. In: *The Metabolic Basis of Inherited Disease,* 3rd ed. (J. B. Stanbury, J. C. Wyngaarden, and D. S. Fredrickson, eds.). McGraw-Hill, New York, pp. 1033–1050.

Beard, A. W. 1959. The association of hepatolenticular degeneration with schizophrenia. *Acta Psychiatr. Neurol. Scand.* **34,** 411–428.

Bearn, A. G., and Kunkel, H. G. 1954. Abnormalities of copper metabolism in Wilson's disease and their relationship to the aminoaciduria. *J. Clin. Invest.* **33,** 400–409.

Beck, A. B. 1941. Studies on copper content of milk of sheep and of cows. *Aust. J. Exp. Biol. Med. Sci.* **19,** 145–150.

Bennets, H. W., and Chapman, F. E. 1937. Copper deficiency in sheep in Western Australia: A preliminary account of the etiology of enzootic ataxia of lambs and an anemia of ewes. *Aust. Vet. J.* **13,** 138–149.

Bird, D. W., Savage, J. E., and O'Dell, B. L. 1966. Effect of copper deficiency and inhibitors on the amine oxidase activity of chick tissues. *Proc. Soc. Exp. Biol. Med.* **123,** 250–254.

Blomfield, J., McPherson, J., and George, C. R. P. 1969. Active uptake of copper and zinc during haemodialysis. *Brit. Med. J.* **2,** 141–145.

Blomfield, J., Dixon, S. R., and McCredie, S. A. 1971. Potential hepatotoxicity of copper in recurrent hemodialysis. *Arch. Intern. Med.* **128,** 555–569.

Bohre, G. R., Huisman, J., and Lifferink, H. F. L. 1965. Acute copper poisoning aboard a ship. *Ned. Tijdschr. Geneeskd.* **109,** 978–979.

Boutigny, P. H. 1833. De la presence du cuivre dans le ble et dans un grand nombre d'autres substances. *J. Chim. Med.* **9,** 147–160.

Bowland, J. P., Braude, R., Chamberlain, A. G., Glascock, R. F., and Mitchell, K. G. 1961. The absorption, distribution and excretion of labelled copper in young pigs given different quantities, as sulphide, orally or intravenously. *Brit. J. Nutr.* **15,** 59–71.

Brady, F. O., Monaco, M. E., Forman, H. J., Schutz, G., and Feigelson, P. 1972. On the role of copper in activation of and catalysis by tryptophan-2, 3-dioxygenase. *J. Biol. Chem.* **247,** 7915–7922.

Braude, R., Mitchell, K. G., and Pittman, R. J. 1973. A note on cuprous chloride as a feed additive for growing pigs. *Anim. Prod.* **17,** 321–323.

Broman, L. 1967. The function of ceruloplasmin—a moot question. In: *Molecular Basis of Some Aspects of Mental Activity,* Vol. 2 (O. Walaas, ed.). Academic Press, New York, p. 131.

Bucholz, D. F. 1818. Analyse eines merkwurdigen Kupfererzes von Poinik in Ungarn. *Schweigeer. J.* **XXII,** pp. 43–50.

Buffoni, F., and Blaschko, H. 1964. Benzylamine oxidase and histaminase: Purification and crystallization of an enzyme from pig plasma. *Proc. R. Soc. London Ser. B* **161,** 153–167.

Bush, J. A., Mahoney, J. P., Gubler, C. J., Cartwright, G. E., and Wintrobe, M. M. 1956a. Studies on copper metabolism. *J. Lab. Clin. Med.* **47,** 898–906.

Bush, J. A., Jensen, W. N., Athens, J. W., Ashenbrucker, H., Cartwright, G. E., and Wintrobe,. M. M. 1956b. Studies on copper metabolism. XIX. The kinetics of iron metabolism and erythrocyte life span in copper-deficient swine. *J. Exp. Med.* **103,** 701–712.

Butler, E. J. 1963. The influence of pregnancy on the blood, plasma and caeruloplasmin copper levels of sheep. *Comp. Biochem. Physiol.* **9,** 1–12.

Cairns, J. E., Williams, H. P., and Walshe, J. M. 1969. "Sunflower cataract" in Wilson's disease. *Brit. Med. J.* **3,** 95–96.

Carlton, W. W., and Henderson, W. 1965. Studies in chickens fed a copper deficient diet supplemented with ascorbic acid, reserpine and diethylstilbestrol. *J. Nutr.* **85,** 67–72.

Carlton, W. W., and Kelly, W. A. 1969. Neural lesions in the offspring of female rats fed a copper deficient diet. *J. Nutr.* **97,** 42–52.

Carrico, R. J., and Deutsch, H. F. 1970. The presence of zinc in human cytocuprein and some properties of the apoprotein. *J. Biol. Chem.* **245,** 723–727.

Cartwright, G. E. 1950. Copper metabolism in human subjects. In: *A Symposium on Copper Metabolism* (W. D. McElroy and B. Glass, eds.). Johns Hopkins Press, Baltimore, pp. 274–314.

Cartwright, G. E., and Wintrobe, M. M. 1964a. Copper metabolism in normal subjects. *Amer. J. Clin. Nutr.* **14,** 224–232.

Cartwright, G. E., and Wintrobe, M. M. 1964b. The question of copper deficiency in man. *Amer. J. Clin. Nutr.* **15,** 94–110.

Cartwright, G. E., Gubler, C. J., and Wintrobe, M. M. 1954. Studies on copper metabolism. XI. Copper and iron metabolism in the nephrotic syndrome. *J. Clin. Invest.* **33,** 685–698.

Cartwright, G. E., Markowitz, H., Shields, G. S., and Wintrobe, M. M. 1960. Studies on copper metabolism. XXIX. A critical analysis of serum copper and ceruloplasmin concentrations in normal subjects, patients with Wilson's disease, and relatives of patients with Wilson's disease. *Amer. J. Med.* **28,** 555–563.

Cartwright, G. E., Markowitz, H., Shields, G. S., and Wintrobe, M. M. 1962. Studies on copper metabolism. XXIX. A critical analysis of serum copper in normal subjects, patients with Wilson's disease and relatives of patients with Wilson's disease. *Amer. J. Med.* **28,** 555–563.

Cavell, P. A., and Widdowson, E. M. 1964. Intakes and excretions of iron, copper, and zinc in the neonatal period. *Arch. Dis. Child.* **39,** 496–501.

Chou, W. S., Savage, J. E., and O'Dell, B. L. 1968. Relation of monoamine oxidase activity and collagen cross-linking in copper-deficient and control tissues. *Proc. Soc. Exp. Biol. Med.* **128,** 948–952.

Church, A. H. 1869. Researches on turacin, an animal pigment containing copper. *Philos. Trans. R. Soc. London* **159,** 627–636.

Church, A. H. 1892. Turacin, a remarkable animal pigment containing copper. *Roy. Inst. Proc.* **14,** 44–49.

Chuttani, H. K., Gupta, P. S., Gulati, S., and Gupta, D. W. 1965. Acute copper sulfate poisoning. *Amer. J. Med.* **39,** 849–854.

Clemetson, A. 1966. Chronic copper poisoning in sheep. *Aust. Vet. J.* **42,** 34.

Cohen, E., and Elvehjem, C. A. 1934. The relation of iron and copper to the cytochrome and oxidase content of animal tissue. *J. Biol. Chem.* **107,** 97–105.

Cordano, A., and Graham, G. G. 1966. Copper deficiency complicating severe chronic intestinal malabsorption. *Pediatrics* **38,** 596–604.

Cordano, A., Baertl, J. M., and Graham, G. G. 1964. Copper deficiency in infancy. *Pediatrics* **34,** 324–336.

Cox, D. H., and Harris, L. H. 1960. Effect of excess dietary zinc on iron and copper in the rat. *J. Nutr.* **70,** 514–520.

Craine, J. E., Daniels, G. H., and Kaufman, S. 1973. Dopamine- β-hydroxylase: The subunit structure and anion activation of the bovine adrenal enzyme. *J. Biol. Chem.* **248,** 7838–7844.

Cuadros, A., and Hirsch, J. G. 1972. Copper on intrauterine devices stimulates leukocyte exudation. *Science* **175,** 175–176.

Cumings, J. N. 1959. *Heavy Metals and the Brain.* Charles C. Thomas, Springfield, Illinois, pp. 3–71.

Cunningham, I. J. 1931. CXLI. Some biochemical and physiological aspects of copper in animal nutrition. *Biochem. J.* **25,** 1267–1294.

Curzon, G., and O'Reilly, S. 1960. A coupled iron ceruloplasmin oxidation system. *Biochem. Biophys. Res. Commun.* **2,** 284–286.

Danks, D. M., Cambell, P. E., Stevens, B. J., Mayne, V., and Cartwright, E. 1972a. Menkes' kinky hair syndrome: An inherited defect in copper absorption with widespread effects. *Pediatrics* **50,** 188–201.

Danks, D. M., Campbell, P. E., Walker-Smith, J., Stevens, B. J., Gillespie, J. M., Blomfield, J., and Turner, B. 1972b. Menkes' kinky-hair syndrome. *Lancet* **1,** 1100–1102.

Davenport, S. J. 1953. Health hazards of metals. 1. Copper. *U.S. Bur. Mines Inf. Circ.* **7666,** 1–114.

Davis, P. N., Norris, L. C., and Kratzer, F. H. 1962. Interference of soybean proteins with the utilization of trace minerals. *J. Nutr.* **77,** 217–223.

Deiss, A., Lee, G. R., and Cartwright, G. E. 1970. Hemolytic anemia in Wilson's disease. *Ann. Intern. Med.* **73,** 413–418.

Denny-Brown, D. 1964. Hepatolenticular degeneration (Wilson's disease). *N. Engl. J. Med.* **270,** 1149–1156.

Dick, A. T. 1954. Studies on the assimilation and storage of copper in crossbred sheep. *Aust. J. Agric. Res.* **5,** 511–544.

Dick, A. T., and Bull, L. B. 1945. Some preliminary observations on the effect of molybdenum on copper metabolism in herbivorous animals. *Aust. Vet. J.* **21,** (3), 70–72.

DiPaolo, D. V., Kanfer, J. N., and Newberne, P. M. 1974. Copper deficiency and the central nervous system. Myelination in the rat: Morphological and biochemical studies. *J. Neuropathol. Exp. Neurol.* **33,** 226–236.

Dreosti, I. E., and Quicke, G. V. 1968. Blood copper as an indicator of copper status with a note on serum proteins and leucocyte counts in copper-deficient rats. *Brit. J. Nutr.* **22,** 1–7.

Dunlap, W. M., James, G. W., III., and Hume, D. M. 1974. Anemia and neutropenia caused by copper deficiency. *Ann. Intern. Med.* **80,** 470–476.

Everson, G. J., Shrader, R. E., and Wang, T. 1968. Chemical and morphological changes in the brains of copper-deficient guinea pigs. *J. Nutr.* **96,** 115–125.

Fay, J., Cartwright, G. E., and Wintrobe, M. M. 1949. Studies on free erythrocyte protoporphyrin, serum iron, serum iron-binding capacity and plasma copper during normal pregnancy. *J. Clin. Invest.* **28,** 487–491.

Fell, G. S., Smith, H., and Howie, R. A. 1968. Neutron activation analysis for copper in biological material applied to Wilson's disease. *J. Clin. Pathol.* **21,** 8–11.

Fomon, S. J. 1974. *Infant Nutrition,* 2nd. ed. Saunders, Philadelphia, p. 363.

Fredericq, L. 1878. Sur l'organisation et la physiologie du poulpe *(Octopus vulgars). Arch. Zool. Exp.* **7,** 535–583.

Fridovich, I. 1972. Superoxide radical and superoxide dismutase. *Accounts Chem. Res.* **5,** 321–326.

Frommer, D. J. 1972. The measurement of biliary copper secretion in humans. *Clin. Sci.* **42,** 26P.

Frykholm, K. O., Frithiof, L., Fernstrom, A. I. B., Moberger, G., Blohm, S. G., and Bjorn, E. 1969. Allergy to copper derived from dental alloys as a possible cause of oral lesions of lichen planus. *Acta Derm.-Venereol. (Stockholm)* **49,** 268–281.

Gaber, B. P., and Aisen, P. 1970. Is bivalent iron bound to transferrin? *Biochim. Biophys. Acta* **221,** 228–233.

Gallagher, C. H., Reeve, V. E., and Wright, R. 1973. Copper deficiency in the rat: Effect on the ultrastructure of hepatocytes. *Aust. J. Exp. Biol. Med. Sci.* **51,** 181–189.

Gallop, P. M., Blumenfeld, O. O., and Seifter, S. 1972. Structure and metabolism of connective tissue proteins. *Annu. Rev. Biochem.* **41,** 617–672.

Gilsanz, V., Barrera, A., and Anaya, A. 1960. The renal biopsy in Wilson's disease. *Arch. Inter. Med.* **105,** 758–761.

Goldfischer, S., and Sternlieb, I. 1968. Changes in the distribution of hepatic copper in relation to the progression of Wilson's disease (hepatolenticular degeneration). *Amer. J. Pathol.* **53,** 883–901.

Goldstein, N. P., Ewert, J. C., Randall, R. V., and Gross, J. B. 1968. Psychiatric aspects of Wilson's disease (hepatolenticular degeneration): Results of psychomotor tests during long-term therapy. *Amer. J. Psychiatry* **124,** 1555–1561.

Goodman, J. G., and Dallman, P. R. 1969. Role of copper in iron localization in developing erythrocytes. *Blood* **34,** 747–753.

Gopalan, C., Reddy, V., and Mohan, V. S. 1963. Some aspects of copper metabolism in protein–calorie malnutrition. *J. Pediatr.* **63,** 646–649.

Graham, G. G., and Cordano, A. 1969. Copper depletion and efficiency in the malnourished infant. *John's Hopkins Med. J.* **124,** 139–150.

Graham, G. G., and Cordano, A. 1976. Copper deficiency in human subjects. In: *Trace Elements in Human Health and Disease,* Vol. I (A. S. Prasad, ed.). Academic Press, New York, pp. 363–372.

Grant-Frost, D. R., and Underwood, E. J. 1958. Zinc toxicity in the rat and its interrelation with copper. *Aust. J. Exp. Biol. Med. Sci.* **36,** 339–346.

Gregoriadis, G., and Sourkes, T. 1967. Intracellular distribution of copper in the liver of the rat. *Canad. J. Biochem.* **45,** 1841–1851.

Gubler, C. J., Lahey, M. E., Chase, M. S., Cartwright, G. E., and Wintrobe, M. M. 1952. Studies on copper metabolism. III. The metabolism of iron in copper-deficient swine. *Blood* **7,** 1075–1092.

Hagenfeldt, K. 1972. Intrauterine contraception with the copper-T device. *Contraception* **6,** 37–54.

Halsted, J. A., Hackley, B. M., and Smith, J. C., Jr. 1968. Plasma-zinc and copper in pregnancy and after oral contraceptives. *Lancet* **2,** 278–279.

Hanna, C., and Fraunfelder, F. P. 1973. Lens capsule change after intraocular copper. *Ann. Ophthalmol.* **5,** 9–22.

Harless, E. 1847. Ueber das blaue Blut einiger wirbellosen Thiere und dessen Kupfergehalt. *Arch. Anat. Physiol. Wiss. Med.* **14,** 148–156.

Harris, E. D., Gonnerman, W. A., Savage, J. E., and O'Dell, B. L. 1974. Connective tissue amine oxidase. II. Purification and partial characterization of lysyl oxidase from chick aorta. *Biochim. Biophys. Acta.* **341,** 332–344.

Hart, E. B., Steenbock, H., Waddell, J., and Elvehjem, C. A. 1928. Iron in nutrition: Copper as a supplement to iron for hemoglobin building in the rat. *J. Biol. Chem.* **77,** 797–812.

Heilmeyer, L., Keiderling, W., and Struve, C. 1941. *Kupfer and Eisen als körpereigene Wirkstoffe und ihre Bedeutung beim Krankheitsgeschehen.* Fischer, Jena, Germany, pp. 1–132.

Herman, G. E., and Kun, D. 1961. Intracellular distribution of copper in rat liver and its response to hypophysectomy and growth hormone. *Exp. Cell. Res.* **22,** 257–263.

Hill, C. H., and Matrone, G. 1962. Copper and zinc interrelations in poultry nutrition. In: *Proceedings of the 12th World Poultry Congress (Sydney) 1962,* pp. 219–222, Waverly Press, Baltimore.

Hill, C. H., and Starcher, B. 1965. Effect of reducing agents on copper deficiency in the chick. *J. Nutr.* **85,** 271–274.

Holmberg, C. G., and Laurell, C.-B. 1947. Investigations in serum copper I. Nature of serum copper and its relation to the iron-binding protein in human serum. *Acta Chem. Scand.* **1,** 944–950.

Holmberg, C. G., and Laurell, C. B. 1948. Investigations in serum copper. II. Isolation of the copper containing protein, and a description of some of its properties. *Acta Chem. Scand.* **2,** 550–556.

Holmberg, C. G., and Laurell, C. B. 1951. Investigations in serum copper. III. Caeruloplasmin as an enzyme. *Acta Chem. Scand.* **5,** 476–480.

Holtzman, N. A., Elliott, D. A., and Heller, R. H. 1966. Copper intoxication: Report of a case with observations on ceruloplasmin. *N. Engl. J. Med.* **275,** 347–352.

Holtzman, N. A., Charache, P., Cordano, A., and Graham, G. G. 1970. Distribution of serum copper in copper deficiency. *Johns Hopkins Med. J.* **126,** 34–42.

Holtzman, N. A., Graham, G. G., and Bucknall, W. E. 1973. Role of copper and copper-dependent ferroxidases in hematopoeisis. *Proc. IIIéme Symp. Internat. sur la maladie de Wilson,* Paris.

Hopper, S. H., and Adams, H. S. 1958. Copper poisoning from vending machines. *Public Health Rep* **73,** 910–914.

Howell, J. McC., and Davison, A. N. 1959. The copper content and cytochrome oxidase activity of tissues from normal and swayback lambs. *Biochem. J.* **72,** 365–367.

Ishimura, Y., and Hayaishi, O. 1973. Noninvolvement of copper in the L-tryptophan-2,3-dioxygenase reaction. *J. Biol. Chem.* **248,** 8610–8612.

Johnson, N. C., Kheim, T., and Kountz, W. B. 1959. Influence of sex hormones on total serum copper. *Proc. Soc. Exp. Biol. Med.* **102,** 98–99.

Jones, M. S., and Jones, O. T. G. 1969. The structural organization of heme synthesis in rat liver mitochondria. *Biochem. J.* **113,** 507–514.

Josephs, H. W. 1931. Treatment of anemia in infants with iron and copper. *Bull. Johns Hopkins Hosp.* **49,** 246–258.

Karpel, J. T., and Peden, V. H. 1972. Copper deficiency in long-term parenteral nutrition. *J. Pediatr.* **80,** 32–36.

Kelly, W. A., Kesterson, J. W., and Carlton, W. W. 1974. Myocardial lesions in the offspring of female rats fed a copper deficient diet. *Exp. Mol. Pathol.* **20,** 40–56.

Kimmel, J. R., Markowitz, H., and Brown, D. M. 1959. Some chemical and physical properties of erythrocuprein. *J. Biol. Chem.* **234,** 46–50.

Klein, W. J., Jr., Metz, E. N., and Price, A. R. 1972. Acute copper intoxication: A hazard of hemodialysis. *Arch. Intern. Med.* **129,** 578–582.

Konovalov, N. V. 1960. *Hepatocerebral Dystrophy.* Medgiz, Moscow.

Krebs, H. A. 1928. Über das Kupfer im menschlichen Blutserum. *Klin. Wochenschr.* **7,** 584–585.

Kunath, B. 1969. Zur Psychopathologie der hepatozerebralen Degeneration. *Fortschr. Neurol. Psychiatr. Ihrer Grenzgeb.* **37,** 91–106.

Lahey, M. E., Gubler, C. J., Chase, M. S., Cartwright, G. E., and Wintrobe, M. M. 1952. Studies on copper metabolism; hematologic manifestations of copper deficiency in swine. *Blood* **7,** 1053–1074.

Lea, C. M., and Luttrell, V. A. 1965. Copper content of hair in kwashiorkor. *Nature (London)* **206,** 413.

Lee, G. R., Cartwright, G. E., and Wintrobe, M. M. 1968a. Heme biosynthesis in copper-deficient swine. *Proc. Soc. Exp. Biol. Med.* **127,** 977–981.

Lee, G. R., Nacht, S., Lukens, J. N., and Cartwright, G. E. 1968b. Iron metabolism in copper-deficient swine. *J. Clin. Invest.* **47,** 2058–2069.

Lee, G. R., Nacht, S., Christensen, D., Hansen, S. P., and Cartwright, G. E. 1969. The contribution of citrate to the ferroxidase activity of serum. *Proc. Soc. Exp. Biol. Med.* **131,** 918–923.

Lee, G. R., Williams, D. M., and Cartwright, G. E. 1976. Role of copper in iron metabolism and heme biosynthesis. In: *Trace Elements in Human Health and Disease,* Vol. I (A. S. Prasad, ed.). Academic Press, New York, pp. 373–390.

Lippes, J., Zielenzny, M., and Sultz, H. 1973. The effect of copper on loop A. *J. Reprod. Med.* **10,** 166–170.

Magee, A. C., and Matrone, G. 1960. Studies on growth: Copper metabolism of rats fed high levels of zinc. *J. Nutr.* **72,** 233–242.

Mann, T., and Keilin, D. 1938. Haemocuprein and hepatocuprein, copper protein compounds of blood and liver in mammals. *Proc. R. Soc. London Ser. B* **126,** 303–315.

Manzler, A. D., and Schreiner, A. W. 1970. Copper-induced acute hemolytic anemia: A new complication of hemodialysis. *Ann. Inter. Med.* **73,** 409–412.

Markowitz, H., Cartwright, G. E., and Wintrobe, M. M. 1959. Studies on copper metabolism. XXVII. The isolation and properties of an erythrocyte cuproprotein (erythrocuprein). *J. Biol. Chem.* **234,** 40–45.

Martin, G. M., Derr, M. A. and Benditt, E. P. 1964. Ceruloplasmins of several animal species: Comparison of electrophoretic mobilities and substrate specificity. *Lab. Invest.* **13,** 282–287.

McCord, J. M., and Fridovich, I. 1969. Superoxide dismutase: An enzymic function for erythrocuprein (hemocuprein). *J. Biol. Chem.* **244,** 6049–6055.

McDonald, I., and Warren, P. J. 1961. The copper content of the liver and hair of African children with kwashiorkor. *Brit. J. Nutr.* **15,** 593–596.

McHargue, J. S. 1925. The association of copper with substances containing the fat-soluble A vitamin. *Amer. J. Physiol.* **72,** 583–594.

McHargue, J. S. 1926. Further evidence that small quantities of copper, manganese and zinc are factors in the metabolism of animals. *Amer. J. Physiol.* **77,** 245–255.

McIntyre, N., Clink, H. M., Levi, A. J., Cumings, J. N., and Sherlock, S. 1967. Hemolytic anemia in Wilson's disease. *N. Engl. J. Med.* **276,** 439–444.

McMullen, W. 1971. Copper contamination of soft drinks from bottles pourers. *Health Bull. Edinburgh* **29,** 94–96.

Menkes, J. H., Alter, M., Steigleder, G. K., Weakley, D. R., and Sung, J. H. 1962. A sex-linked recessive disorder with retardation of growth, peculiar hair and focal cerebral and cerebellar degeneration. *Pediatrics* **29,** 764–779.

Mills, C. F., and Williams, R. B. 1962. Copper concentration and cytochrome oxidase and ribonuclease activities in the brains of copper deficient lambs. *Biochem. J.* **85,** 629–632.

Milne, D. B., and Weswig, P. H. 1968. Effect of supplementary copper on blood and liver copper-containing fractions in rats. *J. Nutr.* **95,** 429–433.

Misra, H. P., and Fridovich, I. 1972. The role of superoxide anion in the autoxidation of epinephrine and a simple assay for superoxide dismutase. *J. Biol. Chem.* **247,** 3170–3175.

Mitchell, H. H., and Hamilton, T. S. 1949. The dermal excretion under controlled environmental conditions of nitrogen and minerals in human subjects, with particular reference to calcium and iron. *J. Biol. Chem.* **178,** 345–361.

Mondovi, B., Rotilio, G., Costa, M. T., Finazzi-Agro, A., Chiancone, E., Hansen, R. E., and Beinert, H. 1967. Diamine oxidase from pig kidney: Improved purification and properties. J. Biol. Chem. **242,** 1160–1167.

Morrison, D. B., and Nash, T. P. 1930. The copper content of infant livers. *J. Biol. Chem.* **88,** 479–483.

Moustgaard, J., and Hojgaard-Olsen, N. J. 1951. *Nord. Veterinaermed.* **3,** 763–779.

Narayanan, A. S., Siegel, R. C., and Martin, G. R. 1974. Stability and purification of lysyl oxidase. *Arch. Biochem. Biophys.* **162,** 231–237.

Neal, W. M., Becker, R. B., and Shealy, A. L. 1931. A natural copper deficiency in cattle rations. *Science* **74,** 418–419.

Nielsen, A. L. 1944a. On serum copper. III. Normal values. *Acta. Med. Scand.* **118,** 87–91.

Nielsen, A. L. 1944b. On serum copper. IV. Pregnancy and parturition. *Acta. Med. Scand.* **118,** 92–96.

O'Dell, B. L. 1976. Biochemistry and physiology of copper in vertebrates. In: *Trace Elements in Human Health and Disease,* Vol. I (A. S. Prasad, ed.). Academic Press, New York, pp. 391–413.

O'Dell, B. L., Hardwick, B. C., Reynolds, G., and Savage, J. E. 1961. Connective tissue defect resulting from copper deficiency. *Proc. Soc. Exp. Biol. Med.* **108,** 402–405.

Okereke, T., Sternlieb, I., Morell, A. G., and Scheinberg, I. H. 1972. Systemic absorption of intrauterine copper. *Science* **177,** 358–360.

O'Reilly, S., Weber, P. M., Oswald, M., and Shipley, L. 1971. Abnormalities of the physiology of copper in Wilson's disease. III. The excretion of copper. *Arch. Neurol. (Chicago)* **25,** 28–32.

Osaki, S. 1966. Kinetic studies of ferrous ion oxidation with crystalline human ferroxidase (ceruloplasmin). *J. Biol. Chem.* **241,** 5053–5059.

Osaki, S., and Walaas, O. 1967. Kinetic studies of ferrous iron oxidation with crystalline human ferroxidase. II. Rate constants at various steps and formation of a possible enzyme–substrate complex. *J. Biol. Chem.* **242,** 2653–2657.

Osaki, S., Johnson, D. A., and Frieden, E. 1966. The possible significance of the ferrous oxidase activity of ceruloplasmin in normal human serum. *J. Biol. Chem.* **241,** 2746–2751.

Osborn, S. B., and Walshe, J. M. 1967. Studies with radioactive copper (^{64}Cu and ^{67}Cu) in relation to the natural history of Wilson's disease. *Lancet* **1,** 346–350.

Paine, C. H. 1968. Food-poisoning due to copper. *Lancet* **2,** 520.

Partridge, S. M. 1969. Elastin, biosynthesis and structure. *Gerontologia* **15,** 85–100.

Passouant, P., Mirouze, J., Mary, P., Baldy-Moulinier, M., and Mahini, P. 1969. Epilepsie de type psycho-moteur manifestation évolutive d'un cas maladie de Wilson. *J. Med. Montpellier* **4,** 147–149.

Passwell, J., Cohen, B. E., Ben Bassat, I., Ramot, B., Shchory, M., and Lavi, U. 1970. Hemolysis in Wilson's disease: The role of glucose-6-phosphate dehydrogenase. *Isr. J. Med. Sci.* **6,** 549–554.

Pimentel, J. C., and Marques, F. 1969. "Vineyard sprayer's lung": A new occupational disease. *Thorax* **24,** 678–688.

Pinnell, S. R., and Martin, G. R. 1968. The crosslinking of collagen and elastin: Enzymatic conversion of lysine in peptide linkage to α-amino-adipic-δ-semialdehyde (allysine) by an extract from bone. *Proc. Natl. Acad. Sci. U.S.A.* **61,** 708–716.

Pomerantz, S. H. 1963. Separation, purification and properties of two tyrosinases from hamster melanoma. *J. Biol. Chem.* **238,** 2351–2357.

Porter, H. 1970. Neonatal hepatic mitochondrocuprein: The nature, submitochondrial localization, and possible function of the copper accumulating physiologically in the liver of newborn animals. In: *Trace Element Metabolism in Animals* (C. F. Mills, ed.). Livingstone, Edinburgh and London, pp. 237–247.

Porter, H., Wiener, W., and Barker, M. 1961. The intracellular distribution of copper in immature liver. *Biochim. Biophys. Acta* **52,** 419–423.

Prasad, A. S., Oberleas, D., Lei, K. Y., Moghissi, K. S., and Stryker, J. C. 1975. Effect of oral contraceptive agents on nutrients. I. Minerals *Amer. J. Clin. Nutr.* **28,** 377–384.

Prasad, A. S., Ortega, J., Brewer, G. J., Oberleas, D., and Schoomaker, E. B. 1976. Trace elements in sickle cell disease. *J. Amer. Med. Assoc.* **235,** 2396–2398.

Prasad, A. S., Brewer, G. J., Schoomaker, E. B., and Rabbani, P. 1978. Hypocupremia induced by large doses of zinc therapy in adults. *J. Amer. Med. Assoc.* (in press).

Prohaska, J. R., and Wells, W. W. 1974. Copper deficiency in the developing rat brain: A possible model for Menkes' steely hair disease. *J. Neurochem.* **23,** 91–98.

Ragan, H. A., Nacht, S., Lee, G. R., Bishop, C. R., and Cartwright, G. E. 1969. Effect of ceruloplasmin on plasma iron in copper-deficient swine. *Amer. J. Physiol.* **217,** 1320–1323.

Reinhold, J. G., Kfoury, G. A., Ghalambor, N. A., and Bennett, J. C. 1966. Zinc and copper concentrations in hair of Iranian villagers. *Amer. J. Clin. Nutr.* **18,** 294–300.

Reinhold, J. G., Kfoury, G. A., and Thomas, T. A. 1967. Zinc, copper and iron concentrations in hair and other tissues: Effects of low zinc and low protein intake in rats. *J. Nutr.* **92,** 173–182.

Reynolds, E. S., Tannen, R. L., and Tyler, H. R. 1966. The renal lesion in Wilson's disease. *Amer. J. Med.* **40,** 518–527.

Rimington, C. 1939. Porphyrins and their relation to metabolism of blood pigments. *Proc. R. Soc. Med.* **32,** 1268–1275.

Roche-Sicot, J., Sicot, C., Feldmann, G., Rueff, B., and Benhamou, J. P. 1973. The syndrome of acute intravascular hemolysis and acute liver failure as a first manifestation of Wilson's disease. *Digestion* **8,** 447.

Roensch, L. F., Savage, J. E., and O'Dell, B. L. 1972. Purification and characterization of tropoelastin from copper deficient chick aorta. *Fed. Proc. Fed. Amer. Soc. Exp. Biol.* **31,** 480 (abstract).

Roeser, H. P., Lee, G. R., Nacht, S., and Cartwright, G. E. 1970. The role of ceruloplasmin in iron metabolism. *J. Clin. Invest.* **49,** 2308–2417.

Rosen, E. 1949. Copper within the eye: With the report of a case of typical sunflower cataract involving the posterior capsule of the left eye. *Amer. J. Ophthalmol.* **32,** 248–252.

Röttger, H. 1950. Kupfer bei Mutter und Kind. *Arch. Gynaekol.* **177,** 650–660.

Rucker, R. B., and Goettlich-Rieman, W. 1972. Properties of rabbit aorta amine oxidase. *Proc. Soc. Exp. Biol. Med.* **139,** 286–289.

Rucker, R. B., and O'Dell, B. L. 1971. Connective tissue amine oxidase. I. Purification of bovine aorta amine oxidase and its comparison with plasma amine oxidase. *Biochim. Biophys. Acta* **235,** 32–43.

Rucker, R. B., Parker, H. E., and Rogler, J. C. 1969. Effect of copper deficiency on chick bone collagen and selected bone enzymes. *J. Nutr.* **98,** 57–63.

Russ, E. M., and Raymunt, J. 1956. Influence of estrogens on total serum copper and caeruloplasmin. *Proc. Soc. Exp. Biol. Med.* **92,** 465–466.

Sacks, A., Levine, V. E., Hill, F. C., and Hughes, R. C. 1943. Copper and iron in human blood. *Arch. Intern. Med.* **71,** 489–501.

Salmon, M. A., and Wright, T. 1971. Chronic copper poisoning presenting as pink disease. *Arch. Dis. Child.* **46,** 108–110.

Sandberg, L. B., Weissman, N., and Smith, D. W. 1969. The purification and partial characterization of a soluble elastin-like protein from copper-deficient porcine aorta. *Biochemistry* **8,** 2940–2945.

Sass-Kortsak, A. 1965. Copper metabolism. *Adv. Clin. Chem.* **8,** 1–67.

Scheinberg, I. H., and Gitlin, D. 1952. Deficiency of ceruloplasmin in patients with hepatolenticular degeneration (Wilson's disease). *Science* **116,** 484–485.

Scheinberg, I. H., and Sternlieb, I. 1959. The liver in Wilson's disease. *Gastroenterology* **37,** 550–564.

Scheinberg, I. H., and Sternlieb, I. 1965. Wilson's disease. *Annu. Rev. Med.* **16,** 119–134.

Scheinberg, I. H., and Sternlieb, I. 1969. Metabolism of trace metals. In: *Duncan's Diseases of Metabolism, Endocrinology and Nutrition,* Vol. II, 6th ed. (P. K. Bondy, ed.). Saunders, Philadelphia, pp. 1321–1334.

Scheinberg, I. H., and Sternlieb, I. 1976. Copper toxicity and Wilson's disease. In: *Trace Elements in Human Health and Disease,* Vol I (A. S. Prasad, ed.). Academic Press, New York, pp. 415–438.

Schroeder, H. A., Nason, A. P., Tipton, I. H., and Ballassa, J. J. 1966. Essential trace metals in man: Copper. *J. Chronic Dis.* **19,** 1007–1034.

Schubert, W. K., and Lahey, M. E. 1959. Copper and protein depletion complicating hypoferremic anemia of infancy. *Pediatrics* **24,** 710–733.

Schulman, S. 1968. Wilson's disease. In: *Pathology of the Nervous System,* Vol. 1 (J. Minckler, ed.). McGraw-Hill, New York, pp. 1139–1152.

Semple, A. B., Parry, W. H., and Phillips, D. E. 1960. Acute copper poisoning: An outbreak traced to contaminated water from a corroded geyser. *Lancet* **2,** 700–701.

Shapiro, J., Morell, A. G., and Scheinberg, I. H. 1961. A copper-protein of human liver. *J. Clin. Invest.* **40,** 1081.

Shields, G. S., Markowitz, H., Klassen, W. H., Cartwright, G. E., and Wintrobe, M. M. 1961. Studies on copper metabolism. XXXI. Erythrocyte copper. *J. Clin. Invest.* **40,** 2007–2015.

Shields, G. S., Coulson, W. F., Kimball, D. A., Carnes, W. H., Cartwright, G. E., and Wintrobe, M. M. 1962. Studies on copper metabolism. XXXII. Cardiovascular lesions in copper deficient swine. *Amer. J. Pathol.* **41,** 603–621.

Siegel, R. C., Pinnell, S. R., and Martin, G. R. 1970. Crosslinking of collagen and elastin: Properties of lysyl oxidase. *Biochemistry* **9,** 4486–4490.

Sjollema, B. 1933. Kupfermangel als Ursache von Krankheiten bei Pflanzen und Tieren. *Biochem. Z.* **267,** 151–156.

Sjollema, B. 1937. Kupfermangel als Ursache von Tier-krankheiten. *Biochem. Z.* **295,** 372–376.

Smith, C. K., and Mattson, R. H. 1967. Seizures in Wilson's disease. *Neurology* **17,** 1121–1123.

Smith, D. W., Weissman, N., and Carnes, W. H. 1968. Cardiovascular studies on copper deficient swine. XII. Partial purification of a soluble protein resembling elastin. *Biochem. Biophys. Res. Commun.* **31,** 309–315.

Smith, H. 1967. The distribution of antimony, arsenic, copper and zinc in human tissue. *J. Forensic Sci. Soc.* **7,** 97–102.

Sourkes, T. L. 1972. Influence of specific nutrients on catecholamine synthesis and metabolism. *Pharmacol. Rev.* **24,** 349–359.

Starcher, B., and Hill, C. H. 1965. Hormonal induction of ceruloplasmin in chicken serum. *Comp. Biochem. Physiol.* **15,** 429–434.

Sternlieb, I. 1966. The Kayser–Fleischer ring. *Med. Radiogr. Photogr.* **42,** 14–15.

Sternlieb, I. 1972. Evolution of the hepatic lesion in Wilson's disease (hepatolenticular degeneration). In: *Progress in Liver Diseases,* Vol. IV (H. Popper and F. Schaffner, eds.). Grune & Stratton, New York, pp. 511–525.

Sternlieb, I., and Scheinberg, I. H. 1963. The diagnosis of Wilson's disease in asymptomatic patients. *J. Amer. Med. Assoc.* **183,** 747–750.

Sternlieb, I., and Scheinberg, I. H. 1964. Penicillamine therapy in hepatotenticular degeneration. *J. Amer. Med. Assoc.* **189,** 748–754.

Sternlieb, I., and Scheinberg, I. H. 1968. Prevention of Wilson's disease in asymptomatic patients. *N. Engl. J. Med.* **278,** 352–359.

Sternlieb, I., and Scheinberg, I. H. 1974. Wilson's disease. In: *The Liver and Its Diseases* (F. Schaffner, S. Sherlock, and C. M. Leevy, eds.). Stratton Intercontinental Medical Book Corp., New York, pp. 328–336.

Sternlieb, I., Morell, A. G., Tucker, W. D., Greene, M. W., and Scheinberg, I. H. 1961. The incorporation of copper into ceruloplasmin *in vivo:* Studies with copper-64 and copper-67. *J. Clin. Invest.* **40,** 1834–1840.

Sternlieb, I., Scheinberg, I. H., and Walshe, J. M. 1970. Bleeding oesophageal varices in patients with Wilson's disease. *Lancet* **1,** 638–641.

Sternlieb, I., van den Hamer, C. J. A., Morell, A. G., Alpert, S., Gregoriadis, G., and Scheinberg, I. H. 1973. Lysosomal defect of hepatic copper excretion in Wilson's disease (hepatolenticular degeneration). *Gastroenterology* **64,** 99–105.

Strickland, G. T., and Leu, M. L. 1975. Wilson's disease: Clinical and laboratory manifestations in 40 patients. *Medicine (Baltimore)* **54,** 113–137.

Strickland, G. T., Beckner, W. M., Leu, M. L., and O'Reilly, S. 1969. Copper-67 studies in Wilson's disease patients and their families. *Clin Res.* **17,** 396.

Sturgeon, P., and Brubaker, C. 1956. Copper deficiency in infants: A syndrome characterized by hypocupremia, iron deficiency anemia, and hypoproteinemia. *AMA J. Dis. Child.* **92,** 254–265.

Sussman, W., and Scheinberg, I. H. 1969. Disappearance of Kayser–Fleischer rings: Effects of penicillamine. *Arch. Ophthalmol.* **82,** 738–741.

Suttle, N. F., and Mills, C. F. 1966a. Studies of the toxicity of copper to pigs. 1. Effects of oral supplements of zinc and iron salts on the development of copper toxicosis. *Brit. J. Nutr.* **20,** 135–148.

Suttle, N. F., and Mills, C. F. 1966b. Studies of the toxicity of copper to pigs. 2. Effect of protein source and other dietary components on the response to high and moderate intakes of copper. *Brit. J. Nutr.* **20,** 249–261.

Sykes, B. C., and Partridge, S. M. 1972. Isolation of a soluble elastin from lathyritic chicks. *Biochem. J.* **130,** 1171–1172.

Tatum, H. J. 1973. Metallic copper as an intrauterine contraceptive agent. *Amer. J. Obstet. Gynecol.* **117,** 602–618.

Thiers, R. E., and Vallee, B. L. 1957. Distribution of metals in subcellular fractions of rat liver. *J. Biol. Chem. 226, 911–920.*

Tönz, O., Furrer, H. U., and Bangerter, U. 1971. Kupferinduzierte Hämolyse bei Morbus Wilson. *Schweiz. Med. Wochenschr.* **101,** 1800–1802.

Trachtenberg, D. I. 1972. Allergic response to copper—its possible gingival implications. *J. Periodontol.* **43,** 705–707.

Underwood, E. J. 1977. *Trace Elements in Human and Animal Nutrition,* 4th ed. Academic Press, New York., pp. 56–108.

Vallee, B. L. 1954. The time course of serum copper concentrations of patients with myocardial infarctions. *Matabolism* **1,** 420–434.

Van Campen, D. R. 1966. Effects of zinc, cadmium, silver and mercury on the absorption and distribution of copper-64 in rats. *J. Nutr.* **88,** 125–130.

van Ravesteyn, A. H. 1944. Metabolism of copper in man. *Acta Med. Scand.* **118,** 163–196.

Vilter, R. W., Bozian, R. C., Hess, E. V., Zellner, D. C., and Petering, H. G. 1974. Manifestations of copper deficiency in a patient with systemic sclerosis on intravenous hyperalimentation. *N. Engl. J. Med.* **291,** 188–191.

Wahal, P. K., Mittal, V. P., and Bansal, O. P. 1965. Renal complications in acute copper sulphate poisoning. *Indian Pract.* **18,** 807–812.

Walshe, J. M. 1966. Wilson's disease: A review. In: *Biochemistry of Copper* (J. Peisach, P. Aisen, and W. E. Blumberg, eds.). Academic Press, New York, pp. 475–498.

Weisiger, R. A., and Fridovich, I. 1973. Superoxide dismutase: Organelle specificity. *J. Biol. Chem.* **248,** 3582–3592.

Williams, D. M., Christensen, D. D., Lee, G. R., and Cartwright, G. E. 1974. Serum azide-resistant ferroxidase activity. *Biochim. Biophys. Acta* **350,** 129–134.

Willms, B., Blume, K. G., and Löhr, G. W. 1972. Hämolotische Anämie bei Morbus Wilson (Hepatolentikuläre Degeneration). *Klin. Wochenschr.* **50,** 995–1002.

Wilson, S. A. K. 1912. Progressive lenticular degeneration: A familial nervous disease associated with cirrhosis of the liver. *Brain* **34,** 295–509.

Wintrobe, M. M. 1961. *Clinical Hematology,* 5th ed. Lea and Febiger, Philadelphia, p. 141.

Wintrobe, M. M. 1974. *Clinical Hematology,* 7th ed. Lea and Febiger, Philadelphia, pp. 150–152.

Wintrobe, M. M., Cartwright, G. E., and Gubler, C. J. 1953. Studies on the function and metabolism of copper. *J. Nutr.* **50,** 395–419.

Wolff, S. M. 1964. Renal lesions in Wilson's disease. *Lancet* **1,** 843–845.

Yamada, H., and Yasunobu, K. T. 1962. Monoamine oxidase. II. Copper, one of the prosthetic groups of plasma monoamine oxidase. *J. Biol. Chem.* **237,** 3077–3082.

Zipper, J. A., Tatum, H. J., Pastene, L., Medel, M., and Rivera, M. 1969. Metallic Cu as an intrauterine contraceptive adjunct to the "T" device. *Amer. J. Obstet. Gynecol.* **105,** 1274–1278.

Zipursky, A., Dempsey, H., Markowitz, H., Cartwright, G. E., and Wintrobe, M. M. 1958. Studies on copper metabolism. XXIV. Hypocupremia in infancy. *AMA J. Dis. Child.* **95,** 148–158.

CHAPTER 3

FLUORIDE

INTRODUCTION

Interest in the biological significance of fluoride was at first confined to its toxic effects on animals, following the discovery of chronic endemic fluorosis of man and farm stock in several countries in 1931 (Underwood, 1977). The beneficial effect of fluoride on the incidence of dental caries was recognized in 1901 following the observation of Eager (1901) that children with mottled enamel were relatively free from dental decay. A quantitative relationship between caries incidence and fluoride in drinking water was first shown by Dean (1942), who conducted a survey of 21 cities in the United States. Later studies by Hodge (1950) indicated that the optimal level of fluoride in the drinking water for dental health was 1 ppm.

Although fluoride at a level of 1 ppm in drinking water or in various topical applications is known to be a safe and effective cariostatic agent (Marthaler, 1967; Caldwell and Thomas, 1970), its mode of action, optimal time–dose relationship, and interactions with other elements have not been sufficiently clarified. Whereas other trace elements have been reported to have cariostatic properties, fluoride is without question the most effective (Navia, 1970; Navia *et al.,* 1976). It is believed that fluoride exerts its anticariogenic action by enzyme inhibition of cariogenic bacteria in dental plaque.

BIOCHEMISTRY

Fluoride is known to affect the activity of several enzymes. Excess fluoride decreases the fatty acid oxidase activity of the rat kidney and partially inhibits the intestinal lipase activity (Sievert and Phillips, 1959). The overall utilization of fatty acid is impaired due to fluorosis.

A decrease in the glycogen turnover rate and lowered activity of glucose-6-phosphate dehydrogenase in the liver have been reported in fluoritic rats (Carlson and Suttie, 1966). These effects, however, may be due to an altered feeding pattern of the animals due to fluorosis. Fluoride has been reported to inhibit the growth and glycolysis of cultured strain of L-mouse fibroblasts, probably due to a depression in the activity of enolase and a shift in the ratio of NAD to NADH (Suttie *et al.,* 1974).

In a long-term experiment in dairy heifers, excessive accumulation of fluoride in bone was associated with osseous abnormalities and increased alkaline phosphatase activity in the bone (Miller and Shupe, 1962). The biochemical changes noted above however do not adequately explain the physiological and pathological effects of fluoride on human tissue.

METABOLISM

Fluoride from inorganic sources is quickly absorbed and distributed throughout the body. While some fluoride crosses the gastric mucosa, most is quickly absorbed from the small intestine. As much as 95% of the total body fluoride is probably incorporated into skeletal and dental tissues. Distribution of fluoride within the bone varies, and it is higher in cancellous than in compact bone. Growing bones are more biologically active and appear to incorporate fluoride more readily (Weidmann and Weatherell, 1970). Fluoride tends to accumulate in soft tissues with ectopic calcification (Call *et al.,* 1965; Navia *et al.,* 1976; Smith *et al.,* 1960).

Fluoride is found in bone and tooth apatite (Eanes and Posner, 1970), substituting for hydroxyl groups at selected sites in the apatite lattice. Pure fluorapatite is rarely found, because if all the hydroxyl positions in the apatite were exchanged for fluoride, its concentration in the fluoroapatite formed would be 3.8%, and most bone and enamel does not approach such a value, with the exception of shark enamel, which seems to contain fluoroapatite (Glas, 1962). No evidence has been reported to indicate that CaF_2 is present in the skeleton, although it has been found in enamel topically treated with fluoride. This molecule is easily lost from the surface, although the fluoride associated with apatite structures remains in the enamel (Baud and Bang, 1970; Navia *et al.,* 1976).

Body fluids such as saliva, bile, and blood contain concentrations of fluoride ranging from 0.1 to 0.2 ppm. These levels vary according to the fluoride intake in the diet and drinking water. Dietary fluoride is highly dependent on whether or not the area is fluoridated. In fluoridated areas, the dietary fluoride content exclusive of the drinking water has been reported to range from 1.7 to 3.4 mg/day (Kramer *et al.,* 1974), and in nonfluoridated areas, the fluoride intake was found to be about 1 mg/day (Navia *et al.,* 1976).

Generally, the mammary gland and the placenta appear to act as barriers that interfere with fluoride transfer to the milk or the fetus (Zipkin and Babeaux, 1965), although Armstrong *et al.* (1970) did question the existence of such a placental barrier. Fluoride is usually excreted through the kidneys, but up to 10% may be eliminated in the feces. Some fluoride may be excreted through sweat glands, but this amount is difficult to determine, and it depends on factors such as temperature and activity of the individual. Fluoride excretion is rapid, and a large percentage of an orally or parenterally administered dose is excreted within a few hours (Muhler *et al.*, 1966; Navia *et al.*, 1976).

Foods high in fluoride (Underwood, 1977) include sea foods (5–10 μg/g) and tea (100 μg/g). Cereal and other grains contain 1–3 μg/g. Cow's milk usually contains 1–2 μg/g (dry basis). An important source of fluoride is fluoridated drinking water.

CLINICAL EFFECTS OF FLUORIDE SUPPLEMENTATION

A low level of fluoride in drinking water and consequent decreased concentration in bone has been associated with osteoporosis (Leone *et al.*, 1954). It was postulated that osteoporosis and Paget's disease might be controlled by the administration of fluoride in doses as high as 100 mg/day (Rich *et al.*, 1964). Studies in rats (Lane and Steinberg, 1973) in which fluoride was compared to diphosphonates in its ability to inhibit osteoporosis of disuse indicated no beneficial effect of fluoride. Studies in which pigs were used as animal models (Spencer *et al.*, 1971) indicated that there were no intrinsic differences in strength of cortical bone from femora of swine on rations with or without fluoride (Navia *et al.*, 1976).

Hodge and Smith (1968) concluded that in humans, the beneficial effects of fluoride were not clearly established, although a reduction of bone pain and urinary calcium excretion had been documented in multiple myeloma. Riggs *et al.* (1972) suggested that sodium fluoride together with calcium supplements might stimulate formation of normal bone, although more work is needed to establish the effectiveness of these substances in metabolic bone diseases (Navia *et al.*, 1976).

The cariostatic effect of fluoride for humans has been clearly demonstrated in epidemiological studies of persons consuming water that contained an optimal level of 1 or 2 ppm of fluoride (Arnold *et al.*, 1962; Ast *et al.*, 1956). Although water fluoridation is an effective public health measure that should be "the cornerstone of any national program of dental caries prevention" (Horowitz, 1973), there are also other approaches to using this valuable element in caries control (Navia *et al.*, 1976).

During fetal life, when the deciduous teeth are actively mineralizing, it is possible to make fluoride available. Fluoride is made available to the suckling infant if the mother has a sufficiently high fluoride intake. Zipkin and Babeaux (Babeaux and Zipkin, 1966; Zipkin and Babeaux, 1965) reviewed the subject of maternal transfer of fluoride and concluded that the placenta acts as a barrier, limiting the availability of maternal fluoride to the fetal tissues, and that milk contains a low concentration of fluoride (0.1–0.2 ppm F) that does not increase significantly even with a dietary intake of fluoride as high as 5 mg/day (Navia *et al.,* 1976). No additional benefits from the maternal ingestion of fluoridated water were found if the offspring also ingested fluoridated water from birth (Carlos *et al.* 1962; Horowitz and Heifetz, 1967).

Animal studies that were directed to evaluating the systemic effects of fluoride on caries were inconclusive because more than one developmental period was examined (Stookey *et al.,* 1962; König *et al.,* 1960; Shaw and Sognnaes, 1954; Navia *et al.,* 1976). Some of the mechanisms that have been suggested to explain the cariostatic properties of fluoride are: (1) alteration of tooth crown morphology; (2) formation of large, perfect crystals of apatite; (3) stimulation of processes at the enamel surface; (4) decreased solubility of enamel; and (5) decreased bacterial enzymatic activity. Most likely, each of these mechanisms is responsible in some measure for the cariostatic effect of fluoride.

The results of studies of the effects of fluoride on caries in humans have not enabled investigators to distinguish clearly between preeruptive and posteruptive effects of this element. In a recent paper, Aasenden and Peebles (1974) studied a group of children from nonfluoridated communities who had ingested a 0.5 mg fluoride supplement/day from 1 week to 4 months after birth until 3 years of age and then continued on a 1 mg/day supplement until 10 years of age, when oral examinations were done. This group was compared with children from the same communities who had not received fluoride and with a group of children with a lifetime exposure to fluoridated water. Comparison of mean scores of decayed and filled surfaces per child for all teeth and for first molars between the three groups (fluoride-supplemented, fluoridated-water-exposed, and nonsupplemented subjects), indicated the scores to be 1 : 2 : 5. These authors also evaluated the incidence and severity of enamel fluorosis and found the mean fluorosis index to be twice as high in the group supplemented with fluoride (0.88) as in the group that received fluoridated water throughout life (0.40). In the supplemented group, 14% had moderate lesions, whereas only 2.2% had these lesions in the group drinking fluoridated water (Navia *et al.,* 1976).

This human study shows the combined pre- and posteruptive effects of fluoride and does not attempt to separate them. Thus, the net reduction in caries is the result of the addition of these two effects of fluoride. In view of the higher incidence of enamel fluorosis reported in the human study, it is possible that a greater beneficial effect might have been seen if the fluoride administration had started immediately before eruption and continued thereafter, rather than a continuous supplementation throughout in the earlier preeruptive stage. Studies with experimental animal models suggest a definite advantage in providing fluoride immediately before eruption, when its uptake is greatest, and continuing this administration during the early posteruptive maturation period (Navia *et al.,* 1968, 1976). This approach would avoid possible deleterious effect during the period of greatest ameloblast activity, and would still increase fluoride concentration in the outer enamel surface. This would make fluoride available to strengthen the resistance of the tooth (Navia, 1973) by influencing the maturation process of enamel, pellicle formation, and bacterial plaque metabolism on the enamel surface (Bowen and Hewitt, 1974; Navia *et al.,* 1976).

The posteruptive administration of fluoride in the drinking water offered to weanling rats decreased the severity of carious lesions (Navia *et al.,* 1976). Molars of these rats were found to contain a substantial level of fluoride (0.160 μg/g) in comparison with the level in control rats (0.013 μg F/g). Fluoride given preeruptively during the time of tooth mineralization also increased the fluoride level of the tooth, although it did not make the molar caries-resistant. Actually, the caries susceptibility increased at higher doses of fluoride. These data suggest that fluoride content of molars is not the only factor responsible for the cariostatic effect. Results from this study support the concept that posteruptive administration of fluoride is most beneficial, especially if it includes the time when the tooth is actually emerging into the oral cavity (Navia *et al.,* 1976). At this time, even a short exposure of the molars to fluoride is capable of conferring a lasting protection against caries. Madsen and Edmonds (1964) fed a diet supplemented with sodium fluoride to weanling cotton rats for only 2 days (12 and 13 days of age), when first molars of this strain of rats start to erupt. At 40 days of age, a significant reduction in molar caries scores between treated rats and untreated controls was noted. Only the newly erupted first molars were protected significantly by early fluoride treatment. A similar response to another cariostatic agent, sodium trimetaphosphate, was noted when it was offered immediately following tooth eruption (Navia *et al.,* 1968, 1976).

Fluoride may have an additional role in absorption or utilization of other dietary nutrients. Fluoride can enhance the intestinal absorption of iron (Ruliffson *et al.,* 1963). Fluoride has been shown to activate other enzyme systems, most notably adenyl cyclase (Drummond *et al.,* 1971). Thus, a wider role of fluoride is possible in human metabolism.

In summary, administration of supplemented fluoride should be considered and evaluated at times when the tooth is erupting or has recently erupted, inasmuch as it is at these times that the cariostatic effects are found to be most dramatic. The administration of supplemental fluoride before tooth eruption is not effective and is possibly even detrimental, particularly when other trace elements are given concomitantly (Navia *et al.*, 1976). Hunt and Navia (1975) have shown repeatedly that when elements previously supposed to have cariostatic properties are administered along with fluoride during tooth formation, there is an enhancement of enamel hypoplasia that makes the molars highly susceptible to caries. The interaction shown to exist between trace elements and fluoride (Buttner, 1963) is important and should be investigated further. Local administration of frequent doses of fluoride to the erupted tooth appears to be an ideal approach to ensure maximum effectiveness of this highly beneficial element to dental health (Navia *et al.*, 1976).

CLINICAL EFFECTS OF FLUORIDE EXCESS

Mottled teeth due to fluorosis are characterized by chalky white patches distributed irregularly over the surface of the teeth, with a secondary infiltration of yellow to brown staining. Enamel is weak, and in severe cases, there is loss of enamel with "pitting," which gives the tooth surface a corroded appearance. Mottled enamel is seen in permanent teeth, and it develops during the formation of teeth.

Fully formed enamel of adult teeth is unaffected by fluorosis, and deciduous teeth are affected only at high fluoride intake when other signs of fluorosis are evident (Underwood, 1977).

In areas with highly fluoridated water ($>$ 8 ppm fluoride), not only is there a high incidence of severe mottled enamel, but also disturbances in ossification and systemic signs of fluorosis can develop. Osteosclerosis, calcification of ligaments and tendinous insertions, and crippling deformities such as kyphosis, stiffness of the spine, and bony exostoses may be seen in adults residing for 30 to 40 years in endemic areas. Genu valgum (knock knee) has been reported to occur in subjects between the ages of 10 and 25 years in endemic areas of southern India and South Africa. The etiology of this rare syndrome of fluoride toxicity and the reason for its recent disappearance are not well understood. Low-calcium and high-molybdenum dietary intake may have played additional roles in the overall clinical effects of fluorosis in these areas (Underwood, 1977).

REFERENCES

Aasenden, R., and Peebles, T. C. 1974. Effect of fluoride supplementation from birth on human deciduous and permanent teeth. *Arch. Oral Biol.* **19**, 321–326.

Armstrong, W. D., Singer, L., and Makowski, E. L. 1970. Placental transfer of fluoride and calcium. *Amer. J. Obstet. Gynecol.* **107**, 432–434.

Arnold, F. A., Likins, R. C., Russell, A. L., and Scott, D. B. 1962. Fifteenth year of Grand Rapids fluoridation study. *J. Amer. Dent. Assoc.* **65,** 780–785.

Ast, D. B., Smith, D. J., Wachs, B., and Cantwell, K. T. 1956. Newburgh–Kingstone caries–fluroine study XIV. Combined clinical and roentgenographic dental findings after 10 years of fluoride experience. *J. Amer. Dent. Assoc.* **52,** 314–325.

Babeaux, W. L., and Zipkin, I. 1966. Dental aspects of the prenatal administration of fluoride. *J. Oral Ther. Pharmacol.* **3,** 124–135.

Baud, C. A., and Bang, S. 1970. Electron probe and X-ray diffraction microanalyses of human enamel treated *in vitro* by fluoride solutions. *Caries Res.* **4,** 1–13.

Bowen, W. H., and Hewitt, M. J. 1974. Effect of fluoride on extracellular polysaccharide production by *Streptococcus mutans*. *J. Dent. Res.* **53,** 627–629.

Buttner, W. 1963. Action of trace elements on the metabolism of fluoride. *J. Dent. Res.* **42,** 453–460.

Caldwell, R., and Thomas, J. 1970. Application of chemical agents for the control of dental caries. In: *Dietary Chemical vs. Dental Caries, Adv. Chem. Ser. No. 94*. American Chemical Society, Washington, D.C., pp. 161–180.

Call, R. A., Greenwood, D. A., LeCheminant, W. H., Shupe, J. L., Nielsen, H. M., Olson, L. E., Lamborn, R. E., Mangleson, F. L., and Davis, R. V. 1965. Histological and chemical studies on effects of fluoride in man. *Public Health Rep.* **80,** 529–538.

Carlos, J. P., Gittelsohn, A. M., and Haddon, W. 1962. Caries in deciduous teeth in relation to maternal ingestion of fluoride. *Public Health Rep.* **77,** 658–660.

Carlson, J. R., and Suttie, J. W. 1966. Pentose phosphate pathway enzymes and glucose oxidation in fluoride-fed Rats. *Am. J. Physiol.* **210,** 79–83.

Dean, M. T. 1942. In: *Fluorine and Dental Health* (F. R. Moulton, ed.). American Association for the Advancement of Science, Washington, D.C., pp. 6–11, 23–31.

Drummond, G. I., Severson, D. L., and Duncan, L. 1971. Adenyl cyclase: Kinetic properties and nature of fluoride and hormone stimulation. *J. Biol. Chem.* **246,** 4166–4173.

Eager, J. M. 1901. Denti di Chiaie. *Public Health Rep.* **16,** 2576–2577.

Eanes, E. D., and Posner, A. S. 1970. Structure and chemistry of bone mineral. In: *Biological Calcification: Cellular and Molecular Aspects* (H. Schraer, ed.). Appleton-Century-Crofts, New York, pp. 1–26.

Glas, J. E. 1962. Studies on the ultrastructure of dental enamel. VI. *Odont. Rev.* **13,** 315–326.

Hodge, H. C. 1950. Concentration of fluorides in drinking water to give point of minimum caries with maximum safety. *J. Amer. Dent. Assoc.* **40,** 436–439.

Hodge, H. C., and Smith, F. A. 1968. Fluorides and man. *Annu. Rev. Pharmacol.* **8,** 395–408.

Horowitz, H. S. 1973. Fluoride: Research on clinical and public health applications. *J. Amer. Dent. Assoc.* **87,** 1013–1018.

Horowitz, H. S., and Heifetz, S. B. 1967. Effects of prenatal exposure to fluoridation on dental caries. *Public Health Rep.* **82,** 297–304.

Hunt, C. E., and Navia, J. M. 1975. Preeruptive effects of molybdenum, boron, strontium, and fluorine on dental caries in the rat. *Arch. Oral Biol.* **20,** 497–501.

König, K. G. von, Marthaler, T. M., Schait, A., and Mühlemann, H. R. 1960. Karieshemmung durch Fluor in Wasser, Milch and Futter und Skelettfluorspeicherung im Rattenversuch bei Verabreichung während und nach Abschluss der Zahnentrücklung. *Schweiz. Monatsschr. Zahnheilkd.* **70,** 290–314.

Kramer, L., Osis, D., Wiatrawski, E., and Spencer, H. 1974. Dietary fluoride in different areas in the United States. *Amer. J. Clin. Nutr.* **27,** 590–594.

Lane, J. M., and Steinberg, M. E. 1973. The role of diphosphonates in osteoporosis of disuse. *J. Trauma* **13,** 863–869.

Leone, N. C., Shimkin, M. B., Arnold, F. A., Stevenson, C. A., Zimmerman, E. R., Geiser, P. A., and Lieberman, J. E. 1954. Medical aspects of excessive fluoride in a water supply. *Public Health Rep.* **69,** 925–936.

Madsen, K. O., and Edmonds, E. J. 1964. Prolonged effect on caries of short term fluoride treatment. I. Sensitivity of newly erupted cotton rat molars to dietary fluoride. *Arch. Oral Biol.* **9,** 209–217.

Marthaler, T. M. 1967. The value in caries prevention of other methods of increasing fluoride ingestion, apart from fluoridated water. *Int. Dent. J.* **17,** 606–618.

Miller, G. W., and Shupe, J. L. 1962. Alkaline bone phosphatase activity as related to fluoride ingestion by dairy cattle. *Amer. J. Vet. Res.* **23,** 24–31.

Muhler, J. C., Stookey, G. K., Spear, L. B., and Bixler, D. 1966. Blood and urinary fluoride studies following the ingestion of single doses of fluoride. *J. Oral Ther. Pharmacol.* **2,** 241–260.

Navia, J. M. 1970. Effects of minerals on dental caries. In: *Dietary Chemical vs. Dental Caries. Adv. Chem. Ser.* **94.** American Chemical Society, Washington, D.C., pp. 123–160.

Navia, J. M. 1973. Prevention of dental caries: Agents which increase tooth resistance to dental caries. *Int. Dent. J.* **22,** 427–440.

Navia, J. M., Lopez, H., and Harris, R. S. 1968. Cariostatic effects of sodium trimetaphosphate when fed to rats during different stages of tooth development. *Arch. Oral Biol.* **13,** 779–786.

Navia, J. M., Hunt, C. E., First, F. B., and Narkates, A. J. 1976. Fluoride metabolism: Effect of pre-eruptive or posteruptive fluoride administration on rat caries susceptibility. In: *Trace Elements in Human Health and Disease,* Vol. II (A. S. Prasad, ed.). Academic Press, New York, pp. 249–268.

Rich, C., Ensick, J., and Ivanovich, P. 1964. The effects of sodium fluoride on calcium metabolism of subjects with metabolic bone diseases. *J. Clin. Invest.* **43,** 545–556.

Riggs, B. L., Jowsey, J., Kelly, P. J., and Hoffman, D. L. 1972. Treatment for postmenopausal and senile osteoporosis. *Med. Clin. North Amer.* **56,** 989–997.

Ruliffson, W. S., Burns, L. V., and Hughes, J. S. 1963. The effect of fluorine ion on Fe-59 iron levels in blood of rats. *Trans. Kansas Acad. Sci.* **66,** 52–58.

Shaw, J. H., and Sognnaes, R. F. 1954. Experimental rat caries. V. Effect of fluorine on the caries-conduciveness of a purified ration. *J. Nurt.* **53,** 207–214.

Sievert, A. H., and Phillips, P. H. 1959. Metabolic studies on the sodium fluoride-fed rat. *J. Nutr.* **68,** 109–120.

Smith, F. A., Leone, N. C., and Hodge, H. C. 1960. The effects of absorption of fluoride. V. Chemical determination of fluoride in human soft tissues following prolonged ingestion of fluoride at various levels. *AMA Arch. Ind. Health* **21,** 330–337.

Spencer, G. R., El-Sayed, F. I., Kroening, G. H., Pell, K. L., Shoup, N., Adams, D. F., Franke, M., and Alexander, J. E. 1971. Effects of fluoride, calcium, and phosphorus on porcine bone. *Amer. J. Vet Res.* **21**(11), 1751–1774.

Stookey, G. K., Osborne, J., and Muhler, J. C. 1962. Effects of pre- and postnatal fluoride on caries. *Dent. Prog.* **2,** 137–140.

Suttie, J. W., Dieschet, M. P., Quissell, D. O., and Young, K. L. 1974. In: *Trace Element Metabolism in Animals,* Vol. 2 (W. G. Hoekstra *et al.,* eds.). University Park Press, Baltimore, pp. 327–337.

Underwood, E. J. 1977. *Trace Elements in Human and Animal Nutrition.* Academic Press, New York, pp. 347–374.

Weidmann, S. M., and Weatherell, J. A. 1970. Distribution of fluoride; distribution in hard tissue. In: *Fluorides and Human Health. WHO Monogr. Ser.* No. 59, Geneva, Switzerland, pp. 104–128.

Zipkin, I., and Babeaux, W. L. 1965. Maternal transfer of fluoride. *J. Oral Ther. Pharmacol.* **1,** 652–665.

CHAPTER 4

IODINE

INTRODUCTION

The ancient Greeks used burnt sponges empirically in the treatment of human goiter. This knowledge led the French physician Coindet to use iodine salts for the treatment of goiter (Coindet, 1820). A systematic investigation of this concept was undertaken by Chatin, between the years 1850 and 1876 (Chatin, 1850–1854). He determined the natural occurrence of iodine in air, water, soils, and foods from various localities and compared his results with the incidence of goiter. Chatin concluded that the occurrence of goiter was associated with a deficiency of environmental iodine and recommended that the water supply in goitrous districts be enriched with this element.

During the second half of the 19th century, iodine was shown to be concentrated in the thyroid gland and to be reduced in concentration in the thyroid in persons from endemic goiter regions. In 1899, these findings were confirmed by Oswald (1899), and thyroglobulin was identified. In 1919, Kendall (1919) isolated from the thyroid gland a crystalline compound containing 65% iodine that he claimed was the active principle and which he named thyroxine. Subsequently, it was shown that thyroxine is a tetraiodo derivative of a compound of phenol and tyrosine, or tetraiodothyronine, and its synthesis was accomplished (Underwood, 1977).

During the first quarter of this century, investigations in several countries established clearly that endemic goiter in man was due to deficiency of iodine in the food and water supplies of the affected regions. The first large-scale trial of iodine supplementation in man was carried out between 1916 and 1920 in the schools of Ohio. Similar prophylactic measures were soon initiated in goitrous areas in other countries with such success that iodized salt soon became a widely recognized form of control.

Endemic goiter was subsequently shown to occur with varying intensity in many countries and on every continent, with the actual number of goitrous individuals in the world estimated in 1960 at close to 200 million. Women and children appear to be more affected than adult males. In certain countries, notably the United States, Switzerland, and New Zealand, the intensity of the disease declined markedly as a result of the use of iodized salt, although there is some evidence of a rise in goiter incidence in certain areas of the United States in recent years, presumably associated with a decline in the sale of iodized as compared with noniodized salt.

METABOLISM AND BIOCHEMISTRY

The body of a healthy human adult probably contains a total of 10–20 mg iodine, of which 70–80% is concentrated in the thyroid gland. The concentration of iodine in the skeletal muscles is less than one one-thousandth of that in the thyroid. The level of iodine in the ovaries is 3–4 times that in the muscles, and is usually higher than that in most other extrathyroid tissues, other than the bile, hair, pituitary gland, and salivary glands. The iodine-concentrating mechanisms of the salivary gland appear to be similar to those of the thyroid. Significant concentrations of iodine also occur in the orbitary fat and the orbicular muscle of the eye.

Iodine occurs in tissues as organically bound iodine and as inorganic iodide. The latter is usually present in most tissues in extremely low concentrations, near the range of 1–2 μg/100 g. In the saliva, the iodine is almost entirely in the inorganic form.

The concentrations of organically bound iodine are small in tissues other than the thyroid. A level of about 5 μg/100 g appears to be normal for muscle, with higher levels in the ovaries. Most of the organic iodine of the tissues consists of thyroxine bound to protein, together with widely distributed minute concentrations of other compounds, including triiodothyronine. Muscle iodine concentrations decrease in hypothyroidism and increase in hyperthyroidism.

In mammals, the normal healthy thyroid contains 0.2–0.5% of iodine on a dry basis, giving an average total of 8–12 mg in the adult human gland. This amount may be reduced to as low as 1 mg or less in endemic goiter.

Iodine exists in the thyroid as inorganic iodide, mono- and diiodotyrosine, thyroxine, triiodothyronine, polypeptides containing thyroxine, thyroglobulin, and probably other compounds. The iodinated amino acids are bound with other amino acids in peptide linkage to form thyroglobulin, the unique, iodinated protein of the thyroid gland that is the chief constituent of the colloid filling the follicular lumen. Thyroglobulin is a glycoprotein with a molecular weight of 650,000. It represents 90% of the total iodine of the gland.

IODINE IN BLOOD

Iodine exists in normal blood in both inorganic and organic forms. Inorganic iodide concentrations are too low for direct determination, and the range is 0.08–0.60 μg/100 ml, with values below 0.08 indicating iodine deficiency and values above 1 μg/100 ml suggesting exogenous iodine administration.

The organic iodine of the blood, which does not occur in the erythrocytes, is present mainly as thyroxine bound to the plamsa proteins. Only a very small proportion, about 0.05%, is free in human serum. Up to 10% of the organic iodine of the plasma is made up of several iodinated substances, including tri- and diiodothyronine and minute concentrations of other compounds that most likely are tissue metabolites of thyroxine. Thyroglobulin occurs only in pathological states involving damage to the thyroid gland, and the iodotyrosines do not normally appear in the peripheral circulation. On the other hand, triiodothyronine is secreted into the blood by the thyroid.

The protein-bound iodine of the serum (serum PBI) or the butanol-extractable iodine of the serum (serum BEI) corresponds well with the circulating thyroid hormone level, and various methods have been developed to measure serum PBI and serum BEI. The PBI levels in the serum vary significantly with species, age, pregnancy, and level of thyroid activity.

Serum PBI levels rise significantly during human pregnancy. As early as the third week of pregnancy, the levels rise to the upper part of the normal range or higher, suggesting hyperthyroidism. This rise is not attended, however, by any clinical evidence of excessive thyroid activity.

Increased serum PBI values are highly characteristic of hyperthyroidism and decreased values are indicative of hypothyroidism in man. Caution in interpreting results is necessary, since misleadingly high PBI values can occur when pharmaceutical iodine preparations have been previously administered. If the thyroidal radioiodine uptake is also high, hyperthyroidism can be diagnosed with more confidence.

IODINE IN MILK

The concentration of iodine in milk is influenced by the stage of lactation and dietary iodine intakes. Iodine is unique among the trace elements for the ease with which it passes the mammary barrier and in the extent to which the level in the milk is influenced by variations in dietary iodine intakes. The iodine content of milk is reduced below normal in goitrous regions, and the determination of iodine in milk has been proposed as a convenient means of establishing the iodine status of an area and of providing an index of endemic goiter incidence.

Cow's colostrum is much higher in iodine than true milk, and in late lactation, there is a fall in concentration. Kirchgessner (1959) reported a mean value of 264 ± 100 μg/liter for colostrum, compared with 98 ± 82 for milk.

IODINE IN THYROID

In human subjects, the only known role of iodine is the synthesis of the thyroid hormones—thyroxine and triiodothyronine. The activity of the thyroid is regulated by a negative feedback mechanism involving the pituitary and the hypothalamus. The hypothalamus secretes the thyrotropin-releasing factor (TRF), a peptide that reaches the adenohypophysis via the portal vessels of the pituitary stalk and provokes secretion of the thyroid-stimulating hormone (TSH) by the b_2 cells. TSH is a glycoprotein with a molecular weight of about 25,000 that stimulates the gland to release its hormones and to trap iodide. The thyroid hormones, in turn, inhibit the release of both TRF by the hypothalamus and TSH by the pituitary, and in this way keep the plasma level of the thyroid hormones normal. Triiodothyronine, which has about 4 times the potency of thyroxine, is also stronger in inhibiting TSH secretion.

ABSORPTION AND EXCRETION

Iodine occurs in foods largely as inorganic iodide and in this form is absorbed from all levels of the gastrointestinal tract. Other forms of inorganic iodine are reduced to iodide prior to absorption. Iodide administered orally is absorbed rapidly and almost entirely from the gastrointestinal tract, with very little being excreted in the feces. Iodinated amino acids are well absorbed as such, although more slowly and not as completely as iodide. A proportion of their iodine may be lost in the feces in organic combination, and the remainder is broken down and absorbed as iodide.

Iodine is excreted mainly in the urine, with smaller amounts appearing in the feces and the sweat. Fecal iodine excretion in normal adults ranges from 6.7 to 42.1 μg/day. Follis (1964) set a urinary level of 50 μg I/g creatinine as the tentative lower limit of normal for adolescents, with 32.5 μg/g as the corresponding figure for children 5–10 years old, and 75 μg/g for adult males. Koutras (1968) considers a urinary iodine excretion below 40 μg/day as suggestive of iodine deficiency in man, if renal iodide clearance is normal.

INTERMEDIARY METABOLISM

The total iodide pool consists of the iodide present in the extracellular space, together with the red blood cells and certain areas of selective concentration, such as the thyroid and the salivary glands and, to a lesser extent, the gastric glands and dense connective tissue. Equilibrium within the total iodide pool is reached very rapidly.

Despite its high iodine content and the efficiency with which it traps iodine, the thyroid gland contributes little to the iodide pool, the reason being that the binding into organic form is so rapid, except when the process is blocked by administration of antithyroid agents. Significant quantities of iodide are also trapped by the salivary glands, apparently by mechanisms resembling those of the thyroid. Since salivary iodide is not converted into organic form and is usually all reabsorbed, this process represents little net loss to the iodide pool.

Iodide Pool

The iodide pool is continuously replenished from three sources: exogenously from the diet, endogenously from the saliva, and from the breakdown of iodine hormones produced by the thyroid. Iodide is continuously lost from this pool by the activities of the thyroid, kidneys, and salivary glands, which compete for the available iodine. Koutras (1968) represented iodine metabolism as a metabolic cycle consisting of three main pools: the plasma inorganic iodide, the intrathyroidal iodine pool, and the pool comprising the hormonal or protein-bound iodine of the plasma and the tissues. The rates of removal of iodide from the first of these pools by the thyroid and the kidneys are expressed as thyroidal and renal clearances, calculated as organ accumulation of iodide per unit time divided by plasma iodide concentration. In healthy humans, total clearance from the iodide pool occurs at the rate of approximately 50 ml/min or 3 liters/hr, to which the kidneys contribute about two thirds and the thyroid about one third. If the volume of the total iodide pool is taken as 25 liters, the rate of turnover is approximately 12%/hr. In normal man, the renal iodide clearance is very constant at about 35 ml/min over all ranges of plasma iodide examined. In fact, there is no renal homeostatic mechanism to keep the plasma iodide level constant. Thyroid clearance, by contrast, is sensitive to changes in plasma iodide concentration and varies greatly with the activity of the gland. The thyroid in normal persons clears an average of 10–20 ml/ min, whereas in exophthalmic goiter or Grave's disease, a clearance of 100 ml/min is usual and over 1000 ml/min is possible. The measurement of thyroid ^{131}I clearance is a valuable diagnostic aid in hyperthyroidism, but is much less sensitive as a diagnostic test in myxedema. In goitrous cretins with congenital inability of the thyroid to trap iodide, the salivary glands are similarly affected and the saliva/plasma iodide ratio is less than unity. This ratio can therefore be used diagnostically where this type of dyshormonogenesis is suspected, but has no such value in patients with iodine deficiency goiter, or in patients with goiter and a normal plasma iodide level (Underwood, 1977).

The intrathyroidal iodine pool involves a series of consecutive steps in the synthesis of the thyroid hormones. First, the iodide brought to the gland in the plasma is trapped by an energy-requiring active mechanism that can be blocked by perchlorate- and thiocyanate-type antithyroid agents. This iodide is oxidized to elemental iodine, or to a similar reactive form, as a preliminary to its incorporation into organic combination by a peroxidase. The more reactive iodine combines with the tyrosine residues and thyroglobulin to form 3-monoiodotyrosine and 3,5-diiodotyrosine. This reaction takes place near the boundary between follicular cells and follicular lumen, with the same enzyme system probably acting as iodide–peroxidase and as tyrosine–iodinase. This reaction can be blocked by a great number of antithyroid substances of the thiouracil type and also by iodide itself in high concentrations. The ability of the thyroid gland to trap iodide is not reduced by such agents. Two diiodotyrosine molecules combine to form one molecule of thyroxine, or one mono- and one diiodotyrosine combine to form one molecule of triiodothyronine. These are stored in the colloid bound to thyroglobulin. The normal human thyroid gland contains about 8–12 mg of iodine, mainly in the form of two iodotyrosine and two iodothyronine molecules bound in this way. In a recent study of pancreatin hydrolysates of normal human thyroids, the distribution of the iodine was found to be 16.1% as iodide, 32.7% as monoiodotyrosine, 33.4% as diiodotyrosine, 16.2% as thyroxine, and 7.6% as triiodothyronine (Underwood, 1977).

The thyroid hormones are released through proteolysis of thyroglobulin by a protease system that yields both iodotyrosines and thyroactive thyronines. The normal human thyroid has been estimated to secrete 51.6 μg iodine daily as thyroxine and 11.9 μg as triiodothyronine. The iodotyrosines liberated from the proteolysis of thyroglobulin, unlike the iodothyronines, are not secreted into the circulation, but instead are deiodinated by an enzyme called "deiodinase" or "dehalogenase." The iodine thus released is not lost from the gland, but is reutilized for hormone synthesis.

The human thyroid must trap about 60 μg iodide daily to ensure an adequate supply of hormones. This is achieved primarily by adjustment of the thyroidal iodide clearance rate.

The circulating thyroid hormones, which comprise the third metabolic iodine pool as stated by Koutras (1968), occur mostly bound to a thyroxine-binding globulin, to prealbumin, and to albumin itself, with only about 0.05% of the thyroxine normally present in the free state. It is for this reason that the serum PBI corresponds so well with the circulating thyroid hormone level. According to Rall *et al.* (1964), approximately 10% of the circulating thyroxine and 56% of the circulating triiodothyronine are metabolized in man daily. Once these hormones enter the tissues, approximately 80% is broken down by several deiodinating enzymes, with the iodine so liberated returning to the iodide pool, thus completing the iodide cycle.

Disturbances in the peripheral metabolism of thyroxine occur in some forms of thyroid disease in man. Nicoloff and Dowling (1968) were able to demonstrate increased hepatic incorporation of labeled thyroxine, with an increased rate of deiodination, in Graves' disease, while in patients with primary hypothyroidism, hepatic incorporation and the rate of deiodination were reduced. The pathogenetic basis of these changes is unknown, but it seems that the amount of labeled thyroxine incorporated in the liver is directly related to the deiodination rate of that organ.

NATURE AND MODE OF ACTION OF THYROID HORMONES

Several different compounds possess thyroidal activity equal to or in excess of that of thyroxine. Thus, in comparison with thyroxine (3,5,3′,5′-tetraiodothyronine), 3,5,3′-triiodothyronine is 3–5 times as active, depending on the dose used; 3,3′-diiodothyronine is similar in potency; 3,5-diiodo-3′,5′-dibromothyronine is almost as active; and 3,5,3′-triiodothyropropionic acid is 300 times more active in accelerating amphibian metamorphosis (Michel, 1956). On the other hand, 3,3′,5′-triiodothyronine has only one one-twentieth of the activity of thyroxine or one one-hundredth of that of its isomer. The following generalizations can be made: The thyronine nucleus (Fig. 3) is essential to any activity; iodine substitution in the inner aromatic ring is needed for substantial activity; partial replacement of iodine by bromine results in little loss of activity; an alanine side chain is not essential; and whatever the aliphatic side chain on the nucleus, a 3,5,3′-substitution in the rings ensures maximal activity (Underwood, 1971).

The mechanism of action of thyroid hormone at the tissue level is still obscure. Many enzymes in various tissues are affected by variations in thyroid activity, or by treatment of the animal with thyroactive substances, but direct involvement of thyroxine or triiodothyronine in an enzyme system needed for the energy-transforming processes of the cells has not been demonstrated. These hormones have been shown to increase the initial rate of oxidation of succinate by submitochondrial particles of rat liver, associated with increased efficiency of phosphorylation. The active forms of the hormones at the cellular level can actually be elaborated in the cells. Thus, 3,5,3′-triiodothyropyruvic acid and 3,3,3′-triiodothyroacetic acid, both of which occur in the tissues, are as effective as thyroxine, in promoting the metamorphosis of tadpoles, and the latter has an immediate effect in raising the BMR of rats. This compound, however, quickly loses its effect and does not lead to a rise in the BMR of myxedema patients (Underwood, 1977).

Adminstration of thyroid hormone increases the size, number, and metabolic activity of mitochondria in mammalian skeletal muscle (Gustafsson *et al.*, 1965). It has been proposed that activation of ATP utilization by transmembrane Na^+ pumping may be one of the primary mediators in the

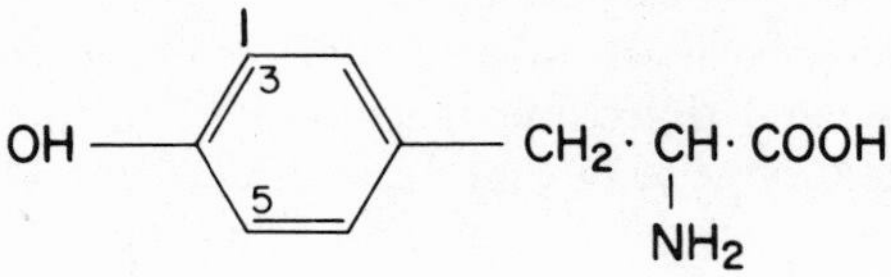

I
3
OH — — $CH_2 \cdot CH \cdot COOH$
5
NH_2

3-Monoiodotyrosine

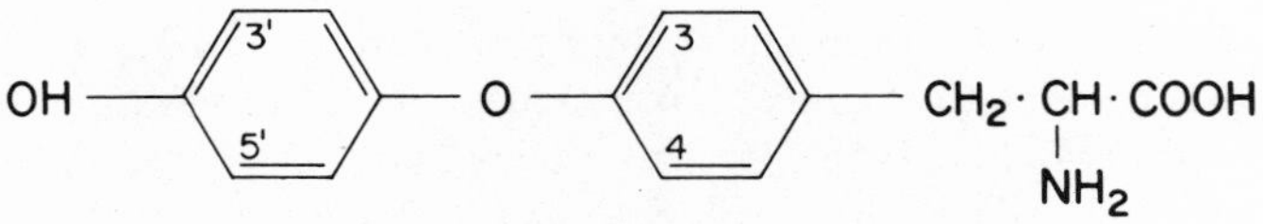

3' 3
OH — — O — — $CH_2 \cdot CH \cdot COOH$
5' 4
NH_2

Thyronine
[4-(4'-Hydroxyphenoxy) phenylalanine]

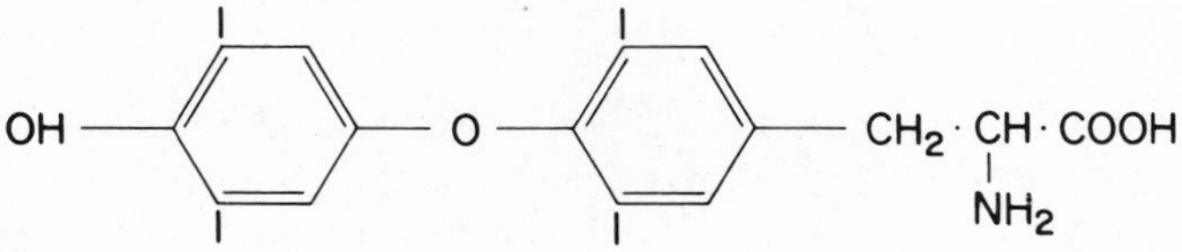

I I
OH — — O — — $CH_2 \cdot CH \cdot COOH$
I I
NH_2

Thyroxine
(3,3',5,5'-Tetraiodothyronine)

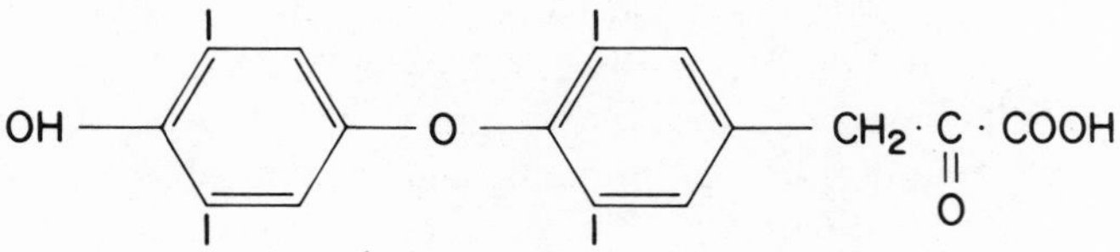

I I
OH — — O — — $CH_2 \cdot C \cdot COOH$
I I
O

3,5,3'-Triiodothyropyruvic acid

Fig. 3. Structural formulas of monoiodotyrosine, the thyronine nucleus, thyroxine, and triiodothyropyruvic acid. From Underwood (1971).

calorigenic response to T_3 and T_4 (Ismael-Beigi and Edelman, 1971). More than 90% of the increment in the oxygen consumption in the liver and muscle of euthyroid rats produced by injections of T_3 and T_4 could be attributed to increased energy use by the Na^+ pump. Ouabain eliminated the effect of T_3 on liver slices by inhibition of Na^+ transport.

It has been suggested that the primary effect of thyroid hormone is on the control of gene expression, but the precise mode of action has not been demonstrated. High-affinity saturable binding sites for ^{125}I-labeled T_3 and T_4 that function as receptors for thyroid hormones have been demonstrated (Samuels and Tsai, 1973; Samuels *et al.*, 1974a,b). Further studies are needed to define the action of thyroid hormone at the cellular level.

IODINE DEFICIENCY AND THYROID FUNCTION

The rate of energy exchange and the quantity of heat liberated by an organism at relative rest are elevated in subjects with hyperthyroidism and reduced below normal in those with hypothyroidism. After total thyroidectomy, the BMR gradually falls to approximately one-half normal and may be raised again by the administration of thyroactive substances. The calorigenic action of the thyroid hormones can be demonstrated by measuring the oxygen consumption of excised tissues. Liver, kidney, muscle, and other tissues from iodine-deficient or thyroidless animals consume less oxygen than normal, while these tissues from hyperthyroid animals consume more oxygen than normal.

The changes in cellular oxidation are accompanied by disturbances in the metabolism of water, salts, proteins, carbohydrates, and lipids. In hypothyroidism, the retention of water and salt is increased and the plasma volume is considerably reduced. Administration of thyroid hormone, or of iodine where the hypofunctioning thyroid results from iodine deficiency, induces a pronounced water and salt diuresis and an increase in plasma volume. Hypothyroid states are accompanied by above-normal, and hyperthyroid states by subnormal, serum cholesterol levels in man.

The thyroid hormone is essential for growth during early life in all mammals and birds. Total thyroidectomy induces severe dwarfism in rats or birds, whereas athyreosis in human infants leads to cretinism, which occurs in severely goitrous regions. In these regions, iodine administration during adolescence increases the rate of growth and also reduces the incidence of goiter.

Endemic goiter is often associated with an incidence of feeblemindedness and deaf-mutism in children. Human hypothyroidism is characterized by mental sluggishness and apathy, and hyperthyroidism by emotional instability, nervousness, and irritability, accompanied usually by muscle tremors and hyperactivity of the sweat glands.

In humans, colloid goiter frequently develops at puberty, and hyperthyroidism is sometimes precipitated at the menopause. Goitrous cretins are usually sterile, invariably fail to develop normal sexual vigor, and demonstrate a delayed maturation of the genitalia. Thyroidectomy at an early age is followed, in all species, by a long period during which the gonads and secondary sex organs remain in an infantile condition.

IODINE REQUIREMENTS

The minimum dietary requirement of man or other species is difficult to assess because of considerable individual variability and the effects of the environment, including the nature of the rest of the diet. Calculations based on average daily urine losses give an adult human requirement of 60–120 μg/day (Underwood, 1977).

The iodine content of drinking water usually reflects the iodine content of the soil and rocks of a particular region and hence of the locally grown foods. This content has been correlated with the incidence of goiter in many areas ever since the pioneering studies of Chatin over a century ago. Kupzis (1932) found that the water supplies in goitrous areas in Latvia ranged from 0.1 to 2.0 μg I/liter, compared with 2–15 μg I/liter for nongoitrous areas. Young *et al.* (1936) reported that the drinking water in villages in England, where the incidence of goiter in humans was assessed at 56%, averaged 2.9 μg I/liter, compared with 8.2 μg I/liter in other villages where the goiter incidence was only 3%. In general, however, less than 10% of the total daily intake of iodine is supplied by the drinking water.

Animal products, such as milk or eggs, can be much richer in iodine when they come from animals consuming iodine-enriched diets. On average diets, hen's eggs contain about 4–10 μg iodine, most of which is located in the yolk. The iodine content of foods of marine origin is much higher than that of any other class of foodstuffs. The edible flesh of sea fish and shellfish may contain 300–3000 ppb on a fresh basis, compared with 20–40 ppb for freshwater fish. The order of magnitude of iodine concentrations of other classes of foods (in parts per billion on a fresh edible basis) is as follows: fresh fruits, 20; leafy and root vegetables, 30; cereal grains, 40; meats, 40; milk and milk products, 40; eggs, 90.

Compulsory iodization of domestic salt is the most economical, convenient, and effective means of mass prophylaxis in most goitrous regions and is now carried out as a public health measure in many countries.

GOITROGENIC SUBSTANCES

Goitrogens are substances that are capable of producing thyroid enlargement by interfering with thyroid hormone synthesis. The pituitary responds by increasing its output of TSH, which induces hypertrophy in the gland in an effort to increase thyroid hormone production.

The first clear evidence of a goitrogen in food was obtained by Chesney *et al.* (1928) (Underwood, 1971). Rabbits fed a diet that consisted mainly of fresh cabbage developed goiters that could be prevented by a supplement of 7.5 mg iodine per rabbit per week. "Cabbage goiter" was subsequently demonstrated in other animal species, and goitrogenic activity was reported for a wide range of vegetable foods, including virtually all cruciferous plants. Astwood *et al.* (1949) isolated and identified a new compound named "goitrin" (L-5-vinyl-2-thiooxalidone) from rutabaga and showed that the goitrogenic activity of *Brassica* seeds could be largely accounted for by the presence of this compound in combined form (progoitrin).

Goitrin occurs in the edible portions of most *Brassica* species, but is not responsible for the entire goitrogenicity of all foods. Other thioglycosides with antithyroid activity have been found in cruciferous plants, and similar activity has been associated with the presence of cyanogenetic glucosides in white clover. The latter owe their potency to the conversion of the HCN into thiocyanate in the tissues. Thiocyanate is a goitrogenic agent that acts by inhibiting the selective concentration of iodine by the thyroid. Its action is reversible by iodine, while that of goitrin, which acts by limiting hormonogenesis in the gland, is either not reversible by such means or is only partly so. The number of goitrogens of this latter type is large, and most of them possess the thiouryelene radical. All of them act by inhibiting the iodination of tyrosine, probably through inhibition of the thyroidal peroxidase, and appear to affect the conversion of mono- to diiodotyrosine (DIT) to a greater extent than the iodination of tyrosine to form monoiodotyrosine (MIT), thus leading to an increased MIT/DIT ratio in the thyroid (Underwood, 1977).

Goitrogens are widely employed in the treatment of thyrotoxicosis in man. Those in clinical use include methyl and propyl thiouracil, carbimazole, and methimazole. The derivatives of aminobenzene, phenylbutazone, and paraamino-salicylates are also used. Iodide itself, in large doses, may act as an antithyroid agent in thyrotoxicosis, and this form of therapy was common before goitrogenic drugs were available.

The actual significance of natural goitrogens in the production of human goiter is unclear. Clements (1960), working in Australia, showed that milk from cows consuming certain cruciferous plants in the graze contains a potent goitrogen, the effect of which on children could not be overcome by the feeding of 10 mg KI per week. This result suggests that the goitrogen is of the goitrin or thiouracil type. Goitrogens have also been found in the milk of cows fed cruciferous fodder in both England and Finland. These interesting and important observations certainly deserve further study and clinical evaluation.

IODINE TOXICITY

The prolonged administration of large doses of iodine to normal persons markedly reduces thyroidal iodine uptake. This is the antithyroidal or goitrogenic effect, referred to previously, which can be used in the treatment of thyrotoxicosis. Iodide goiter and hypothyroidism rarely occur from this cause, although there is a region in Japan in which the consumption of large quantities of iodine with the diet is reported to be the cause of endemic goiter (Underwood, 1977).

The effects of iodine doses several times greater than those likely to be obtained from ordinary diets were examined in a series of experiments with several species carried out by Arrington *et al.* (1965). Significant species differences in tolerance to high intakes of iodide were shown to exist. In all species studied, the tolerance was high, i.e., relative to normal dietary iodine intakes, pointing to an extremely wide margin of safety for this element. Adult female rats fed 500, 1000, 1500, and 2000 ppm of iodine, as KI, from 0 to 35 days prepartum, showed increasing neonatal mortality of the young with increasing levels of iodine, but the effects of the lowest level of supplemental iodine fed were slight when compared with those receiving no supplemental iodine. Histological examination of mammary gland tissue from females fed iodine indicated that milk secretion was either absent or markedly reduced. The fertility of male rats fed 2500 ppm iodine from birth to 200 days of age seemed to be unimpaired.

The mechanism by which the excess iodine affects egg production and embryonic mortality, or reproduction in female rats and rabbits, is not clearly understood. Preliminary experiments conducted by Marcilese *et al.* (1968) indicate that thyroxine production is not impaired in hens fed high levels of iodine. However, the growing ova were shown to have a marked ability to concentrate iodine from the high doses administered. This finding is in keeping with the earlier demonstration of the specific incorporation of orally administered radioiodine into hens' eggs and follicles. Ova continued to develop in hens not laying, and many ova were found to be regressing. It has been suggested that development ceases and regression takes place when a threshold amount of iodine reaches the ova.

REFERENCES

Arrington, L. R., Taylor, R. N., Jr., Ammerman, C. B., and Shirley, R. L. 1965. Effects of excess dietary iodine upon rabbits, hamsters, rats and swine. *J. Nutr.* **87,** 394–398.

Astwood, E. B.. Greer, M. A., and Ettlinger, M. G. 1949. 1,5-Vinyl-2-thiooxalidone, an antithyroid compound from yellow turnip and from *Brassica* seeds. *J. Biol. Chem.* **181,** 121–130.

Chatin, A. 1852. Présence de l'iode dans l'air, les eaux, le sol et les produits alimentaires des alpes, de la France et du Piedmont. *Arch. Gen. Med. (Paris),* 4th series, **28,** 245–248.

Chesney, A. M., Clawson, T. A., and Webster, B. 1928. Endemic goitre in rabbits. I. Incidence and characteristics. *Bull. Johns Hopkins Hosp.* **43,** 261–277.

Clements, F. W. 1960. Naturally occurring goitrogens. *Brit. Med. Bull.* **16,** 133–137.

Coindet, J. F. 1820. Découverte d'un nouveau remède contre le goitre. *Ann. Chim. Phys.* **15,** 49–59.

Follis, R. H., Jr. 1964. Patterns of urinary iodine excretion in goitrous and nongoitrous areas. *Amer. J. Clin. Nutr.* **14,** 253–268.

Gustafsson, R., Tata, J. R., Lindberg, O., and Ernste, L. 1965. The relationship between the structure and activity of rat skeletal muscle mitochondria after thyroidectomy and thyroid hormone treatment. *J. Cell. Biol.* **26,** 255–278.

Ismail-Beigi, F., and Edelman, I. S. 1971. The mechanism of the calorigenic action of thyroid hormone stimulation of Na plus + K plus-activated adenosine triphosphatase activity. *J. Gen Physiol.* **57,** 710–722.

Kendall, E. C. 1919. Isolation of the iodine compound which occurs in the thyroid. *J. Biol. Chem.* **39,** 125–147.

Kirchgessner, M. 1959. Interactions between different elements in colostrum and milk. *Z. Tierphysiol. Tierernaehr. Futtermittelkd.* **14,** 270–277.

Koutras, D. A. 1968. In: *Activation Analysis in the Study of Mineral Metabolism in Man.* I.A.E.A., Vienna.

Kupzis, J. 1932. Die Jodfrage in Lettland in Zusammenhange mit dem Kropfe. *Z. Hyg. Infektionskr.* **113,** 551–573.

Marcilese, N. A., Harms, R. H., Valsecchi, R. M., and Arrington, L. R. 1968. Iodine uptake by ova of hens given excess iodine and effect upon ova development. *J. Nutr.* **94,** 117–120.

Michel, R. 1956. Recent progress in the physiology and biochemistry of thyroid hormones. *Amer. J. Med.* **20,** 670–683.

Nicoloff, J. T., and Dowling, J. T. 1968. Studies of peripheral thyroxine distribution in thyrotoxicosis and hypothyroidism. *J. Clin. Invest.* **47,** 2000–2015.

Oswald, A. 1899. Die Eiweisskörper der Schilddruse. *Hoppe-Seyler's Z. Physiol. Chem.* **27,** 14–49.

Rall, J. E., Robbins, J., and Lewallen, C. G. 1964. The thyroid. In: *The Hormones,* Vol. 5 (G. Pincus, K. V. Thimann, and E. B. Astwood, eds.). Academic Press, New York, pp. 159–439.

Samuels, H. H., and Tsai, J. S. 1973. Thyroid hormone action in cell culture: Demonstration of nuclear receptors in intact cells and isolated nuclei. *Proc. Natl. Acad. Sci. U.S.A.* **70,** 3488–3492.

Samuels, H. H., Tsai, J. S., and Casanova, J. 1974a. Thyroid hormone action: *In vitro* demonstration of putative receptors in isolated nuclei and soluble nuclear extracts. *Science* **184,** 1188–1191.

Samuels, H. H., Tsai, J. S., Casanova, J., and Stanley, F. 1974b. Thyroid hormone action: *In vitro* characterization of solubilized nuclear receptors from rat liver and cultured GH 1 cells. *J. Clin. Invest.* **54,** 853–865.

Underwood, E. J. 1971. *Trace Elements in Human and Animal Nutrition,* 3rd ed. Academic Press, New York, pp. 218–258.

Underwood, E. J. 1977. *Trace Elements in Human and Animal Nutrition,* 4th ed. Academic Press, New York, pp. 271–301.

Young, M., Crabtree, M. G., and Mason, E. M. 1936. The relationship of the iodine contents of water, milk and pasture to the occurrence of endemic goitre in two districts of England. *Med. Res. Counc. (G. Brit.) Spec. Rep. Ser.* **217,** 7–13.

CHAPTER 5

IRON

INTRODUCTION

Iron was considered to be of celestial origin in ancient civilizations of the Eastern Mediterranean area. The "metal of heaven" was used in Egypt and Mesopotamia for therapeutic purposes. The oldest manuscript, the Ebers Papyrus, an Egyptian pharmacopea dating around 1500 B.C., describes two remedies that contained iron. The ancient Hindus (500 B.C.) also used iron therapeutically.

Iron compounds enjoyed popularity among medical practitioners in the Greco-Roman period, and it appears that Hippocrates used iron therapeutically. The therapeutic indications for iron during the Roman era included alopecia, acne, dermatitis, wounds, hemorrhoids, gout, pulmonary diseases, diarrhea, vomiting, weakness, edema, fever, and cystitis (Fairbanks *et al.,* 1971). In an authoritative medical encyclopedia prepared by Avicenna in the 10th century, a detailed description of the effects of iron was included. In the 17th century, there emerged a rational role for iron as a specific therapy for a disease known as chlorosis. Although the first description of chlorosis was given by Lange in 1554, a systematic account was provided by Lazarus Riverius in 1640. He enumerated ten major manifestations of chlorosis, pallor (sometimes of a lead color, blue or green), edema, heaviness of body and limbs, dyspnea, palpitation, headache, rapid pulse, unusually sound or prolonged sleep, a loathing of "wholesome meat," and lastly cessation of the menses. He recognized the primary importance of poor nutrition and recommended use of iron in chlorosis. Sydenham in 1681, however, is properly credited with having identified iron as a specific remedy for chlorosis.

Although iron became an accepted method of treatment of chlorosis, the mechanism of its action remained in doubt. At the close of the 19th century, however, Bunge regarded therapy with inorganic iron as purely suggestive, without any physiological or pharmacological significance. His views were accepted, and undoubtedly this acceptance delayed the acquisition of knowledge with respect to the role of iron in human metabolism.

In 1893, Stockman demonstrated clearly a response in hemoglobin due to iron administration in chlorotic women. He also assayed the iron content of a variety of diets and concluded that the iron content of diets consumed by chlorotic women was less than that in diets consumed by normal women.

During the latter part of the 19th century, medicine underwent the first stage of scientific revolution. Johann Duncan employed the microscope for the study of peripheral blood in 1867 and concluded that every single blood cell of chlorotic women contained less pigment in comparison with healthy subjects. The study of blood morphology developed rapidly thereafter, and by 1889, Hayem confirmed hypochromia and microcytosis as characteristic blood findings in chlorosis.

Although Whipple and Robscheit-Robbins held previously that inorganic iron was of no benefit in hypochromic anemia, in 1925 (Whipple and Robscheit, 1925), they studied a series of dogs rendered anemic by repeated phlebotomies and concluded that animals receiving iron and liver regenerated hemoglobin in appreciable amounts. On the basis of these observations, liver was administered to patients with pernicious anemia, resulting in one of the major discoveries of modern medicine. In 1932, Heath *et al.* (1932) unequivocally demonstrated that inorganic iron is incorporated quantitatively into hemoglobin. The studies of Heath *et al.* (1932) were confirmed by the painstaking and elaborate iron-balance studies of Reimann *et al.* (1937), and these studies finally settled the long-lived controversy as to whether iron is absorbed and utilized in the anemia of chronic blood loss.

In the mid 1920's, several groups of investigators studied plasma iron simultaneously. Fontès and Thivolle (1925) were first to identify a nonhemoglobin iron protein in normal horse serum, the concentration of which decreased in the course of anemia induced by venesection. The studies of Barkan (1933) and those of Moore *et al.* (1937) pointed clearly to the plasma iron as the major form of transport iron. Heilmeyer and Plötner (1937) studied serum iron extensively in health and disease. Many clinical disorders were shown to be associated with low serum iron. Based on their studies, a modern concept of iron metabolism accounting for observed clinical phenomena emerged.

McCance and Widdowson (1937) concluded from their studies that: (1) once iron was absorbed, its excretion was very minimal and was not controlled either by the gastrointestinal tract or by the kidneys; (2) the plasma iron was in equilibrium with tissue iron; (3) the level of plasma iron influenced the rate of iron absorption; and (4) the intestine somehow regulated the rate of iron absorption.

Radioactive iron first became available in 1938. The use of this isotope contributed enormously to the understanding of iron metabolism. Hahn *et al.* (1939) were soon able to show that in nonanemic dogs, very little iron was absorbed, and that approximately 90% of the amount of iron absorbed by anemic dogs was promptly taken up by bone marrow and incorporated into hemoglobin. These workers also observed that the larger the dose of iron, the lower was the percentage absorbed in the anemic dog. They commented that the need of the body for iron in some manner determined the absorption of this element. They also postulated a receptor substance in the bowel mucosa, which might readily become saturated and thus limit iron absorption. The nature of the receptor was not known, but the possibility that this may be a protein or more specifically a material such as ferritin or apoferritin capable of taking up a limited amount of iron from the intestinal lumen and in turn passing it on to the plasma when the iron level was lowered was suggested.

In 1946, Granick (1946) adopted and extended the hypothesis of ferritin as the mucosal regulator of iron absorption. This hypothesis, known as the "mucosal block" theory, became widely accepted as the physiological mechanism of regulation of iron absorption. According to this hypothesis, iron entering the mucosal cells is converted to ferritin iron. This ferritin iron is in equilibrium with small amounts of ferrous ions in the cells, and the ferrous ions are in equilibrium with the plasma Fe^{3+}. When the body is depleted of iron and the plasma iron is lowered, the iron from the mucosa begins to move out into the bloodstream. The "physiological saturation" of the mucosal cells with respect to ferrous ions is maintained until part or all of the ferritin iron is converted to ferrous iron. Further iron depletion leads to a fall in the ferrous iron below its "saturation" value in the mucosal cells, and once this occurs, the radioactive iron administered orally begins to be absorbed. This hypothesis envisioned a mucosal block that was absolute or nearly so. As will be discussed later, it is clear now that by some unknown mechanism, there normally is attenuation of iron absorption as the iron dose increases, but no absolute block exists.

A basic approach to the biochemistry of iron began with the investigations of Keilin and others in the 1920's. These studies established that iron, through its presence in the hemoprotein enzymes, the cytochromes, is vitally concerned with oxidative mechanisms of all living cells. Subsequently, iron-containing flavoprotein enzymes were discovered (Mahler and Elowe, 1953; Richert and Westerfeld, 1954). It became clear that iron is intimately involved in oxygen utilization by the tissues as well as in oxygen transport as part of the hemoglobin molecule. Subsequent studies have now established that iron deficiency and diseases involving disturbances in iron metabolism are relatively common in human populations.

BIOCHEMISTRY

The transition metals, including iron, share two properties of great importance in biology (Worwood, 1977): (1) their ability to exist in more than one relatively stable oxidation state and (2) their ability to form many complexes. Examples of iron-containing proteins are (1) simple iron protein (ferrodoxins); (2) hemoproteins: hemoglobin and myoglobin, which are involved as oxygen carriers; cytochromes, which are important for oxidative phosphorylation [iron behaves as an electron donor from substrates to molecular oxygen with simultaneous generation of adenosine triphosphate (ATP)]; (3) iron-sulfur proteins, which are proteins with either acid-labile sulfide or cysteinyl sulfur; examples are aconitase, adrenodoxin, succinate dehydrogenase, NADH dehydrogenase, and xanthine oxidase; (4) transferrin and lactoferrin, which are iron-binding proteins involved in the transport of iron; (5) ferritin, which is the soluble iron-storage protein found in all cells; and (6) hemosiderin, which refers to iron that is demonstrable by staining tissues with potassium ferrocyanide. The granules of hemosiderin contain anything from closely packed and well-oriented ferritin molecules to amorphous deposits of iron. The origin of hemosiderin, its function as an iron store, and its relationship with ferritin are not clearly understood.

Ferrodoxins are simple iron-proteins that occur in all photosynthesizing cells and are usually associated with chloroplasts (Fig. 4). The molecular weight ranges between 6,000 and 30,000, and the protein contains 2–7 atoms of iron per molecule. Ferrodoxins play a very important role in the complex process of photosynthesis. Electrons (and hydrogen) are displaced from water to ferredoxin, with the consequent release of oxygen (Fairbanks *et al.*, 1971):

$$H_2O + \text{ferredoxin}_{ox.} \xrightarrow[\text{chloroplasts}]{\text{sunlight}} \text{ferredoxin}_{red.} + O_2$$

In turn, reduced ferredoxin may participate in such synthetic reactions as these:

$$\text{Ferredoxin}_{red.} + CO_2 \rightarrow (CH_2O)_x + \text{ferredoxin}_{ox.}$$
$$\text{Ferredoxin}_{red.} + \text{acetyl CoA} + CO_2 \rightarrow \text{pyruvate} + \text{CoA} + \text{ferredoxin}_{ox.}$$
$$\text{Ferredoxin}_{red.} + NADP_2 \rightarrow NADPH_2 + \text{ferredoxin}_{ox.}$$

It has been shown that reduced ferredoxin is also involved in fixation of atmospheric nitrogen into ammonia by the bacterium *Clostridium pasteurianum:*

$$\text{Ferrodoxin}_{\text{red.}} + N_2 \rightarrow NH_3 + \text{ferredoxin}_{\text{ox.}}$$

During evolution, as oxygen was generated by photosynthesis, the change in the atmosphere encouraged the evolution of more complex biological systems. Aerobic glycolysis permitted a more efficient capture of hydrocarbon energy. Thus, there evolved a biochemical stepladder by which the energy stored in covalent bonds could be passed back to oxygen, with the regeneration of carbon dioxide and water. This stepladder required

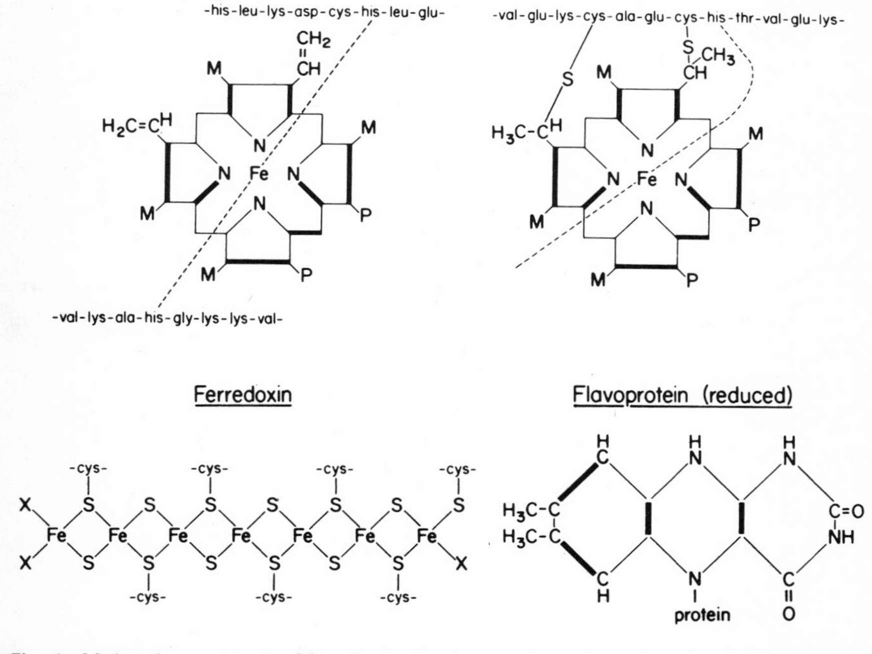

Fig. 4. Molecular structure of four iron-proteins, as they are understood at present. (M) methyl; (P) propionic acid. Hemoglobin and cytochrome *c* are typical heme-proteins. In each, heme is linked to a polypeptide chain through histidyl residues (by two in hemoglobin and by one or two in cytochrome *c*). Additionally, cytochrome *c* has very stable disulfide bonds between heme and cysteinyl residues. Ferredoxin, a biologically ancient and relatively simple iron-protein, may be basically a chain of repeating iron–sulfur linkages bound to a simple protein. The structure of ferrodoxin is not yet fully understood. A general model for iron-flavoproteins does not include iron in the region of the flavin moiety. In these illustrations, double bonds are shown as heavy bars and single bonds as fine lines. From Blomstrom *et al.* (1964).

substances that could be reversibly oxidized and reduced and that could be retained within a highly specialized structure of the cell, the mitochondrion. This need was met by the evolution of a group of protein-containing iron–porphyrin complexes—the cytochromes. The cytochromes function with cytochrome oxidase (copper-dependent enzyme) as the end of a stepladder of electron donors in the tricarboxylic acid (Krebs) cycle, as in this simplified example (Fairbanks *et al.,* 1971):

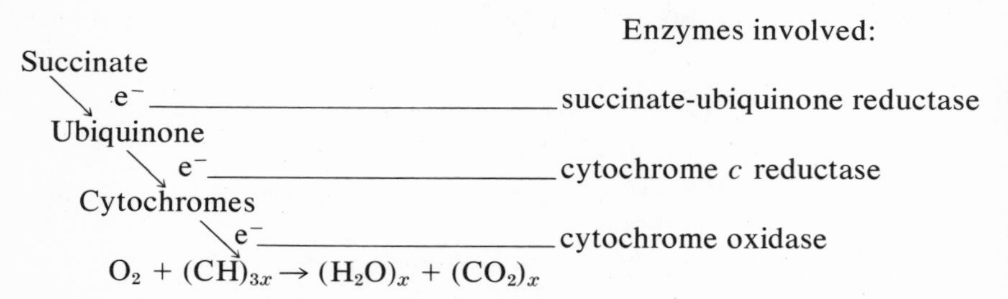

The role of iron in the Krebs cycle is very significant, inasmuch as all of 24 enzymes in this cycle contain iron as an active part of the molecule or require iron as a cofactor.

As the concentration of oxygen in the atmosphere increased, living cells required protection from the noxious effect of the hydrogen peroxide spontaneously formed from O_2 and H_2O. For this protection, other iron–porphyrin–protein complexes developed. These are peroxidases and catalases:

$$2\,H + H_2O_2 \xrightarrow{\text{peroxidase}} 2\,H_2O$$

$$2\,H_2O_2 \xrightarrow{\text{catalase}} 2\,H_2O + O_2$$

These enzymes are widely present in plant and animal tissues (Fairbanks *et al.,* 1971).

The development of the tricarboxylic acid cycle resulted in oxygen dependence of most forms of life. This dependence led to the appearance of mechanisms for entrapment and storage of oxygen. Hemoglobin, which appeared early in evolution, has a single tetrameric molecule and is well suited for adjusting the delicate equilibrium between entrapment and release of oxygen, carbon dioxide, and hydrogen ions (Fairbanks *et al.,* 1971).

Another enzyme, xanthine oxidase, an iron-flavoprotein enzyme responsible for the conversion of hypoxanthine and xanthine to uric acid, depends on iron for its enzymatic function. Iron is an activator of tryptophan pyrrolase (Feigelson and Greengard, 1961), and is an electron carrier in mitochondria.

Cyanide exerts its effects by complexing with iron-containing enzymes, particularly cytochrome oxidase, and thereby inhibiting their activity. Within seconds to minutes after the ingestion or inhalation of cyanide, inactivation of iron enzymes results in giddiness, hyperpnea, headaches, palpitations, cyanosis, and unconsciousness. Convulsions may precede death. High doses are fatal within a few minutes.

Enzyme iron is the smallest iron compartment, but it is very important to life. The iron enzymes may be classified as heme-protein (containing an iron–porphyrin complex), iron-flavoproteins (containing iron and a quinone like ring), and enzymes requiring iron as a cofactor. Examples of these enzymes are: heme-proteins—cytochromes *a, b, c,* c_1, a_3, cytochrome *c* oxidase, lipoxidase, catalase, tryptophan pyrrolase, hemogentisic oxidase, and peroxidases; iron-flavoproteins—cytochrome *c* reductase, succinate dehydrogenase, acyl CoA dehydrogenase, NADH dehyrogenase, and xanthine oxidase; enzymes requiring iron as cofactor—aconitase and succinate dehydrogenase.

The ubiquitous cytochromes function as reversible acceptors–donors of electrons. They function more or less as cofactors, rather than as enzymes. All are heme-proteins with iron in the trivalent state. The molecular structure of cytochrome *c* has been established for several species (Ehrenberg and Theorell, 1955; Fitch and Margoliash, 1967; Margoliash *et al.,* 1959; Paléus *et al.,* 1955; Tuppy and Paléus, 1955). The heme moiety of cytochrome *c* is essentially the same as that of hemoglobin, except that the vinyl side chains are reduced in cytochrome *c* and it is linked with the protein by stable thioether bonds. In cytochrome *c,* the heme component appears to be deeply embedded in the protein. Cytochrome *c* has a molecular weight of about 13,000. The protein component is a single, essentially nonhelical strand of approximately 110 amino acid residues (Fairbanks *et al.,* 1971; Fitch and Margoliash, 1967).

In the cytochromes and other heme-proteins, iron is a part of the prosthetic group at the active site of the molecule. In other iron enzymes, the function of the iron is less clear. Xanthine oxidase is a complex flavoprotein that contains, besides flavin at its active site, both iron and molybdenum. The flavin, molybdenum, and iron compounds seem to function as an internal pathway of electron transport (Handler *et al.,* 1964). In the simpler flavoprotein enzymes, iron may not be a part of the active prosthetic group.

For succinate dehydrogenase, iron is essential both as a constituent of the enzyme molecule and as free ionic iron. Aconitase, on the other hand, seems to require only loosely bound iron. Removal of the iron results in inactivation of aconitase. The role of iron in aconitase seems to be that of chelating or binding the substrate (citrate, *cis*-aconitase, or isocitrate) in such a manner as to facilitate its hydration or dehydration.

Collagen proline hydroxylase, an enzyme necessary for the hydroxylation of protein and collagen biosynthesis, has been shown to require Fe^{2+}, in addition to ascorbic acid and α-ketoglutarate (Udenfriend, 1970). There is no evidence at present, however, to suggest that collagen synthesis is impaired in patients with iron deficiency.

Although most iron enzymes are probably indispensable to life, this is not universally so. One example of an iron enzyme that is not essential for life is catalase. In a rare mutation, catalase may be totally absent from all tissues. Patients with acatalasemia are often clinically well, although they may have gangrene in the oral cavity (Fairbanks *et al.,* 1971).

It was once thought that "parenchymal iron" is inviolate in states of iron depletion in mammalian species. Careful studies have now shown that the activities of several iron enzymes are markedly affected by variations in total body iron content (Fairbanks *et al.,* 1971).

METABOLISM

Among the organs and tissues of the body, the liver and spleen usually contain the highest iron concentration, followed by the kidney, heart, skeletal muscles, pancreas, and brain, which normally represent only one half to one tenth of the concentration in liver and spleen. In man, the liver has a high storage capacity for iron, and the total iron content of the liver may rise to 10 g in certain disease states. In the final stages of hemochromatosis, as much as 50 g of iron may accumulate in the body (Drabkin, 1951). Conversely, the iron content of these tissues and of the bone marrow is reduced below normal in iron deficiency and hemorrhagic anemia.

IRON IN BLOOD

Iron occurs in blood as hemoglobin in the erythrocytes and as transferrin bound in the plasma, in a ratio of nearly 1000 to 1. Minute amounts of nonheme iron also occur in the erythrocytes of human blood.

Hemoglobin

Hemoglobin is a complex of globin and four ferroprotoporphyrin (heme) moieties. It was first synthesized by Fischer and Zeile in 1929 (Fischer and Zeile, 1929), and later a three-dimensional picture of the molecule, with its four attached hemes and the nature of the bond between iron and globin, was established (Ingram *et al.*, 1956). In this combination, iron is stabilized in the ferrous state, which allows it to be reversibly bonded to oxygen, thus permitting hemoglobin to function as an oxygen carrier. The molecular weight of hemoglobin is approximately 65,000, of which the average iron content is 0.34%.

The synthesis of heme and its attachment to globin take place in the later stages of red cell development in the bone marrow. The production of the two parts of the molecule probably occurs simultaneously.

Numerous studies (Allen and Jandl, 1960; Bessis and Breton-Gorius, 1959; Donati *et al.*, 1966; Goldberg, A., 1959; Jandl and Katz, 1963; Jandl *et al.*, 1959; Katz, 1965; Noyes *et al.*, 1964) have offered evidence that the predominant pathway of entry of iron into the erythrocyte precursor is by transitory binding of transferrin to the erythrocyte membrane, followed by the release of the iron and its uptake by the cell (Fig. 5) (Fairbanks *et al.*, 1971). During the process of incorporation of iron into hemoglobin in the reticulocytes, the first step is the binding of the transferrin to the cells (Jandl and Katz, 1963; Morgan and Laurell, 1963).

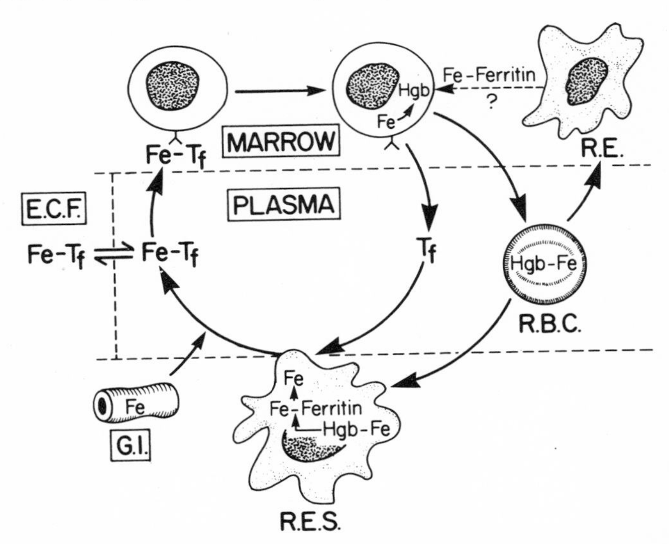

Fig. 5. Transport of iron to erythrocyte membrane. Transferrin (T_f) binds briefly to the membrane and releases its load of iron. The iron is then rapidly taken up by the normoblast and incorporated into heme. Transferrin returns to the plasma, where it is available to take up unbound iron. The transfer of ferritin from reticuloendothelial cells to normoblasts (upper right corner) may also contribute iron for hemoglobin synthesis, but this seem to be a minor mechanism. From Katz (1965) by permission.

The transferrin-binding occurs in two stages: (1) an initial, rapid, temperature-insensitive stage that is probably one of adsorption to the cell membrane; and (2) a slower, temperature-dependent stage that results in a firm union of the transferrin to the cell (Morgan, 1964a). Morgan and Appleton (1969) reported that in the second stage, the transferrin molecules actually pass into the cell by the most likely process of pinocytosis and are not exclusively localized to the cell-membrane receptors as previously believed. Although most of the iron used for hemoglobin synthesis comes from the plasma transferrin, a portion of the iron released from the red cell destruction in the phagocytic cells of the bone marrow can be used directly for this purpose without going through the plasma cycle (Bessis and Breton-Gorius, 1957; Morgan and Baker, 1969; Underwood, 1977).

Binding of transferrin appears to be specific for membranes of erythrocyte precursors. Approximately 50,000 transferrin molecules may be bound to the membrane of each reticulocyte. There is evidence that the reticulocyte preferentially binds transferrin carrying two atoms of iron per molecule (Fairbanks *et al.*, 1971).

Transferrin-binding by the reticulocyte membrane may require an active metabolic process (Jandl and Katz, 1963). Inhibition of metabolism by chemicals reduces the uptake of iron from transferrin, as does treatment of reticulocytes with trypsin (Jandl and Katz, 1963).

The release of iron from transferrin and its transport within the immature erythroid cell to the mitochondria for hemoglobin synthesis is poorly understood. Dissociation of iron does not occur spontaneously, nor does it occur merely by reduction of Fe(III) bound to transferrin, as is commonly believed. Protonic attack on the anion (carbonate or bicarbonate) may be involved in releasing the Fe(III) from its tight attachment to transferrin (Aisen and Brown, 1977). Whether or not an intracellular carrier is involved in the delivery of iron to the site of mitochondrial heme synthesis remains unsettled. Within the normoblast, iron can be visualized by electron microscopy as located in mitochondria, where it exists in an amorphous aggregate called a "ferruginous micelle." Iron seems to pass through the normoblast cytoplasm in the form of a low-molecular-weight complex.

Heme Synthesis

Figure 6 shows an abbreviated scheme for heme synthesis, giving the essential enzymes and illustrating which steps occur within the mitochondria and which occur outside the mitochondria. The initial reaction in heme synthesis is the combination of succinyl-CoA with glycine to form δ-aminolevulinic acid. This reaction is catalyzed by the enzyme δ-aminolevulinic acid synthetase (ALA-S), which is a mitochondrial enzyme. The next step involves combination of the two δ-aminolevulinic acid molecules into porphobilinogen (PBG). This reaction is catalyzed by the enzyme δ-aminolevulinic acid dehydrase (ALA-D). This reaction occurs in the cytoplasm of the cell. The inhibition of this enzymatic step causes an increased urinary excretion and an increase in the blood level of δ-aminolevulinic acid. The next step in the heme synthesis pathway is a combination of four porphobilinogens to form uroporphyrinogen. These reactions occur extramitochondrially and are synthesized by the enzymes synthetase (URO-S) and cosytnthetase (URO-CoS). The next step is the synthesis of

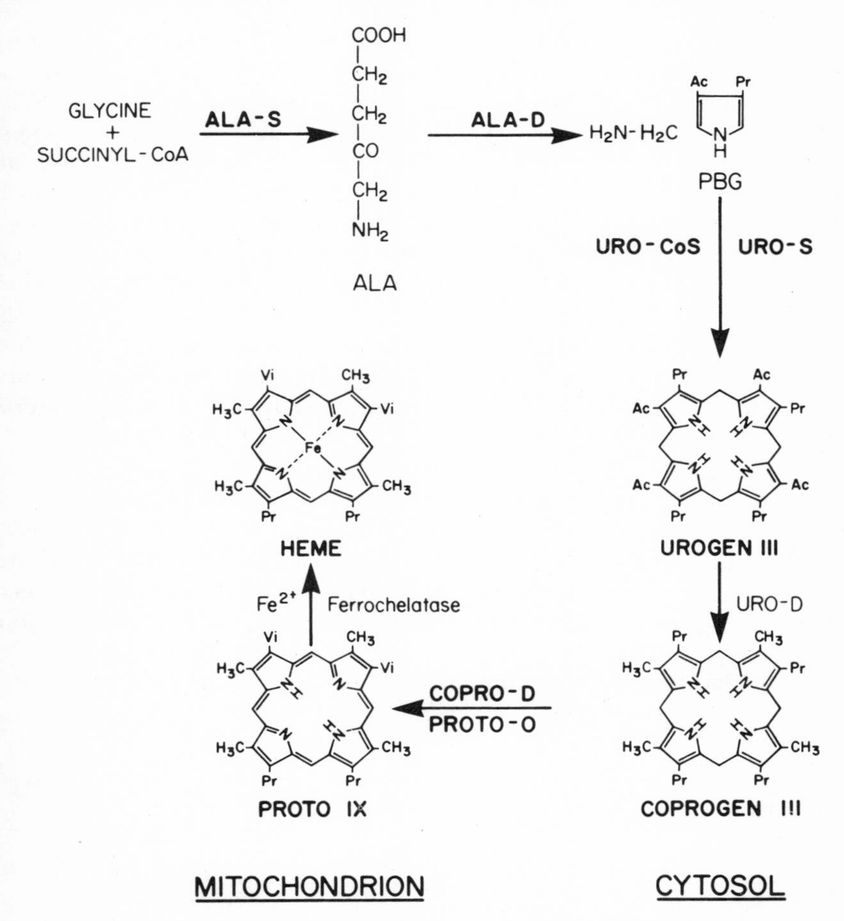

Fig. 6. Heme biosynthetic pathway. (Ac) CH_2COOH; (Pr) $(CH_2)_2COOH$; (Vi) $CH{=}CH_2$; (URO-D) uro-decarboxylase; (COPRO-D) copro-decarboxylase. From Gidari and Levere (1977). Reproduced with permission.

coproporphyrinogen and its conversion to protoporphyrin IX (PROTO IX), which occurs intramitochondrially, catalyzed by COPRO-D and an oxidase (PROTO-O). The final step is the addition of ferrous iron to protoporphyrin to form heme, a reaction catalyzed by the enzyme ferrochelatase (Green *et al.,* 1958; Rimington, 1959; Underwood, 1977). Impaired synthesis of heme due to copper deficiency, probably related to a decreased activity of cytochrome oxidase, a copper-dependent enzyme, has been reported recently (Williams, D. M., *et al.,* 1976). The role of cytochrome oxidase is to reduce Fe(III) to Fe(II), prior to its incorporation in the protoporphyrin molecule.

The level of hemoglobin varies with age, sex, nutrition, state of health, pregnancy, lactation, and environment. In man, the level falls from about 18–19 g/100 ml at birth to about 12 g/100 ml at 3–4 months. This level is matintained until the child is 1 year old, when a slow rise to adult values (13–15 g/100 ml) normally occurs. The hemoglobin levels increase at puberty in males, and the higher hemoglobin levels of the male continue throughout the life span. This difference is most likely a real sex difference, since a significant rise to the level of males does not take place after menopause or hysterectomy, when menstrual blood losses do not occur (Underwood, 1977; Vahlquist, 1950).

Hemoglobin concentrations decrease in late pregnancy, partially due to hydremia (Bond, 1948; de Leuuw *et al.,* 1966; Dieckmann and Wegner, 1934; Gemzell *et al.,* 1954), but iron deficiency is frequently a contributory factor.

Serum Iron

The iron in serum was shown by Holmberg and Laurell (1947) to be completely bound to transferrin (Schade *et al.,* 1949). Serum iron concentrations for human subjects are presented in Table II. Following incubation

Table II. Serum Iron, Total Iron-Binding Capacity (TIBC), and Percentage Saturation in Adult Humans[a]

Species and condition	Number of cases	Serum iron (μg/100 ml)	TIBC (μg/100 ml)	Mean saturation (%)
Normal male	35	127 (67–191)	333 (253–416)	33
Normal female	35	113 (63–202)	329 (250–416)	37
Iron-deficiency anemia	35	32 (0–78)	482 (304–705)	7
Late pregnancy	106	94 (22–185)	532 (373–712)	18
Hemochromatosis	14	250 (191–290)	263 (205–330)	96
Infections	11	47 (30–72)	260 (182–270)	20

[a]From Underwood (1977).

of ^{59}Fe with pooled native human serum *in vitro,* ultrafiltrable iron was determined to be 5–7.5% of the total serum iron at different levels of iron albumin molar ratios (Prasad and Oberleas, 1971). Under similar conditions, approximately 2% of iron was ultrafiltrable when predialyzed serum was used. In physiological concentrations, additions of amino acids to predialyzed serum increased ultrafiltrable ^{59}Fe to levels similar to that observed for native human serum. Histidine and lysine showed significant effects in this regard. Amino acids competed effectively with albumin and only to a lesser degree with transferrin for binding of iron, suggesting a tighter affinity of iron for transferrin (Prasad and Oberleas, 1971).

The amino-acid-bound fraction of iron may have an important physiological role in the biological transport of this element across cellular membranes. Although these studies do not deal with the mechanism directly, one may consider that a possible effect of the presence of amino acids in the gut may have been to render iron more diffusible, thus facilitating its passage through the mucosal wall to some extent (Prasad and Oberleas, 1971).

Normally, only 30–40% of the transferrin carries iron, the remainder being known as the latent iron-binding capacity. Representative values for serum iron, TIBC, and percentage saturation in human subjects are presented in Table II. The differences in serum iron in man can be understood if the iron of the serum is conceived as a pool into which iron enters, from which it leaves, and to which it is returned at varying rates for the synthesis and resynthesis of hemoglobin, ferritin, and other ron compounds.

In man, a well-marked diurnal rhythm with respect to serum iron has been established. Vahlquist (1941) found 15 normal men to have a mean serum iron of 135 ± 10.6 μg/100 ml at 8 A.M. and of 99 ± 9.2 μg/100 ml at 6 P.M.. In night workers, the diurnal rhythm is reversed and diminished (Hamilton, L. D., *et al.,* 1950; Patterson *et al.,* 1953). Sleep deprivation in human subjects also results in a gradual decline in serum iron levels, the maximum drop being to half the original levels (Kuhn *et al.,* 1967). Most of the drop in the iron level occurs during the first 48 hr of sleep deprivation, with a slower decline during subsequent intervals. The serum iron levels return to normal in about one week.

STORAGE IRON COMPOUNDS

Ferritin and hemosiderin are two nonheme compounds that occur widely in the tissues, with the highest concentrations normally present in the liver, spleen, and bone marrow. The two compounds are chemically dissimilar, although intimately related in function. Ferritin is soluble in water, whereas hemosiderin is insoluble (Gabrio *et al.,* 1953; Kaldor, 1958).

Ferritin is a brown compound and contains up to 20% of iron (Laufberger, 1937). It consists of a central nucleus of iron surrounded by a shell of protein. The ferritin molecule is polynuclear iron (hydrous ferric oxide-phosphate) coated by an assembly of protein chains (Harrison, 1977; Granick and Michaelis, 1942; Rothen, 1944). The average number of iron atoms per molecule of ferritin is 3000 or less, but ferritin has the storage capacity of 4500 iron atoms per molecule. The iron-free apoferritin consists of a shell 130 Å (13 nm) in outside diameter with a central cavity of 60 Å (6 nm) across. The molecular weight of horse spleen apoferritin is 440,000, and it has 24 subunits of molecular weight 18,500 that are arranged symmetrically.

The inner surface of the apoferritin shell has a ridged appearance with four indentations or pockets in each half molecule. The complementary structure, the "hole" inside apoferritin, made up a solid object represents the iron core of an iron-repleted ferritin molecule. Ferritin has a tetrad appearance.

Iron stimulates the synthesis of apoferritin at a posttranscriptional stage and does not induce synthesis of apoferritin mRNA. Biosynthesis of apoferritin occurs preferentially on free polysomes, although some synthesis on membrane-bound polysomes has also been found.

The physiological mechanisms of ferritin iron release are not well understood at present. The involvement of xanthine oxidase (molybdenum-containing enzyme) or an $NAD^+/NADH^-$-dependent enzyme catalyzing reductive release through the production of $FMNH_2$ has been suggested. Superoxide is also capable of reducing ferritin iron.

The recent development of an immunoradiometric method for quantitating serum ferritin (Addison *et al.*, 1972) has led to its measurement in several clinical conditions. The mean concentration is higher in men than in women. Some investigators have obtained a high degree of correlation between serum ferritin concentration and storage iron (Lipschitz *et al.*, 1974; Siimes *et al.*, 1974).

Hemosiderin is a relatively amorphous compound. It may contain up to 35% iron, consisting mainly of ferric hydroxide condensed into an essentially protein-free aggregate (Shoden and Sturgeon, 1959, 1960, 1961, 1962). It exists in the tissues as a brown, granular, readily stainable pigment.

Histochemical examination of aspirated samples of bone marrow for hemosiderin has been proposed as a reliable index of body iron stores and as a valuable aid in diagnosis of iron-deficiency anemia (Beutler *et al.*, 1958; Stevens *et al.*, 1953). Shoden and Sturgeon (1960) emphasized the value of using both staining and chemical methods that estimate the soluble (ferritin) as well as the insoluble (hemosiderin) forms of storage iron.

The relative distribution of iron between ferritin and hemosiderin in mammals is in all likelihood determined by the total storage iron concentration. Morgan and Walters (1963) concluded from their studies in human necropsies that with total storage iron in liver and spleen below 500 μg/g tissue, more iron was stored as ferritin than as hemosiderin; with levels above 1000 μg/g, more was stored as hemosiderin. In diseases such as hemochromatosis and transfusional siderosis, which are characterized by extremely high levels of iron in the tissues, most of the iron is present as hemosiderin (Drabkin, 1951; Morgan and Walters, 1963).

Animal experiments suggest that the ratio of ferritin to hemosiderin iron may be affected further by the rate of storage. If iron is injected at high rates, or administered in a form such as saccharated iron that is rapidly cleaved from the serum, hemosiderin is deposited rather than ferritin (Underwood, 1977). On the other hand, with equivalent injections of iron dextrose, which remains in the serum for a relatively long time, ferritin production is greater (Shoden and Sturgeon, 1959, 1960, 1962).

The bone marrow and muscles contain considerable amounts of nonheme iron. The storage iron concentration of bone marrow in normal man is approximately 100 μg/g (Hallgren, 1954). Assuming the total active bone marrow weight to be 3000 g, the storage iron content can be calculated to be 300 mg. Although the concentration of nonheme iron in the muscles is low, the total amount is high because of the large muscle mass. The total amount of storage iron in muscle is at least equal to that of the liver. In subjects with iron overload, the iron concentrations in muscles are raised, but to a smaller extent than in the liver.

IRON IN MILK

The average concentration of iron in human milk is 0–5 μg/ml (Cavell and Widdowson, 1964; Feuillen and Plumier, 1952; Morrison, 1952; Pollycove, 1958). The level of iron in colostrum is 3–5 times higher than that in milk.

Iron occurs in milk in combination with protein. An iron-protein compound named ferrilactin, which occurs in small concentrations, has been isolated from human milk. This salmon-red compound, in which the iron is firmly bound, has two iron-binding sites and a molecular weight of 86,000. It is chemically and immunologically distinct from serum transferrin (Derechin and Johnson, 1962; Gordon *et al.*, 1962; Groves, 1960; Johannson, 1960).

FACTORS THAT AFFECT IRON ABSORPTION

The absorption of iron is affected by the age, iron status, and state of health; by conditions within the gastrointestinal tract; by the amount and chemical form of the iron ingested; and by the amounts and proportions of various other components of the diet, both organic and inorganic. In man, the absorption takes place mainly in the duodenum in the ferrous form (Brown and Justus, 1958; Gabrio and Salomon, 1950; Heath and Patek, 1937; Niccum *et al.,* 1953; Stewart *et al.,* 1950). Absorption does not depend on valency alone, since some ferric compounds are more available than some ferrous compounds (Fritz *et al.,* 1970). Ferric salts appear to be less effective for hemoglobin formation in man than ferrous forms (Heath and Patek, 1937; Niccum *et al.,* 1953; Underwood, 1977).

Iron occurs in foods in inorganic forms, in combination with protein, in heme compounds as a constituent of hemoglobin and myoglobin, and in other inorganic complexes. Iron in heme compounds is absorbed directly into the mucosal cells of the intestine without the necessity of release from its bound form. The inorganic forms of iron and the iron-protein compounds need to be reduced to the ferrous state and released from conjugation for effective absorption. These transformations are accomplished by the gastric juice and other digestive secretions (Underwood, 1977).

Amino acids such as histidine and lysine assist in iron absorption (Kroe *et al.,* 1966; Van Campen and Gross, 1969). It has been suggested that a direct reaction between iron and histidine occurs, and that amino acid–iron chelate may be formed and subsequently absorbed. Since histidine is a product of protein hydrolysis in the gastrointestinal tract, it was suggested that the amino acid may be involved in the normal absorption of iron. Organic acids and reducing substrates in foods, such as ascorbic acid and cysteine, may also assist in reducing and releasing food iron (Granick, 1946, 1951). Ascorbic acid reduces ferric to ferrous iron *in vitro,* and the administration of large doses of this acid with iron salts and some foods can increase the efficiency of iron absorption (Hallberg and Sölvell, 1967; Moore and Dubach, 1951; Pirzio-Biroli *et al.,* 1958). Ascorbic acid has no such effect on the absorption of hemoglobin iron.

In 1955, R. J. Walsh *et al.* (1955) showed that significant amounts of iron are absorbed in human subjects. Hallberg and Sölvell (1967), using a double-isotope technique permitting comparisons to be made on the same subjects, found that the iron of hemoglobin and that of ferrous sulfate were equally well absorbed by normal human subjects when equivalent doses were given. The absorption of iron from ferrous sulfate was increased by ascorbic acid and reduced by sodium phytate, whereas the absorption of hemoglobin iron was unaffected by either.

High levels of phosphate reduce iron absorption (Brock and Diamond, 1934). When sodium phytate is added to diets, iron absorption can be reduced in man. High intakes of zinc, cadmium, copper, and manganese also interfere with iron absorption, apparently through competition for protein-binding sites in the intestinal mucosa, and have been shown to raise iron requirements. Settlemire and Matrone (1967a,b) obtained evidence in the rat that zinc reduces iron absorption by interfering with the incorporation of iron into or with its release from ferritin. The increase in iron requirement due to high zinc intakes was augmented by a shortening of the life span of the red blood cells, resulting in a faster turnover of iron.

Only 5–10% of food iron is normally absorbed by man from ordinary diets. This percentage has been demonstrated with labeled foods (Moore, 1955) and with standard foods with small amounts of iron tracer added (Pirzio-Biroli *et al.,* 1958). Absorption of food iron may be increased to twice this level, or more, in children and in iron deficiency. The absorption of hemoglobin iron is also increased in iron deficiency in man, though the increase is less marked than it is with ferrous sulfate (Hallberg and Sölvell, 1967; Underwood, 1977).

Increased absorption of iron occurs in aplastic anemia, hemolytic anemia, pernicious anemia, pyridoxine deficiency, hemochromatosis, and tranfusional siderosis (Cartwright and Wintrobe, 1954; Dubach *et al.,* 1948; Peterson and Ettinger, 1953). Increased iron absorption appears to be related to increased erythropoiesis, depletion of body-iron stores, increased iron turnover, and hypoxia (Bothwell *et al.,* 1958; Braude *et al.,* 1962; Mendel, 1961; Mendel *et al.,* 1963; Weintraub *et al.,* 1964, 1965). Decreased iron absorption has been related to tissue iron overload (Bothwell *et al.,* 1958; Conrad *et al.,* 1964).

MECHANISMS OF IRON ABSORPTION

McCance and Widdowson (1937, 1938) first proposed the concept that iron absorption is controlled by body needs. Later, Hahn *et al.* (1943) advanced the "mucosal block" theory of iron absorption, which was elaborated by Granick (1946, 1951), thus focusing attention on the mucosal cells. According to this theory, the intestinal mucosa absorbs iron during periods of need and rejects it when stores are adequate. Iron taken up by mucosal cells is converted into ferritin, and when the cells become physiologically saturated with ferritin, further absorption is impeded until the iron is released from ferritin and transferred to plasma.

Granick's mucosal block theory of iron absorption was based on an erroneous interpretation of inadequate data. His concept, that the presence of ferritin in the intestinal mucosa prevents iron absorption, has now been discarded. The evidence against this concept is (1) in man, increasing doses of iron cause increased absorption of iron; (2) in guinea pigs, after an oral dose of iron, the peak in plasma iron concentration precedes the maximal formation of ferritin in intestinal mucosal cells, whereas Granick's hypothesis would require that the converse be true; (3) the studies of mucosal ferritin content after oral iron loading have led to very contradictory results, whether the same or different species were examined; and (4) no correlation was found, in man, between rate of iron absorption and nonheme iron content of the intestinal mucosa (Allgood and Brown, 1967; Beutler, 1961; Brown and Rother, 1961, 1963; Charlton *et al.,* 1965; Hartman *et al.,* 1963; Laurell, 1952; Smith, J. A., *et al.,* 1968). On the other hand, parenteral administration of iron in man has been shown to cause an increase in intestinal mucosal iron content that is maximal at the time of a nadir in absorption of orally administered radioactive iron. These observations support the concept of a mucosal regulation of some kind that modulates the rate of absorption of iron to meet physiological needs (Fairbanks *et al.,* 1971).

Later studies by Crosby and Conrad (Conrad and Crosby, 1963; Conrad *et al.,* 1964; Wheby and Crosby, 1963) provided evidence that in the rat, the ultimate regulator of iron absorption is the iron concentration of the epithelial cells of the upper intestine. In normal rats, only a small part of the ingested iron taken up by mucosal cells is transferred to the bloodstream; the remainder stays in the mucosal cells and is lost into the gut lumen when the cells are sloughed from the tips of the intestinal villi. In iron-deficient rats, most of the ingested iron is absorbed directly into the bloodstream, with very little remaining in the mucosal cells. In rats given excessive iron parenterally, the epithelial cells are "loaded from the rear," and are therefore unable to accept the ingested iron. Data reported by Allgood and Brown (1967) indicate that this mechanism may not be applicable to man. The nonheme iron content of the duodenal mucosa of normal subjects did not differ from that of iron-loaded or iron-deficient subjects. Furthermore, there was no correlation with simultaneous measurements of serum iron or with radioiron absorption. These data may indicate species differences with respect to regulation of iron absorption by the gastrointestinal tract (Underwood, 1977). The existence of an iron-transport system involving binding of iron to iron-receptor sites in the plasma membrane of the epithelial cells and interaction of plasma transferrin with these sites with the release of iron has been suggested (Evans and Grace, 1974).

The absorption of hemoglobin iron, unlike that of inorganic iron, is not affected by ascorbic acid, phytate, or nonabsorbable chelating agents. This observation suggests that iron is not released from heme in the gut lumen, but that the complex is taken up directly by the intestinal epithelial cell, subsequently appearing in the plasma in nonheme form (Conrad *et al.,* 1966; Hallberg and Sölvell, 1967; Weintraub *et al.,* 1968). Weintraub *et al.* (1968) demonstrated the presence of an enzymelike substance in the duodenal mucosa of the dog that is capable of releasing iron from hemoglobin *in vitro.* The rate at which the heme-splitting substance works *in vivo* appeared to be increased by the removal of the nonheme-iron end product from the epithelial cell to the plasma. It seems, therefore, that the labile nonheme-iron content of the intestinal cell determines its ability to accept heme from the lumen in dogs, as well as ionized iron from the lumen in rats (Underwood, 1977).

The observation of Dowdle *et al.* (1960) that iron absorption is not passive but demands the energy produced by the Krebs tricarboxylic acid cycle received convincing support from the studies by P. Jacobs *et al.* (1966). In isolated loops of small bowel with artificial circulation, the absorption of iron is reduced by anoxia or by perfusion of the isolated loop with solutions containing inhibitors of the enzymes of the Krebs cycle.

Iron absorption occurs directly into the bloodstream, rather than through the lymphatics. Absorption is most efficient through the upper portion of the small bowel, and there is little or no absorption of iron through the gastric mucosa (Fairbanks *et al.*, 1971).

P. S. Davis *et al.* (1966) found an iron-binding protein (gastroferrin) in normal gastric juice, but not in patients with hemochromatosis. In iron-deficiency anemia caused by blood loss, the concentration of gastroferrin in gastric juice was reduced and returned to normal levels when hemoglobin level became normal. It was proposed that gastroferrin regulates iron absorption. Thus, normal levels would inhibit absorption of excessive intake of iron, and reduced levels would permit enhanced absorption in iron deficiency. Failure to produce gastroferrin may thus be a causal factor in hemochromatosis. No direct support for this hypothesis is present in the literature.

The excess absorption and deposition of iron characteristic of hemochromatosis has been further related to a primary pancreas defect (Biggs, and Davis, 1963, 1966). A. E. Davis and Biggs (1964, 1965) showed that iron absorption can be significantly reduced in hemochromatosis by the addition of a pancreatic extract with the oral dose of iron. The active factor in pancreatic juice has not been characterized, and the physiological importance of the pancreatic secretion in the normal regulation of iron absorption remains to be evaluated (Underwood, 1977).

EXCRETION OF IRON

The limited ability of the body to excrete iron has been confirmed since the original observation of McCance and Widdowson (1937, 1938). The total iron in the feces of normal human adults is usually between 6 and 16 mg/day, depending on the amount of iron ingested. Most of this iron is unabsorbed food iron. The true excretion of iron is between 0.2 and 0.5 mg/day. This iron is derived from desquamated cells and from the bile. Iron occurs in the bile, mostly from hemoglobin breakdown, to the extent of 1 mg/day. Most of this iron is reabsorbed and does not reach the feces. The amount of iron eliminated in the urine varies from 0.2 to 0.3 mg/day on an average basis in an adult human subject. This amount can be increased to as much as 10 mg/day by the injection of chelating agents.

In addition to the iron excreted in the urine and feces, there is a loss of iron in the sweat, hair, and nails, Most of this loss occurs in desquamated cells, but cell-free sweat also contains some iron. On an average, the loss of iron through the skin of a healthy adult is about 0.5 mg/day. This amount is much greater in the tropics, where the volume of sweat can be as much as 5 liters/day (Foy and Kondi, 1957). Dermal losses of iron may be a contributory factor in the high incidence of iron-deficiency anemia in the tropics.

The total quantity of iron lost in the urine, feces, and sweat amounts to 0.6–1.0 mg/day in an average adult male. This is a considerable loss if one considers that no more than 1.0–1.5 mg iron/day is available for absorption from an ordinary well-balanced diet. In women, iron balance is more precarious because they are subject to regular menstrual blood loss from menarche to menopause. Assuming a normal 28-day cycle, it can be calculated that most women between puberty and menopause lose 0.5–0.8 mg iron/day as a result of menstruation. Additionally, loss of iron due to childbirth and lactation imposes further stress on iron balance. Despite the low iron content in milk, the average daily secretion of iron in milk may approximate 0.4 mg/day.

TRANSPORT AND INTERMEDIARY METABOLISM

Once iron traverses the mucosa of the bowel, it enters the bloodstream and is bound to the specific transport protein, transferrin (see Fig. 5). It is conceived that iron moves initially from the plasma to the labile pool, which may represent iron loosely bound to proteins or cell membranes in the tissues of many organs such as liver and bone marrow. Iron loosely bound to the membrane of the developing normoblast may also be a part of the labile pool. Some of the iron in the labile pool returns to the plasma only to leave it again. Some of the iron in the labile pool may move directly into the normoblast and become incorporated into hemoglobin, and some may move directly into tissue or storage iron (Fairbanks *et al.,* 1971).

Transferrin is the main serum protein responsible for the transport of iron (Ehrenberg and Laurell, 1955; Aasa *et al.,* 1963; Fletcher and Huehns, 1967; Morgan *et al.,* 1966). It is a single-chain polypeptide with two active sites, is loaded with metal, and is relatively resistant to thermal and proteolytic treatment. The carbohydrate content is 6%. In addition to iron, transferrin can bind other metals as well. These are chromium(III), manganese(III), cobalt(III), copper(II), and zinc(II).

Transferrin behaves as an iron acceptor from tissues. Release of iron occurs from three major sites: (1) reticuloendothelial cells, (2) hepatocytes, and (3) the intestine. Release of iron from the reticuloendothelial cells, which is approximately 20 mg/day, is usually rapid, but may be interrupted due to inflammation or acute or chronic disorders. Since the iron-protein bond in native transferrin is so strong as to preclude a simple dissociation mechanism for the release of iron, it may well be that the primary event in the physiological removal of iron from the protein is an attack on the anion (carbonate or bicarbonate), following which disruption of the metal–protein bound would readily occur (Aisen and Brown, 1977).

Copper deficiency is known to affect adversely the normal release of iron from cell to plasma. This effect is related to the ferrooxidase activity of the ceruloplasmin that is responsible for the reduction of Fe(III) to Fe(II), whereby the release of iron from the cells is accomplished (see Chapter 2). Whether or not this is the sole mechanism by which copper affects the release of iron from cells remains to be established. A direct role of ceruloplasmin as an iron carrier from cell membrane to transferrin and an indirect function in which it serves as a source of copper for other copper enzymes, or even a mechanism involving some still unknown biological activity of the protein, are some of the other possibilities that need further investigation (Aisen and Brown, 1977). Serum transferrin is increased in pregnancy, acute hypoxia, and iron deficiency due to estrogen and cortisol administration. The synthesis of transferrin is increased in iron deficiency and decreased as a result of fasting and ethanol intake and in protein malnutrition. The catabolic rate of transferrin is increased in infection, nephrosis, and hemolytic anemias.

Release of transferrin after delivery of its iron probably occurs by reversal of the endocytotic process, since there is no evidence that transferrin is destroyed in the process of iron delivery. This release is also energy-dependent and inhibited by SH reagents.

Erythrocyte precursors normally contain a few iron granules. In iron deficiency, when presumably intracellular iron turnover is more rapid, such granules may be seen only rarely (Beutler *et al.,* 1958; Douglas and Dacie, 1953; Hansen and Weinfeld, 1959; Kaplan *et al.,* 1954). In the anemia of chronic infection, the number of iron granules in erythrocytes may also be decreased, although conflicting evidence bearing on this question has been presented (Hansen and Weinfeld, 1959; Morse and Read, 1954). The reticuloendothelial cell holds onto its iron store tenaciously in chronic infection. Electron-microscopic evidence obtained by Bessis and Breton-Gorius (1962) suggests that in chronic infection, the nurse cell is unable to feed its iron to the developing red cell precursors. It may be that in inflammatory diseases, such as chronic infections, there is more than one mechanism by which iron metabolism of the normoblast is impaired. Besides the mechanism proposed by Bessis and Breton-Gorius (1962), impaired release by reticuloendothelial cells of iron from phagocytized effete erythrocytes may decrease the cycling of iron from reticuloendothelial cells to plasma transferrin and thence to the developing normoblast. This would account for the decreased serum iron and the rapid plasma iron transport rate. It would not readily account, however, for the refractiveness to iron therapy characteristically found in these conditions. Thus, there may be an impairment in metabolic function of the erythrocyte precursor itself in addition to a defect in the mechanism of delivery of iron to these cells (Fairbanks *et al.,* 1971).

Iron from effete erythrocytes is split from hemoglobin by reticuloendothelial cells, and most of it returns to the plasma, where it is again bound to transferrin. It is then reutilized for hemoglobin synthesis. This reutilization of the hemoglobin iron of nonviable erythrocytes normally occurs at such a rate that approximately 40% of the iron of senescent erythrocytes is incorporated into hemoglobin within 2 weeks (Noyes *et al.*, 1960). The remainder of the iron derived from hemoglobin catabolism is more slowly released to plasma. The orderly release of iron from effete red cells is an important source of iron for erythropoiesis, since it must balance the approximately 20 mg of iron normally required daily for resynthesis of hemoglobin. Impairment of reutilization of hemoglobin iron occurs in chronic inflammatory disorders, such as infection, sterile abscess, and rheumatoid arthritis; in malignant diseases; and in a few cases of "primary defective iron reutilization." In these disorders, the reticuloendothelial system appears to be unable to release iron to plasma in a normal manner. The effect is a reduction in the amount of iron available for hemoglobin synthesis (Fairbanks *et al.*, 1971).

The total mass of circulating hemoglobin, amounting to 800–900 g in a normal man, is synthesized and destroyed every 120 days. This process liberates approximately 20 mg of endogenous iron daily, which is reutilized for hemoglobin synthesis. The removal of nonviable red cells, the breakdown of the heme moiety, and the release of iron and the return of this iron to the plasma are the responsibility of the reticuloendothelial cells of the liver, spleen, and bone marrow. Only a few red cells are destroyed intravascularly, except in certain hemolytic diseases, so that plasma hemoglobin is an unimportant pathway in normal hemoglobin metabolism.

^{59}Fe studies have shown that plasma iron has a rapid turnover rate, with a normal half-time of only 90–100 min (Pollycove, 1958). In adult man, it has been calculated that 25–40 mg of total iron is transported by plasma every 24 hr, even though only 3–4 mg is present in the total plasma volume at any one time. Exchange of iron with the tissue stores, with myoglobin and the heme enzymes, and with the gastrointestinal tract and the sites of excretion is restricted to a few milligrams daily (Pollycove, 1958). Pollycove (1958) suggested that more iron goes to the bone marrow than the 20–25 mg needed for hemoglobin synthesis, and the excess constitutes a labile marrow pool that is returned to the plasma. The large and rapid flow of plasma iron to the marrow is reflected in the promptness with which the iron released from the red cell destruction in the phagocytic cells of the bone marrow can be used directly for this purpose without going through the plasma cycle (Underwood, 1977). Tagged hemoglobin can be identified in the peripheral blood within 4–8 hr after administration of iron; with 7–14 days, from 70 to 100% of the isotope is found in circulating hemoglobin (Moore and Dubach, 1951, 1956; Underwood, 1977).

The rapid process of incorporation of plasma iron into ferritin in the liver cells is dependent on energy-yielding reactions in these cells for the continued synthesis of ATP, which, together with ascorbic acid, reduces the ferric iron of transferrin to the ferrous state, thus releasing it from transferrin. The release of iron from the hepatic ferritin to the plasma is mediated by xanthine oxidase (molybdenum- and iron-containing enzyme) acting as a dehydrogenase. The reduced enzyme, formed as a result of oxidation of xanthine and hypoxanthine to uric acid, is reoxidized by some of the ferric iron of ferritin. In this process, the ferric iron of ferritin is reduced to the ferrous state. The iron of ferritin then dissociates easily from its bond to protein and is accepted by transferrin (Underwood, 1977). Osaki and Sirivech (1971), however, reported that in liver homogenates, xanthine oxidase substrates did not release iron from ferritin; on the other hand, the reduced riboflavin and riboflavin derivatives may reduce horse spleen ferritin Fe(III) at a rate likely to be physiologically significant (Sirivech *et al.,* 1974). Mobilization of iron from iron stores also requires the presence of the copper-containing enzyme of the plasma, ceruloplasmin (ferroxidase I), as discussed in Chapter 2.

The iron of plasma is deposited in the liver and spleen just as readily in the form of hemosiderin as it is in the form of ferritin, and iron is released from hemosiderin for utilization by the tissues just as readily as it is from ferritin. The mechanism of release of iron from hemosiderin is unknown. There is evidence to suggest that in the rabbit, the iron of transferrin is not incorporated directly into hemosiderin, as it is into ferritin (Shoden and Sturgeon, 1963). In this species, ferritin has to be formed first, so that liver ferritin appears to be the precursor of liver parenchymal cell hemosiderin (Underwood, 1977).

In the liver, spleen, and bone marrow, where sinusoid walls are fenestrated, iron is transferred from the vascular to the extravascular space, without prior dissociation from its firm complex with protein in transferrin. It has also been shown in rats and rabbits that iron remains bound to transferrin during passage through the capillary wall (Morgan, 1963). A different mechanism exists for the transfer of iron from the mother to the fetus. Inasmuch as the placental transfer of transferrin is much less than the transfer of iron (Gitlin *et al.,* 1964; Morgan, 1964b), iron must dissociate from transferrin on the maternal side of the placenta and then be transferred across the placental cells to be reassociated with new transferrin molecules on the fetal side (Underwood, 1977).

SOURCES OF AND REQUIREMENT FOR IRON

Rich sources of iron are the organ meats (liver, kidney, and heart), egg yolk, dried legumes, cocoa, cane molasses, shellfish, and parsley. Poor sources include milk and milk products, white sugar, white flour and bread (unenriched), polished rice, sago, potatoes, and most fresh fruits. Foods of intermediate iron content are the muscle meats, fish and poultry, nuts, green vegetables, and wholemeal bread. Boiling in liberal amounts of water can reduce the levels of iron in vegetables by as much as 20%. The iron content of cereals is reduced by removal of the germ and outer branny layers in the process of milling. In a study of North American wheats and the flours milled from these wheats, the mean iron content of the whole germ was found to be 43 μg/g, and that of the flour, 10.5 μg/g (Czerniejewski *et al.*, 1964; Underwood, 1977).

The overall intake of iron from different diets varies greatly. The average adult diet in the United States was reported to supply 14–20 mg iron daily (Sherman, 1935), whereas in Australia, the adult diet contains 20–22 mg iron daily (*National Health and Medical Research Council Report*, 1945). A typical poor Indian diet was shown to provide only 9 mg iron daily. However, an improved diet containing less milled rice and more pulse and green vegetables could provide as much as 60 mg/day (W.H.O. Bulletin No. 23, 1951). Iron intake is most likely to be inadequate where there is a heavy dependence on low-cost, high-energy foods that are low in iron, which is of low availability. Adequacy of the diet in other respects does not necessarily ensure adequacy in iron. Monsen *et al.* (1967) found that the daily iron intake of 13 young women maintaining their normal eating habits averaged only 9.2 mg when chemically analyzed and 9.9 mg when calculated. This amount is well below the 15 mg/day recommended for such persons, although the diets were stated to be adequate in protein, calcium, vitamins A and C, and the B vitamins. The diet of these women, however, provided only 1600 cal/day. These observations thus emphasize the importance of caloric intake in determining the total iron intake on a daily basis.

With normal men and postmenopausal women, adequacy of iron intake may not pose any problem. Women during the fertile period, however, are in a more precarious position. Food iron consumption may be declining, due to a progressive decrease in total caloric intake and to reduced opportunities for iron contamination as a result of improved cleanliness in handling of foods and a declining domestic use of iron cooking vessels. Some form of iron supplementation is therefore probably necessary. Several forms of iron have been used for fortification of white flour, including reduced iron (ferrous reductase), ferric ammonium citrate, and ferric pyrophosphate. The results of a long-term clinical trial carried out with women consuming bread fortified with ferrous reductase gave no evidence of therapeutic value as judged by changes in hemoglobin levels (Elwood, 1963). This finding contrasted with the significant mean increase shown by women receiving ferrous gluconate in tablet form, and suggested that the iron in the fortified bread was poorly absorbed.

A possible influence on iron intake of the source, as well as the choice, of foods was clear from a study of nutritional anemia in school children in rural areas of Florida (Underwood, 1977). The typical diet of these children provided only 4–6 mg iron/day . The low iron intake was associated with poor food habits and with the consumption of a high proportion of locally grown foods, produced on poor sandy soils. Turnip greens, the most important source of iron to these people, contained only 50–60 μg iron/g when grown on the poor soils, compared with some 250 μg/g on better soils. The anemia was increased in severity by hookworm infestation, in some instances. It was clear, however, that the anemia was due principally to poor food habits and accentuated by the dependence on locally grown materials subnormal in iron content. These anemic children responded well to oral iron therapy.

The demands for iron are greatest during the first 2 years of life, during the period of rapid growth and hemoglobin increase of adolescence, and throughout the childbearing period in women (Underwood, 1977). The iron requirement of the human infant during the first year of life may be as high as 1 mg/day, but probably averages 0.6 mg/day (Josephs, 1959). This rises to 1.5–2.5 mg from puberty onward. At age 15–16 in males, the requirement also increases temporarily due to the rapid growth and hemoglobin accretion that occurs at this time. Estimates of total human requirements, which take all these factors into account, indicate that enough iron must be consumed to permit absorption of approximately 2.0 mg/day by normal menstruating women. A summary of iron requirements for human subjects is given in Table III (Underwood, 1977).

It is difficult to convert these physiological requirements into dietary requirements because of variations among individual subjects in absorptive capacity and among foods in the availability of their iron for absorption.

Table III. Estimated Human Iron Requirements[a]

Subjects	Absorbed iron requirement (mg/day)	Food iron requirement (mg/day)[b]
Normal men and nonmenstruating women	0.5–1	5–10
Menstruating women	0.2–2	7–20
Pregnant women	2–4.8	20–48[c]
Adolescents	1–2	10–20
Children	0.4–1	4–10
Infants	0.5–1.5	1.5 (mg/kg)[d]

[a]Taken from Committee on Iron Deficiency (Underwood, 1977).
[b]Assuming 10% absorption.
[c]This amount cannot be derived from the diet and should be met by iron supplementation during the latter half of pregnancy.
[d]To a maximum of 15 mg.

This difficulty is further complicated by the ability of the body to increase iron absorption during periods of iron deficiency. Normal subjects commonly absorb ~10% and iron-deficient subjects 10–20% of dietary iron. These amounts may vary considerably, however, in different subjects consuming different diets. The following dietary allowances for iron were recommended by the U.S. National Research Council: infants 0.0–0.5 yr, 10 mg; 0.5–1.0 yr, 15 mg; 1–3 yr, 15 mg; 4–6 yr, 10mg; 7–9 yr, 10 mg; 11–18 yr, 18 mg; premenopausal women, 18 mg; menopausal women, 10 mg; and men, 10 mg (*Recommended Dietary Allowances,* 1974).

The most popular vehicle chosen for iron fortification has been white flour, although the potential for fortification of cane sugar with iron and ascorbic acid has been explored (Layrisse *et al.,* 1976). Iron enrichment of flour with 15 mg iron/lb (about 10 mg/lb in bread) was begun in the United States in 1945. This enrichment did not result in reducing the incidence of anemia in women in the United States or in England, where a similar enrichment program was initiated. This failure is due to the low availability of some of the iron compounds used for fortification. Since April 1974, an iron fortification level of 40 mg iron/lb in flour (25 mg iron/lb bread) has been recommended by the U.S. Food and Drug Administration. This move has been questioned on the grounds of efficacy and safety. According to Callender (1973), at the American recommended level of supplementation and the English level of consumption of bread, flour, biscuits, and cake, only 0.84 mg of absorbed iron per day would be contributed from these sources if meat was included at each meal, and only 0.25 mg/day if little or no meat was consumed at each meal. Thus, according to Callender, such a fortification program cannot be expected to do more than prevent some women who are marginally deficient from developing iron deficiency. With respect to the question of safety, many physicians are of the opinion that fortification at the United States level could be hazardous for patients with idiopathic hemochromatosis, Laennec's cirrhosis, or iron-loading anemias, or with unusually high bread intakes (Crosby, 1970, 1977). Swiss and Beaton (1974), in a study from Canada, concluded that an appreciable reduction in the risk of iron deficiency in menstruating women could be achieved by iron fortification of bread, without an exorbitant increase in iron intake by the other groups, but that reduction of risk of deficiency to zero in the target population by iron fortification alone would require much higher levels of fortification "than would seem either prudent or technologically feasible."

Martinez-Torres and Layrisse (1974) concluded that additional iron fortification in the United States would increase total iron absorption up to 1.1 mg in normal women and to 2.1 mg in iron-deficient women. This increase would reduce significantly the frequency of iron-deficiency anemia due to chronic menstrual blood loss.

It is clear that individual treatment programs will be required for patients with hemochromatosis, sideroblastic anemias, and other iron-loading disease states if the iron fortification program is implemented in the United States. Studies are needed to define precisely the effect of the recommended level of fortification on iron balance in subjects with marginal deficiency of iron and those who suffer from iron-loading diseases.

IRON DEFICIENCY

MANIFESTATIONS OF IRON DEFICIENCY

Iron deficiency in human adults is manifested clinically by listlessness and fatigue, palpitation on exertion, and sometimes by a sore tongue, angular stomatitis, dysphagia, and koilonchyia (Darby, 1951). In children, anorexia, depressed growth, and decreased resistance to infection are commonly observed, but the oral lesions and nail changes are rare. Inasmuch as deficiency of zinc in man is known to occur concomitantly with iron deficiency in many parts of the world, and a deficiency of zinc affects growth and gonadal functions adversely, produces esophageal and nail changes, and adversely affects resistance to infection, one may postulate that many of the so-called manifestations of iron deficiency in man may actually be a result of zinc deficiency (Prasad, 1966). Etiological factors responsible for production of zinc deficiency may also affect iron balance adversely. Further studies are thus needed to clarify and separate various tissue effects of iron and zinc deficiencies (Prasad, 1966).

Iron deficiency results in the development of hypochromic, microcytic anemia, accompanied by a normoblastic, hyperplastic bone marrow that contains little or no hemosiderin. In addition, serum iron is decreased and total iron-binding capacity is increased, and there is decreased saturation of transferrin. The presence of hypochromasia and microcytosis is not essential for diagnosis of iron-deficiency anemia because an inadequate iron supply may retard erythropoiesis for some time before these characteristics of red cells are recognized (Bainton and Finch, 1964). A plasma transferrin saturation of 10% or less implies an inadequate supply of iron to the erythroid tissue, which in time is associated with hypochromic, microcytic anemia.

Abnormalities of the gastrointestinal tract, including gastric achlorhydria and associated histological lesions consisting of varying degrees of superficial gastritis and atrophy, have long been observed in iron-deficiency anemia (Hawksley *et al.,* 1934; Lees and Rosenthal, 1958). A loss of plasma proteins into the gut has also been reported in infants with iron-deficiency anemia (Wilson, J. F., *et al.,* 1962). Gastric achlorhydria, impaired absorption of xylose and vitamin A, and steatorrhea were observed in one study in association with iron-deficiency anemia in children. Most of the abnormalities enumerated above were generally absent from children with anemia not due to iron deficiency (Underwood, 1977). In contrast, in older age groups (16–20 yr) of subjects from the Middle East who were chronically and severely iron-deficient, no evidence of malabsorption was obtained, and small-intestinal biopsy failed to reveal any significant changes (Halsted *et al.,* 1955). Thus, the effects of iron deficiency on the gastrointestinal tract are not completely well established and need further investigation.

Formerly, it was believed that anemia was the primary manifestation of iron deficiency and that other heme proteins and iron enzymes were not affected in this condition. Beutler (Beulter, 1957, 1959a,b; Beutler and Blaisdell, 1958, 1960) investigated systematically the heme enzymes in iron deficiency. In iron-deficient rats, a marked decrease in cytochrome *c* was demonstrated in the liver and kidneys, with no reduction in the catalase activity of red cells, a small reduction in cytochrome oxidase in the kidneys, but not in the heart, and a partial depletion of succinic dehydrogenase in the kidneys and heart, but not in the liver. Cytochrome *c* can be reduced to as little as half of normal concentrations in the skeletal muscles, liver, kidney, and intestinal mucosa of young iron-deficient rats, with a smaller reduction in the brain (Dallman, 1969; Dallman and Schwartz, 1965a,b; Salmon, 1962). Catalase activity appears to be very little affected in iron-deficient rats (Cusack and Brown, 1965; Srivastava *et al.,* 1965. Succinic dehydrogenase activity is reduced in the cardiac muscle of iron-deficient rats and chicks (Beutler and Blaisdell, 1958, 1960; Davis, P. N., *et al.,* 1968). The variations in degree of heme-protein depletion in different tissues in response to iron deprivation are not well understood. They are most likely related to organ function, growth rate, cell turnover, and the stability constant of iron for the enzymes in the particular tissues (Underwood, 1977). Although the changes in iron-dependent enzymes as a result of iron deficiency have been well documented, it is not clear whether these changes have any bearing on the clinical manifestations of this disorder.

The iron-deficiency anemia of human infants usually occurs between 4 and 24 months of age (Beal *et al.,* 1962; Sturgeon, 1956a,b). A depletion of iron reserves occurs during the period of rapid growth of the infant, despite the considerable "store" of iron contained in the blood at birth. The blood of the newborn child normally contains 18–19 g hemoglobin/100 ml, which, if the blood volume is taken as 300 ml, represents 180–190 mg iron. This is about 6 times the amount usually stored in the liver (McCance and Widdowson, 1951). At about 6 months of age, the average weight of the baby is 7 kg, and the blood hemoglobin level is 12 g/100 ml. It therefore contains about 280 mg iron in the form of hemoglobin at this time, of which 180–190 mg was present at birth. If this iron, plus the amount stored in the liver and absorbed from the milk, were all retained in the body, it is difficult to visualize iron deficiency arising at all. It has been shown, however, that a significant negative balance of iron occurs in infants due to an excessive fecal loss in the neonatal period (Cavell and Widdowson, 1964). This is an important cause of iron depletion, although how long such excessive fecal loss of iron continues beyond the neonatal period is not established (Underwood, 1977).

A significant increase in hemoglobin levels in infants receiving oral iron supplement has been demonstrated in a number of studies. The regular need for supplementation with medicinal iron, or with iron-fortified foods, has been stressed by several investigators (Beal *et al.,* 1962; Farquhar, 1963; Sturgeon, 1956a,b), even with infants born of nonanemic mothers who have received ample iron during pregnancy. In premature babies and in babies born of frankly anemic mothers, the hemoglobin levels and the liver iron stores may be subnormal, indicating an even greater need for iron supplementation, especially during early infancy (Underwood, 1977).

Iron-deficiency anemia is encountered frequently in adults. In adult men and postmenopausal women, the etiolgical factors are chronic blood loss due to bleeding ulcers, malignancy, or infections such as hookworm infestations. Iron-deficiency anemia is much more common in women than in men because women of fertile age are subject to additional iron losses due to menstruation, pregnancy, and lactation. The incidence or iron deficiency in women has been reported as 20–25% in different studies (Laufberger, 1937; Rybo, 1966). In economically underprivileged groups in both the developed and the developing countries, a high incidence of iron deficiency has been observed, especially during the period of active childbearing and during pregnancy (Bothwell and Finch, 1962; Mukherjee and Mukherjee, 1953). This high incidence is related to a variety of factors, including infection, heavy reliance on foods of vegetable origin in which the iron is poorly available, and excessive sweating in hot climates (Underwood, 1977).

During pregnancy, 350–400 mg iron is lost in the fetus and its adnexa. Although the absorption of iron is increased in pregnancy, this increase is not sufficient to prevent signs of iron deficiency in many women in late pregnancy. In the third trimester of pregnancy, hemoglobin levels normally fall, due partly to an increase in plasma volume and partly, in most instances, to inadequate dietary intake of iron. Supplemental iron has no effect on the hydremia of pregnancy (de Leeuw *et al.,* 1966), but can significantly increase blood hemoglobin levels (de Leeuw *et al.,* 1966; Morgan, 1961; Sturgeon, 1959; Underwood, 1977).

TREATMENT OF IRON DEFICIENCY

Most patients with iron-deficiency anemia can be treated satisfactorily with a readily soluble oral iron preparation providing the equivalent of 180–220 mg iron in three or four daily divided doses. Gastrointestinal symptoms are infrequent, but if they occur, they may be alleviated by decreasing the dosage. There is rarely any justification for the adminsitration of enteric-coated, prolonged-release, or multiple hematinic iron preparations. There are available parenteral iron preparations that have proved useful in the treatment of iron deficiency when there is malabsorption or severe gastrointestinal side effects due to oral iron administration. Parenteral iron therapy poses a higher incidence of toxic reaction. Blood transfusions are not justified in the management of chronic iron-deficiency anemia (Fairbanks *et al.,* 1971).

CLINICAL SYNDROMES ASSOCIATED WITH IRON DEFICIENCY

Iron deficiency may masquerade in various guises, and several syndromes of iron deficiency have been regarded at one time or another as clearly defined clinical entities. In some of the syndromes, there seems to be suggestive evidence of multiple nutritional deficiencies (Fairbanks *et al.,* 1971).

IRON DEFICIENCY WITHOUT ANEMIA

Since the earlier studies of Heilmeyer and Plötner (1937), several other investigators have now confirmed the existence of iron deficiency without anemia (Fielding *et al.,* 1965; Garby *et al.,* 1969a,b; Heinrich, 1968; Jacobs, A., *et al.,* 1965; Maier, 1966; McFarlane *et al.,* 1967). This stage of iron-deficiency anemia is two to three times more prevalent than iron-deficiency anemia. Many investigators believe that iron deficiency may be symptomatic before anemia develops. The usual symptoms are fatigue, headache, dizziness, irritability, and palpitations (Fairbanks *et al.,* 1971).

SIDEROPENIC DYSPHAGIA: THE PLUMMER–VINSON (PATERSON–KELLY) SYNDROME

Sideropenic dysphagia is an unusual syndrome found in association with iron deficiency. Kelly (1919) and Paterson (1919) published observations of this syndrome of dysphagia and postcricoid esophageal stricture. It occured predominantly in middle-aged women. Associated features were "dyspepsia," smooth tongue, fissures at the angles of the mouth, and anemia. A high incidence of esophageal carcinoma was noted in women of this age group, suggestive of a possible relationship to this benign esophageal lesion. Kelly regarded this condition as secondary to inflamation of the intramural autonomic plexi of the esophagus, and for treatment suggested dilatation of the stricture with the esophagoscope (Fairbanks *et al.,* 1971).

Vinson (1922), apparently unaware of these reports, reported 69 cases of "hysterical dysphagia" observed at the Mayo Clinic in 1922. Of these patients, 80% were women. Splenomegaly was noted in 12 cases. X-ray of the esophagus was normal. Vinson believed that the "secondary anemia" was due to nutritional inadequacy. Vinson gave Plummer credit for priority in describing this syndrome (Fairbanks *et al.,* 1971).

Whether iron deficiency leads to web formation or, conversely, dysphagia leads ultimately to iron deficiency cannot be completely resolved at present. However, since in the adult, a reduced iron intake probably requires decades before it leads to iron-deficiency anemia and because dysphagia has been relieved by iron therapy in some cases, it is likely that the dysphagia is the end result of long-standing iron deficiency. Both esophageal web and koilonychia, which are regarded as hallmarks of this syndrome, have been noted to occur in animals with zinc deficiency (Prasad, 1966), whereas these features are not noted as a result of iron deficiency in experimental animals. It is conceivable that in this syndrome, deficiency of both iron and zinc plays a role. This syndrome is very rarely seen in the United States at present. One cannot help but wonder whether the infrequency of this disorder in the United States at present may not reflect a better level of nutrition (Fairbanks *et al.,* 1971).

NUTRITIONAL IRON-DEFICIENCY ANEMIA IN INFANTS ASSOCIATED WITH HYPOPROTEINEMIA AND HYPOCUPREMIA

In 1956, Ulstrom and associates described four infants who presented with pallor, irritability, edema, and hepatosplenomegaly. These children manifested marked hypochromic anemia and decreased serum iron, copper, albumin, and gamma globulin levels. The children responded to transfusion or administration or iron, or both (Fairbanks *et al.,* 1971).

Subsequently, several additional cases were observed. In the majority, there had been a prolonged interval of consumption of a diet restricted entirely to milk. Edema and irritability were observed frequently, and hepatosplenomegaly was present in most cases. All patients had moderate to marked hypochromic microcytic anemia, hypoferremia, hypocupremia, hypoalbuminemia, and hypogammaglobinemia, and growth retardation was noted in more than half the patients in one series. In most cases, these manifestations were corrected by the administration of a normal diet with iron supplements; administration of iron alone corrected all features except the hypocupremia.

Hypocupremia and hypoproteinemia have not been regarded as part of the picture of iron-deficiency anemia of infants. It is believed that some factor(s) in milk may cause anemia as a result of increased gastrointestinal bleeding. Hypoproteinemia and hypocupremia may have been caused by marked gastrointestinal protein loss somehow related to milk intake. Milk itself is a poor source of iron and copper; thus, main dependence on a milk diet may have precipitated deficiency of both iron and copper in the infants. In some cases, a gastrointestinal malabsorption syndrome may have resulted in deficiency of iron, copper, and protein. They did not respond completely to the administration of iron in that hypoproteinemia and hypocupremia were not relieved, but with the addition of copper to the diet, these abnormalities were also corrected (Fairbanks *et al.*, 1971).

PICA

Pica is predominantly a disorder of children and of pregnant women. It was formerly regarded as a part of the symptom complex of chlorosis. More commonly, pica occurs in those of poor socioeconomic status. Surveys of the prevalence of pica in the southern United States revealed that in 1940, at least 25% of poor schoolchildren of rural Mississippi had recently eaten dirt or clay (Gutelius *et al.*, 1962). Of poor pregnant women of rural Mississippi, approximately 40% admitted to being habitual eaters of laundry starch, and 27% admitted habitual clay ingestion. It is also clear that pica is prevalent among infants in underdeveloped countries (Fairbanks *et al.*, 1971).

Although some observations suggested that the perversion of appetite is not relieved specifically by iron, others have indicated a curative effect of iron on this symptom.

Chronic lead poisoning may also occur in children with pica. Since the anemia of lead poisoning is usually hypochromic and microcytic in children, and since, in children with pica and chronic lead poisoning, iron deficiency commonly coexists, the presence of chronic lead poisoning may easily be overlooked. In children who exhibit pica and whose anemia fails to respond to iron therapy, the possibility of lead poisoning should be entertained (Smith, H.D., 1964; Fairbanks *et al.*, 1971).

Minnich *et al.* (1968) showed that ingestion of iron with certain clays results in markedly decreased absorption of iron. Garretson and Conrad (1967) were not able to demonstrate a similar effect from ingestion of laundry starch. The possibility that protein deficiency may have been responsible for the decreased erythropoeisis in those habitually eating laundry starch has been considered.

Clay may also affect the metabolism of other cations. Geophagia (clay-eating) is associated with an interesting syndrome of iron deficiency, hypogonadism, iron-deficiency anemia, and dwarfism (Fairbanks *et al.*, 1971; Prasad, 1966). This syndrome has been attributed to a combined deficiency of iron and zinc. Potassium may also be adsorbed to clay, and weakness and myalgia due to hypokalemia were observed in a young woman who consumed at least three handfuls of clay daily (Mengel *et al.*, 1964). She had severe neurological signs of potassium depletion and a severe iron-deficiency anemia. The severe weakness was alleviated by administration of potassium, and the anemia responded to iron-dextran. The compulsion to eat clay was also abated.

Reynolds *et al.* (1968) found habitual ingestion of ice to be the most common variant of pica, manifested by 23 in 38 consecutive adults with iron-deficiency anemia, and confirmed the curative effect of iron therapy. Coltman (1969) showed that very small doses of iron relieve compulsive ice-eating (pagophagia) long before there is any significant change in hemoglobin concentration. It was speculated that the prompt relief of pagophagia by iron therapy might reflect a change in the enzyme iron compartment (Fairbanks *et al.*, 1971).

SYNDROME OF DWARFISM, ANEMIA, AND HYPOGONADISM (COMBINED WITH IRON AND ZINC DEFICIENCY)

Although growth disturbances have been noted in infants with iron-deficiency anemia (Schubert and Lahey, 1959) these disturbances have been relatively mild and have rarely been recognized in older children. Reimann (1955) catalogued an impressive group of congenital anomalies seen in Turkish patients with severe hypochromic microcytic anemias. Reimann attributed these aberrations primarily to iron deficiency in pregnancy, resulting in severe fetal iron deficits. Among these disorders were mongolism, dental deformities and oral occlusion, deformities of the external ear, syndactyly, clubfoot, and pigmentary disturbance. In the absence of any convincing evidence of an etiological relationship, it seems likely that in most of these cases the iron-deficiency anemia was coincidental. Furthermore, although iron-deficiency anemia of pregnancy is common in the United States, congenital anomalies are not recognized as a consequence of this deficiency. This question has also been studied in female rats kept on iron-deficient diets from birth to gestation (O'Dell *et al.*, 1961). Although offspring were anemic, and most were nonviable, congenital anomalies were not observed. Reimann described one group that deserves further comment: these patients were characterized by retardation of longitudinal growth, asynchronism of developmental and chronological ages, delayed epiphyseal maturation, and hypogonadism. This syndrome was described in detail in young adults from Iran by Prasad *et al.* (1961), and in subsequent studies from Egypt, it was established that the growth retardation and hypogonadism were related to a deficiency of zinc, whereas the anemia was related to iron deficiency (see Chapter 10). Since a deficiency of zinc in pregnant rats results in congenital malformation in fetuses, one may suggest that the congenital anomalies as observed in Turkey by Reimann may indeed have been due to deficiency of zinc in pregnant mothers.

OTHER MISCELLANEOUS DISORDERS ASSOCIATED WITH IRON DEFICIENCY

Iron deficiency may give rise on rare occasions to papilledema as well as other neurological phenomena. These manifestations are usually accompanied by increased cerebrospinal fluid pressure. The mechanism of this phenomenon is obscure. Since iron deficiency results in abnormalities of intracellular enzymes, it may be that increase in intracranial pressure is related to some subtle changes in brain metabolism. If this is true, it is strange that the phenomenon of papilledema affects those with iron-deficiency anemia only rarely, even when the anemia is severe (Fairbanks *et al.,* 1971).

Combined deficiency of iron and folic acid is a common phenomenon, especially in pregnancy. Deficiency of both iron and folic acid may develop after subtotal gastrectomy. In the anemia of protein malnutrition, iron and folic acid deficiencies also occur together frequently.

Some evidence suggests that in those conditions in which iron and folic acid deficiencies are present concomitantly, the folic acid deficiency may not be due to dietary deprivation, but may be a secondary manifestation of iron deficiency. In six male patients with severe iron-deficiency anemia due to hookworm infestation, low serum folate concentration and megaloblastic erythropoiesis were demonstrated (Velez *et al.,* 1966). These abnormalities were corrected by iron therapy during a time in which the patients consumed a diet low in folic acid. On the other hand, in pregnancy at least, the decrease in serum folate concentration is not secondary to iron deficiency. Clearly, more studies are needed to resolve the question whether iron deficiency *per se* may be responsible for disturbance of folic acid metabolism (Fairbanks *et al.,* 1971).

Development of menorrhagia in iron-deficiency anemia leading to a perpetuating cycle of increasingly severe uterine blood loss and increasingly severe anemia has been reported (Haden, 1932; Wintrobe and Beebe, 1933). In 1957, C. Harris (1957) reported a few cases that seemed to support this observation, and suggested that this vicious cycle could be interrupted by the administration of iron. These reports, however, were based on the patient's subjective evaluation of menstrual bleeding, and in a study reported by A. Jacobs and Butler (1965) in which ^{51}Cr-labeled erythrocytes were used to measure blood loss, more menstrual blood loss was documented in iron-sufficient subjects.

In megaloblastic anemias (pernicious anemia, malabsorption syndrome), there is sometimes a double population of cells, one hypochromic microcytic and the other macrocytic. These patients respond to B_{12} or folic acid initially, but soon the hemoglobin reaches a plateau, and then the hypochromic microcytic picture predominates. At this stage, a second response to administration of iron is observed. This phenomenon has been referred to as "dimorphic anemia."

IRON-DEFICIENCY ANEMIA WITH REGIONAL OR SYSTEMIC IRON OVERLOAD: CONGENITAL ATRANSFERRINEMIA

In 1961, Heilmeyer *et al.* (1961) described a 7-year-old girl with severe hypochromic microcytic anemia who had required frequent transfusions since the age of 3 months. The liver and spleen were enlarged, and biopsy of the liver revealed marked hemosiderosis and fibrosis. Bone marrow aspiration revealed erythroid hyperplasia, and only a trace of iron was present. Serum iron and total iron-binding capacity were decreased. By immunoelectrophoresis, transferrin was found to be absent in the plasma. At autopsy, hemosiderosis affecting the myocardium, liver, spleen, kidneys, and pancreas was observed. Decreased plasma transferrin levels were observed in both parents, thus suggesting that in this case, congenital atransferremia represented the homozygous state (Fairbanks *et al.,* 1971). A similar case was reported by Cáp and associates (1968). The propositus was 11 months of age and had a severe hypochromic anemia and low serum iron, and transferrin was shown to be absent in the plasma (Fairbanks *et al.,* 1971).

The paradoxical accumulation of iron in the liver, spleen, kidneys, heart, and pancreas with absence of iron in the bone marrow is perplexing. Perhaps, in the absence of the normal major mechanism for transport of iron to the normoblast, rhopheocytosis becomes the major mechanism of acquisition of iron by the normoblast. Rhopheocytosis might then deplete the bone marrow reticuloendothelial cells of iron while the reticuloendothelial cells of other organs remain saturated with hemosiderin (Fairbanks *et al.,* 1971).

CONGENITAL IRON-DEFICIENCY ANEMIA WITH IRON OVERLOAD OF LIVER AND SPLEEN AND HYPERFERREMIA

Two children, siblings, with an unusual form of congenital hypochromic microcytic anemia were reported by Shahidi and co-workers (Shahidi, 1964; Shahidi *et al.,* 1964). This disorder resembled congenital atransferremia in that there was failure of delivery of iron to the developing normoblast and absence of iron in the bone marrow, despite hemosiderosis of the liver. In these cases, however, the serum iron concentration was increased (170–250 μg/100 ml), and the total iron-binding capacity was in the range of 300–450 μg/100 ml. Transferrin was present in a normal amount. It seems likely that in this disorder, the normal transfer of iron from transferrin to the normoblast membrane may have been defective.

IDIOPATHIC PULMONARY HEMOSIDEROSIS

In this disorder, there is marked hemosiderosis of the lungs, in combination with iron-deficiency anemia. It is predominantly a disease of children, only about one patient in five being more than 16 years old. In children, the disease has no predilection for sex, but two thirds of adults with idiopathic pulmonary hemosiderosis have been males (Fairbanks *et al.,* 1971).

The cause of this disorder is unknown. Allergy to an unspecified inhaled substance, a form of autoimmune disease, or an abnormal formation of the pulmonary alveolar epithelium or elastic fibers are some of the possibilities considered by various investigators to account for this unusual manifestation. Clinical manifestations include cough, failure to gain weight, fatigue, and pallor. Hemoptysis may occur. As the disease progresses, dyspnea and clubbing of the fingers may be observed. In a small number of cases, pulmonary hypertension has been noted. Physical examination may reveal fine rales over both lungs and dullness to percussion over the lower lobes. The liver and spleen may be palpable. Cervical lymphadenopathy may be present.

The course of the disease is variable. Survival from onset may be as short as 2 weeks to as long as many years. Death may be from cardiac decompensation or from pulmonary hemmorrhage. Myocarditis has been observed rarely (Kennedy *et al.,* 1966; Murphy, 1965).

X ray of the chest early in the course of the disease shows patchy, evanescent pulmonary infiltrates. As the disease progresses, miliary stippling of the lung and fine perihilar fibrosis appear, and hilar lymph nodes may be enlarged.

Peripheral blood shows anisocytosis, poikilocytosis, microcytosis, and hypochromia. Eosinophilia may be seen in some cases. Reticulocytes may be increased in number. The serum bilirubin concentration and urobilinogen excretion may be increased due to increased heme catabolism. Scintigraphic studies have shown a marked increase in pulmonary accumulation of ^{59}Fe at 34 days after infection (DeGowin *et al.,* 1968). Urinalysis shows microscopic hematuria, and stools may be positive for occult blood.

A stain of sputum for hemosiderin shows iron-laden macrophages. Pulmonary function tests reveal a decrease in vital capacity, maximum breathing capacity, imparied oxygen diffusion, and low arterial oxygen saturation.

Histologically, the lungs show degeneration, hyperplasia, and desquamation of the epithelial cells of pulmonary alveoli; capillary proliferation and dilatation; vasculitis; thrombosis and embolism; interstitial fibrosis; degeneration of alveolar elastic fibers; sclerosis of pulmonary arteries and veins; and muscular hypertrophy of bronchial arteries. Hyaline membranes may form. Hemosiderosis affects the interstitial phagocytic cells. Electron-microscopic studies have shown changes in the alveolocapillary membrane, consisting of splitting and broadening of the membrane and increased formation of reticular and elastic fibers (Bässler, 1961). Although the bone marrow iron reserve seems to be depleted, hemosiderosis of the spleen and liver has been reported in some cases. In some cases, cardiac and hepatic iron content may be normal (Soergel and Sommers, 1962). Changes in the renal glomeruli have also been observed, Histological studies of pulmonary and renal tissues, after staining with fluorescent anti-immunoglobulin G antibody, have shown fluorescence of basement membranes of both renal glomeruli and alveolar capillaries (Beirne *et al.,* 1968; Fairbanks *et al.,* 1971).

There is no satisfactory therapy available at present for this disease. Iron-deficiency anemia should be treated with oral iron. Adrenocortical steroid therapy seems to have been of benefit in some cases (Matsaniotis *et al.,* 1968). Azathioprine, a purine antimetabolite, was used in one case with good results (Steiner and Nabrady, 1965; Fairbanks *et al.,* 1971).

GOODPASTURE'S SYNDROME

In this disease, glomerulonephritis and recurrent pulmonary hemorrhage appear to be associated (Goodpasture, 1919). Primarily young adult males are affected. Pulmonary infiltrate and severe iron-deficiency anemia occur in this disorder, as in idiopathic pulmonary hemosiderosis. Progressive glomerulonephritis tends to dominate the clinical syndrome. A few patients have exhibited the nephrotic syndrome. Azotemia appears early and commonly leads to death from uremia within a few weeks to a few years (Bloom *et al.,* 1965; MacGregor *et al.,* 1960; Soergel and Sommers, 1962; Weiss *et al.,* 1968). Adrenocortical steroid therapy seems to have been of benefit in some cases. Azathioprine administration was without benefit in one case (Heiner *et al.,* 1962). Hemodialysis was beneficial in one case, and in another, complete recovery was noted (Freeman *et al.,* 1966; Munro *et al.,* 1967). In one case, bilateral nephrectomy followed by kidney transplant and azathioprine immunosuppressive therapy led to a remission of the pulmonary manifestations (Maddock *et al.,* 1967; Fairbanks *et al.,* 1971).

REFRACTORY HYPOCHROMIC ANEMIA ASSOCIATED WITH BENIGN LYMPHOID–PLASMACYTIC TUMORS AND HYPERGLOBULINEMIA

An unusual syndrome has been described in three children who manifested chronic anemia accompanied by hepatosplenomegaly (in two cases), hyperglobulinemia, and the presence of a solitary lymphoid mass. In each case, the anemia was hypochromic and microcytic. Serum iron and total iron-binding capacity were decreased. The hyperglobulinemia was of the polyclonal type, and in one case, predominantly an increase in α_2-globulin was present. Bone marrow examination showed plasmacytosis and erythroid hypoplasia in one case (Lüthi *et al.,* 1968), plasmacytosis and moderate erythroid hypoplasia in the second (Lee, S. L., *et al.,* 1965), and a normal picture in the third (Neerhout *et al.,* 1969). Iron was decreased or absent in marrow aspirate in two subjects, but was increased in one (Lee, S. L., *et al.,* 1965; Lüthi *et al.,* 1968). Liver biopsy in one case revealed marked hemosiderosis (Lüthi *et al.,* 1968). Mediastinal mass on X ray was noted in one case. The presence of mesenteric tumors was noted in two cases. Microscopically, these tumors were pleomorphic, containing lymphocytes, fibroblasts, reticulum cells, and in some areas, marked plasma cell infiltrates. Hemosiderosis of the neoplasm was observed in two cases in which decreased marrow iron content was observed (Fairbanks *et al.,* 1971).

In each of these cases, all manifestations of this syndrome subsided after surgical removal of the tumor. The mechanism by which this syndrome developed remains obscure. However, diversion of iron from plasma and storage pools into the neoplasm may have played a role in two of these patients (Fairbanks *et al.,* 1971).

ACUTE IRON POISONING

Acute iron poisoning in children may follow the ingestion of only a small number of tablets of an iron preparation. It is characterized by vomiting, gastrointestinal hemorrhage, metabolic acidosis, coma and other neurological changes. Therapy of iron poisoning consists of prompt induction of emesis at home, followed by gastric lavage in the hospital. Neutral or mildly basic solutions of sodium phosphate or sodium bicarbonate should be used for lavage. Desferoxamine should be instilled into the stomach and also should be given by the intramuscular route or, if the patient is hypotensive, by slow intravenous infusion. Because early apparent recovery may be followed in several hours or even a few days by rapid deterioration, children being treated for acute iron poisoning should be closely observed for at least 3 days. Late sequelae such as gastric strictures and pyloric stenosis may occur, but are infrequent (Fairbanks *et al.,* 1971).

SIDEROBLASTIC ANEMIAS

The sideroblastic anemias constitute a heterogenous group of disorders. Hyperferremia, a dimorphic or predominantly microcytic hypochromic peripheral blood picture, erythroid hyperplasia with numerous ringed sideroblasts (nonferritin-iron-loaded mitochondria), an increased plasma iron turnover, and ineffective erythropoiesis are some of the characteristic features of these disorders. Frequently, the cause and pathogenesis remain unknown.

A distinction between reticulated siderocytes as seen in the blood of some patients with hemolytic anemia and after splenectomy and nonreticulated siderocytes observed in the peripheral circulation due to a defect in heme synthesis as seen in sideroblastic anemias must be made (Kurth *et al.,* 1969; Deiss and Cartwright, 1970). The granules in reticulated siderocytes consist of cytoplasmic aggregates of ferritin, whereas in the case of nonreticulated siderocytes, the granules consist of nonferritin iron located within the mitochrondria.

Pyridoxine-responsive anemia as originally described by J. W. Harris *et al.* (1956) is also classified under sideroblastic anemias. The clinical features common to these cases are microcytic hypochromic anemia, hyperferremia, hemosiderosis, and a partial or complete response of the anemia to the continued administration of relatively large amounts of pyridoxine despite lack of evidences of a dietary deficiency of pyridoxine in such cases (Raab *et al.,* 1961).

During the past decade, many reports describing sideroblastic anemias have appeared, and several classifications have been proposed (Mollin, 1965; Heilmeyer, 1966; Hines and Grasso, 1970). A practical classification of sideroblastic anemias is as follows (Fairbanks *et al.,* 1971):

Primary
1. Hereditary sideroblastic anemia
2. Acquired idiopathic sideroblastic anemia

Secondary
1. Sideroblastic anemia due to exogenous chemical agents
2. Dietary deficiencies
3. Sideroblastic anemia accompanying systemic diseases

ETIOLOGY

Hereditary Sideroblastic Anemia

A hereditary sideroblastic anemia has been reported by several investigators. In 1945, Cooley (1945) described an apparently sexlinked hypochromic anemia affecting 19 of 29 males in five generations of a single kindred. Rundles and Falls (1946) described two large Michigan kindred with "hereditary (sex-linked?) hypochromic anemia" (Fairbanks *et al.*, 1971).

In 1957, Heilmeyer *et al.* (1957) reported an iron-loading hypochromic anemia with ringed sideroblasts in the bone marrow in identical twin brothers. Their mother and sister had minimal hematological changes, which suggested that they were also affected but to a lesser degree. These workers coined the term "sideroachrestic" anemia and proposed a defect in heme synthesis as the cause of this disorder. The following year, Lukl *et al.* (1958) described five males in one German kinship affected by "hereditary leptocyte anemia." The bone marrow findings reported by these workers were consistent with those described later in hereditary sideroblastic anemia. The inheritance was believed to be sex-linked recessive. Minor erythrocyte abnormalities were seen in the heterozygous women (Fairbanks *et al.*, 1971).

Large English kindreds with this disorder were reported by Losowsky and Hall (1965) and by Elves and co-workers (Bourne *et al.*, 1965; Elves *et al.*, 1966). In these families, the inheritance was well manifested, conforming to the pattern of an X-chromosomelinked gene. Prasad *et al.*, (1968) reported sex-linked hereditary sideroblastic anemia in a large and complex American Negro family. Detailed clinical and genetic studies were performed in this family, which segregated for sex-linked sideroblastic anemia and glucose-6-phosphate dehydrogenase (G-6-PD) deficiency. Males affected with sideroblastic anemia had growth retardation, hypochromic microcytic anemia, elevated serum iron, decreased unsaturated iron-binding capacity, increased ^{59}Fe clearance, low ^{59}Fe incorporation into erythrocytes, normal erythrocyte survival (^{51}Cr), normal hemoglobin electrophoretic pattern, erythroblastic hyperplasia of marrow with increased iron, and marked increase in marrow sideroblasts, particularly ringed sideroblasts. Perinuclear deposition of ferric aggregates was demonstrated to be intramitochondrial by electron microscopy. Female carriers of the sideroblastic gene were normal, but exhibited a dimorphic population of erythrocytes including normocytic and microcytic cells. The bone marrow studies in the female (mother) showed ringed marrow sideroblasts.

Studies of G-6-PD involved the methemoglobin elution test for G-6-PD activity of individual erythrocytes, quantitative G-6-PD assay, and electrophoresis. In the pedigree, linkage information was obtained from a doubly heterozygous woman, four of her sons, and five of her daughters. Three sons were doubly affected, and one was normal. One daughter appeared to be recombinant. The genes appeared to be linked in the coupling phase in the mother. The maximum likelihood estimate of the recombination value was 0.14 (Prasad *et al.*, 1968).

By means of Price–Jones curves, the microcytic red cells in peripheral blood were quantitated in female carriers. The sideroblast count in the bone marrow in the mother corresponded closely to the percentage of microcytic cells in peripheral blood. This example is the second in which the cellular expression of a sex-linked trait has been documented in the human red cells, the first one being G-6-PD deficiency. The co-existence of the two genes in doubly heterozygous females made it possible to study correlations in cell counts; these studies showed a strong positive correlation except in the probably recombinant, in which a reciprocal relation held that indicated that X-inactivation was at least regional, rather than locus by locus (Prasad *et al.*, 1968).

The most common hereditary sideroblastic anemia is both X-linked and pyridoxine-responsive (Bishop and Bethell, 1959; Horrigan and Harris, 1964; Prasad *et al.*, 1968; Vogler and Mingioli, 1965). In certain families, however, an X-linked disorder has been observed that is not responsive to pyridoxine (Lee, G. R., *et al.*, 1968; Weatherall *et al.*, 1970). In another study, the mode of inheritance of pyridoxine-responsive anemia was believed to be autosomal (Cotton and Harris, 1962). On the basis of these reports, Kushner *et al.* (1971) subclassified the hereditary type of sideroblastic anemia into X-linked and autosomal types. Obviously, many more families must be studied in the future to settle the mode of inheritance of the hereditary type of sideroblastic anemia.

Acquired Idiopathic Sideroblastic Anemia

Acquired idiopathic sideroblastic anemia is characterized by chronic anemia and ringed sideroblasts in the bone marrow. There is a lack of evidence for a congenital or hereditary disorder or other etiological factors such as inflammatory or neoplastic disease, nutritional deficiency, or exposure to drugs or toxins known to produce sideroblastic anemia.

Chromosomal changes have been reported in some cases of acquired sideroblastic anemia. These changes have consisted of aneuploidy of chromosomes of the C and G groups (Dameshek, 1965). Because similar changes are often found in acute leukemia, it seems probable that at least some cases of acquired sideroblastic anemia show a common etiological mechanism with acute granulocytic leukemia. Some investigators believe that the distinction between acquired sideroblastic anemia and erythroleukemia is more semantic than real (Dameshek, 1965). On the other hand, we and others have followed several cases of acquired sideroblastic anemia for many years without observing any transition to erythroleukemia. Kushner *et al.* (1971) reported that only 1 patient out of 17 cases of idiopathic sideroblastic anemia had acute myelogenous leukemia as a terminal event. They also surveyed the literature and found 3 examples of acute leukemia out of 61 reported cases of idiopathic refractory sideroblastic anemia. Thus, neoplastic etiology of this disorder does not appear very likely. It has been hypothesized that idiopathic sideroblastic anemia may be a result of a mutation in somatic tissues, in this case the bone marrow, as distinguished from germ tissue (Kushner *et al.,* 1971). Such a mechanism could lead to a proliferating clone of cells that is genetically different from other cell clones in the same individual. Whether or not somatic mutation occurs in man is not known.

We had an elderly white patient who presented as a typical example of primary acquired sideroblastic anemia in 1965 (Tranchida *et al.,* 1973). Three years later, the peripheral blood smear revealed the presence of atypical and immature lymphocytes. Two small palpable lymph nodes were noted in the right axilla, and a possibly enlarged spleen was visualized on intravenous pyelogram in 1969; however, a biopsy specimen of the lymph node failed to show any evidence for malignant lymphoma. In 1970, a monoclonal gammopathy, immunoglobulin G (IgG), subclass G_1, kappa, Gm (afb) and InV (1−) was documented. At that time, the presence of kappa light chain in urine was also noted. The patient died of bronchopneumonia in February 1971. Autopsy revealed malignant lymphoma, poorly differentiated type, involving the lymph nodes and spleen. This unusual development of malignant lymphoma in a patient with primary acquired sideroblastic anemia has not been recorded previously, to the best of our knowledge. Whether or not primary acquired sideroblastic anemia represents a prelymphoplasmaproliferative or other premalignant blood disorder can be settled only by longitudinal studies in a large number of such patients.

Exogenous Chemicals

The ingestion of chemicals that interfere with heme synthesis (e.g., isonicotinic acid hydrazide, pyrazinamide, cycloserine, and lead salts) has led to the development of sideroblastic anemia. Chloramphenicol has also been reported to cause sideroblastic anemia, although this drug is not known to act as a pyridoxine antagonist. Dacie and Mollin (1966) observed sideroblastic anemia in patients taking acetophenetidin (phenacetin) after subtotal gastrectomy (Fairbanks *et al.,* 1971).

Dietary Deficiencies

Dogs fed a pyridoxine-free diet developed a hypochromic sideroblastic anemia (Harris, E. B., *et al.*, 1965). In one human infant given pyridoxine-deficient formula, severe hypochromic microcytic anemia developed (Synderman *et al.*, 1953). In adults, however, pyridoxine deficiency alone has not been reported as the cause of sideroblastic anemia, although administration of desoxypyridoxine (pyridoxine antimetabolite) has resulted in anemia, glossitis, dermatitis, and neurological abnormalities (Vilter *et al.*, 1953). MacGibbon and Mollin (1965) observed a few cases in which combined deficiency of pyridoxine and either vitamin B_{12} or folic acid resulted in sideroblastic anemia. Sideroblastic anemia was reported in patients with chronic alcoholism (Hines, 1969). These patients also had folic acid deficiency, and possibly may have had dietary deficiency of pyridoxine as well. The anemia and sideroblastic appearance of the bone marrow reverted to normal after abstinence from alcohol (Fairbanks *et al.*, 1971).

Sideroblastic Anemia Accompanying Systemic Diseases

Several instances have been reported in which rheumatoid arthritis, other collagen diseases, myxedema, multiple myeloma, metastatic malignancy, leukemia, or polycythemia vera was associated with sideroblastic anemia (Dacie and Mollin, 1966; Heilmeyer, 1966; MacGibbon and Mollin, 1965). It seems probable that in the majority, the anemia was secondary to systemic disease, although the possibility exists that some may have represented the chance occurrence of two independent disorders (Fairbanks *et al.*, 1971).

BIOCHEMICAL CHANGES

The possibility that there may be abnormalities in heme synthesis in sideroblastic anemias was originally proposed by Heilmeyer *et al.* (1957). Subsequent studies have shown that such abnormalities do occur in at least some of the sideroblastic anemias.

In some cases of hereditary sideroblastic anemia, an increase in free erythrocyte coproporphyrin and uroporphyrin has been observed (Gajdos, 1966). The free erythrocyte protoporphyrin is decreased in these cases, suggesting a defect in the coproporphyrinogen oxidase activity (see Fig. 6). In a few cases, conversion of glycine to heme has been found to be impaired, and a defect of ALA-synthetase (ALA-S) has been postulated (Bottomley, 1977).

In the cases of idiopathic sideroblastic anemia, the only consistent finding in the mature erythrocyte has been a mild to moderate increase in the free erythrocyte protoporphyrin level, suggesting inhibition of the ferrochelatase activity (Bottomley, 1977). In five cases of acquired sideroblastic anemia, Bousser *et al.* (1967) showed impaired incorporation of glycine[^{14}C] into heme in erythroblasts. Vogler and Mingioli (1965, 1968) demonstrated, in reticulocytes, decreased formation of heme from ^{14}C-labeled glycine but normal formation of heme from ^{14}C-labeled ALA in one patient with acquired sideroblastic anemia. Thus, a decrease in the activity of ALA-S in their patient was a possible factor accounting for defective heme synthesis. In another case of acquired sideroblastic anemia with dermal photosensitivity, Rothstein *et al.* (1969) showed decreased formation of heme in reticulocytes incubated with ^{59}Fe-labeled ferric chloride and protoporphyrin. These workers postulated a decreased activity of ferrochelatase as a mechanism accounting for their observation. Another possibility considered was that the decrease in the activity of heme synthetase may have been due to a deficiency of a cofactor because the activities of mixtures of their patient's blood and normal blood were greater than would be predicted from summation of the activities of the unmixed samples (Fairbanks *et al.,* 1971).

Vavra and Poff (1967) found, in erythrocytes or hemolysates of 10 patients with acquired idiopathic sideroblastic anemia, no impairment of heme synthesis on incubation with isotopically labeled glycine, ALA, protoporphyrin, or porphobilinogen. Incubation of bone marrow hemolysates with ALA also showed normal activity of ALA-dehydratas (ALA-D) and heme synthetase.

Thus, defects in heme synthesis have not been demonstrated consistently in these disorders. Such abnormalities as have been reported may even be secondary manifestations. In this regard, it is worth noting that depression of heme synthesis has also been reported in thalassemia (Gajdos, 1966; Vavra *et al.,* 1964). In thalassemia, however, the decreased heme synthesis may be secondary to a decreased rate of synthesis of globin chains.

Bishop and Bethell (1959) suggested that an excessive accumulation of iron might in itself inhibit heme synthesis. Excess Fe(III) may inhibit ALA synthesis *in vitro,* but has no effect on ferrochelatase, although phlebotomy in one patient allegedly showed improvement in ferrochelatase activity.

The variable disturbances in specific steps of heme biosynthesis observed in patients with idiopathic sideroblastic anemia may account for the heterogenous picture seen clinically. Enhanced iron absorbtion and altered iron metabolism often dominates the clinical picture. Control of excess body iron accumulation should prove worthwhile in the management of such cases.

Isoniazide, cycloserine, and chloramphenicol are known to cause sideroblastic anemia. Antituberculous drugs decrease the availability of pyridoxal phosphate, which is required for an early step in heme synthesis. Chloramphenicol inhibits RNA synthesis in the bone marrow and inhibits mitochondrial protein (cytochrome and cytochrome oxidase) synthesis. These effects may secondarily affect the ALA-synthesis activity adversely, thus ultimately decreasing heme synthesis.

Lead toxicity is known to affect heme synthesis adversely and thus cause sideroblastic anemia. Several enzymes in the heme-synthesis pathway are affected adversely. Lead inhibits primarily ALA-dehydratase (a zinc-metalloenzyme). Ferrochelatase, uroporphyrinogen-synthetase, ALA-A, and coproporphyrinogen-oxidase are also affected adversely due to lead exposure (Dressel and Falk, 1956; Lichtman and Feldman, 1963; Goldberg, A., *et al.,* 1956). In addition to its effect on heme synthesis, lead may impair erythroid proliferation and affect erythrocyte membrane adversely.

Sideroblastic anemia due to excess alcohol exposure has been reported to occur. Alcohol affects adversely the activities of ferrochelatase and ALA-D. It has been suggested that the adverse effect of alcohol on ALA-D (zinc enzyme) may be due to hyperzincuria, which is observed in chronic alcoholics.

The availability of pyridoxal phosphate (PLP) is decreased due to excess alcohol intake. Impaired phosphorylation of pyroxidine due to a decreased activity of PLP-kinase in alcoholic subjects was observed by Hines (1975). Lumeng and Li (1974), however, found normal activity of PLP-kinase in erythrocytes, although an accelerated degradation of PLP by acetaldehyde-stimulated erythrocyte phosphatase was observed in alcoholic subjects. It was hypothesized that PLP availability for erythropoietic tissue may have been reduced inasmuch as the liver utilization of PLP appears to be enhanced in alcoholics. Chillar *et al.* (1976) also reported a normal PLP-kinase activity in red cells of sideroblastic anemia patients. Thus, whether or not a decreased activity of PLP-kinase has any role to play in the pathogenesis of sideroblastic anemia remains to be settled.

CLINICAL FEATURES

In hereditary sideroblastic anemia, pallor is present from early childhood, although in some patients, the pallor is mild and overlooked until they are adults. Splenomegaly is usually present.

Patients with idiopathic acquired sideroblastic anemia are usually middle-aged or elderly adults. There is no sex predominance. In these patients, there is pallor but no icterus. The spleen is usually not palpable. The anemia may be slight, moderate, or severe. It is usually normochromic. There is no reticulocytosis.

When the sideroblastic anemia is an epiphenomenon of malignancy, rheumatoid arthritis, or other systemic disorders, the manifestations of the primary disease will dominate the clinical picture. Similarly, the clinical manifestations of chronic lead poisoning are often severe and disabling.

Pyrodoxine-responsive anemia was first reported by J. W. Harris *et al.* (1956) in a young male with a hypochromic microcytic anemia. In subsequent reports (Raab *et al.,* 1961; Roath *et al.,* 1964; Spitzer *et al.,* 1966; Verloop *et al.,* 1964; Vuylsteke *et al.,* 1961), there has been a strong predominance of males. A few patients have had glossitis, peripheral neuropathies, and leg cramps. The anemia has been normochromic and normocytic in more than half the cases, but may be hypochromic and microcytic or macrocytic.

PATHOLOGY

Characteristic changes are seen in the peripheral blood and bone marrow. These changes include hypochromic and microcytic anemia in the hereditary type, whereas in the acquired variety, the anemia may be hypochromic, normochromic, normocytic, or macrocytic. Erythrocytes may show hypochromia, anisocytosis, elliptocytosis, poikilocytosis, target cells, and occasional Pappenheimer bodies. Nucleated erythrocytes may be noted in the peripheral blood. A "dimorphic" appearance, with both normal erythrocytes and bizarre, hypochromic erythrocytes, may be seen in the peripheral blood. This mixed pattern is likely to be found in non-anemic, heterozygous female carriers of the gene for hereditary sideroblastic anemia. In other types of sideroblastic anemias, red cell indices may be normal or hypochromic.

Occasionally, there is a shift to the left in the leukocyte differential count. Usually, leukocytes and platelets are normal. Reticulocytes are usually normal in number.

The bone marrow is invariably hyperplastic and displays marked erythroid hyperplasia. There is often some degree of megaloblastic change in erythroid series. Iron stain displays numerous large cytoplasmic granules in normoblasts. The siderotic granules represent mitochondria distended with ferruginous micelles. Normoblasts containing iron granules distributed around the nucleus are called "ringed sideroblasts" and constitute approximately 50–80% of the normblasts in marrow aspirates from patients with sideroblastic anemias.

Hayhoe and Quaglino (Hayhoe and Quaglino, 1960; Quaglino and Hayhoe, 1960) showed that in acute or chronic erythroleukemia accompanied by sideroblastic erythropoiesis, there is marked staining of normoblast cytoplasm by the periodic acid–Schiff (PAS) method. By contrast, in nonerythroleukemic sideroblastic anemias, there is little or no PAS staining or normoblasts (Fairbanks *et al.,* 1971).

Hemosiderosis commonly affects the liver, spleen, lymph nodes, bone marrow, heart, pancreas, thyroid, and adrenal gland. In the liver, hemosiderin deposits occur predominantly in the parenchymal cells and may be accompanied by diffuse fibrotic change seen in hemochromatosis (Byrd and Cooper, 1961; Hines and Harris, 1964; Horrigan and Harris, 1964; Lukl *et al.,* 1958; Vuylsteke *et al.,* 1961).

The serum iron is usually increased, and transferrin is 70–100% saturated. Some investigators have reported low values for cholesterol and total serum lipids in patients with pyridoxine-responsive anemia. The glucose tolerance test (GTT) may be of the diabetic type if iron loading has been severe and prolonged.

Free erythrocyte protoporphyrin and coproporphyrin are normal to increased (Dacie *et al.,* 1959; Heilmeyer, 1966; Lee, G. R., *et al.,* 1966). In one case of idiopathic acquired sideroblastic anemia with dermal photosensitivity, the free erythrocyte protoporphyrin was increased (Rothstein *et al.,* 1969). Serum folate levels are usually low (Hines and Grasso, 1970; MacGibbon and Mollin, 1965). The low serum folate may be due to a relative deficiency of folic acid as a result of increased but ineffective erythropoiesis. In some cases, it is probably due to dietary deficiency such as is seen in alcoholics.

There may be a slight to moderate shortening of erythrocyte survival as measured by the ^{51}Cr technique in some cases (Bickers *et al.,* 1962; Byrd and Cooper, 1961; Horrigan and Harris, 1964; Verloop and Rademaker, 1960; Vuylsteke *et al.,* 1961). In other subjects, the red cell life span is normal. Ferrokinetic studies may disclose a more rapid than normal plasma iron turnover and an increased rate of plasma iron clearance. Ineffective erythropoiesis has been demonstrated in many cases and should be considered characteristic of this group of disorders (Barry, W. E., and Day, 1964; Byrd and Cooper, 1961; Crosby and Sheehy, 1960; Heilmeyer *et al.,* 1957; Horrigan and Harris, 1964; Lee, G. R., *et al.,* 1966; Roath *et al.,* 1964; Verloop and Rademaker, 1960; Vuylsteke *et al.,* 1961). Iron absorbtion as measured by the use of oral ^{59}Fe-labeled ferrous ascorbate greatly exceeds that in normal subjects (Fairbanks *et al.,* 1971).

THERAPEUTIC TEST

Administration of pyridoxine, at least 100 mg daily, orally or parenterally, results in reticulocytosis and partial correction of the anemia in many persons with sporadic or hereditary hypochromic iron-loading anemia. In some cases, hemoglobin may return to normal levels following pyridoxine therapy for several months. In the majority, however, completely normal hemoglobin levels have not been attained despite prolonged therapy. This diagnostic aid defines pyridoxine-responsive anemia and appears to distinguish it from other sideroblastic anemias (Fairbanks *et al.,* 1971).

TREATMENT

The treatment is unsatisfactory. The underlying disease process, if identified, must be treated. Pyridoxine should be administered as a therapeutic trial to all patients with sideroblastic anemia of obscure cause. The dose required is 100–200 mg daily, orally, in divided doses.

Patients who fail to respond to pyridoxine administration or whose response is minimal should, in addition, receive folic acid in a dose of about 100 mg daily by mouth. One should be certain that pernicious anemia has been ruled out before using large doses of folic acid.

In view of the excessive deposition of iron in the tissues of patients with sideroblastic anemias and the possible hazard of hemochromatosis, a program of therapeutic phlebotomy may be justified in some patients.

COURSE AND PROGNOSIS

For some patients, the course is lifelong with little handicap. This is often true of patients with hereditary sideroblastic anemia, although these patients are subject to the complications of hemochromatosis. In the acquired variety, the course of the disease is often prolonged, and many such patients die of causes unrelated to their anemia (Fairbanks *et al.,* 1971).

Some patients with acquired idiopathic sideroblastic anemia ultimately develop acute granulocytic leukemia (Barry, W. E., and Day, 1964; Björkman, 1956), and at least one has shown progression to fatal aplastic anemia (Britton *et al.,* 1968). Acute leukemia as a terminal event was more common in patients with idiopathic sideroblastic anemia with thrombocytopenia in comparison to those with thrombocytosis (Streeter *et al.,* 1977). As mentioned earlier, one of our patients developed monoclonal gammopathy and lymphoproliferative disorder (Tranchide *et al.,* 1973). It seems likely that with prolonged follow-up studies, at least some of these patients will develop hematological malignancies (Fairbanks *et al.,* 1971).

A few patients have been reported to manifest the clinical features commonly associated with hemochromatosis: diabetes mellitus, cardiac arrhythmia, and cirrhosis. Hemochromatosis may pose a serious threat to survival of patients with hereditary sideroblastic anemia, and at least one patient died in early adult life as a result of hepatic decompensation (Fairbanks *et al.,*1971).

Multiple pulmonary embolic disease, postsplenectomy, was the probable cause of death in at least two patients with hereditary sideroblastic anemia (Byrd and Cooper, 1961; Fairbanks *et al.,* 1971; Losowsky and Hall, 1965).

HEMOSIDEROSIS AND HEMOCHROMATOSIS

"Hemosiderosis" refers to conditions in which there is a generalized increase in the iron content of body tissues, particularly of the liver and the reticuloendothelial system but affecting other organs as well, without demonstrable fibrosis. "Hemochromatosis," on the other hand, implies the histological demonstration both of hemosiderosis and of diffuse fibrotic changes in the affected organs (Fairbanks *et al.,* 1971).

An increased iron storage is due to increased intestinal absorption of a normal dietary intake of iron, a marked increase in the quantity of iron ingested, or an exogenous iron overload by the parenteral route. Increased intestinal absorption of a normal dietary iron may be responsible for the excessive iron accumulation found in idiopathic hemochromatosis, occasionally in chronic alcoholism with Laennec's cirrhosis, and in certain types of porphyria. Patients with chronic anemias commonly have enhanced iron absorption, although it is rarely sufficient to lead to hemochromatosis. This is true for some patients with hemolytic anemias, thalassemias, hemoglobinopathies, and the rare disorder of congenital atransferrinemia. Hemochromatosis may also occur in sideroblastic anemias (Fairbanks *et al.,* 1971).

Increase in dietary iron intake appears to be the cause of excessive iron accumulation in a condition occurring in Africa generally known as "Bantu siderosis." In Asia, an unusual disorder or iron metabolism (Kaschin–Beck disease) has been described resulting from excessive iron intake of drinking water. Prolonged ingestion of large doses of medicinal iron and ingestion of alcoholic beverages with high iron content such as wines in Europe and cider and beers in South Africa may contribute to the development of hemochromatosis in some persons (Fairbanks *et al.,* 1971).

Iron overload occurs in patients who receive multiple blood transfusions. It is difficult to ascertain, in patients who receive numerous transfusions, whether the appearance of hemochromatosis represents iron-induced tissue injury or is the result of viral hepatitis (Fairbanks *et al.,* 1971).

IDIOPATHIC HEMOCHROMATOSIS

Idiopathic hemochromatosis is characterized by excessive iron accumulation in the liver and other viscera and by fibrotic changes in the liver.

This disorder is expressed clinically as diabetes mellitus with cutaneous hyperpigmentation and hepatic dysfunction.

Incidence, Age, and Sex Distribution

Idiopathic hemochromatosis has been reported to occur in 1 per 20,000 hospital admissions. Males are affected predominantly, the sex ratio being approximately 10 : 1. The disease is primarily one of middle age and becomes symptomatic in the fifth or sixth decade of life.

Etiology

Theories currently held are (1) hemochromatosis is merely an epiphenomenon of Laennec's cirrhosis (portal or alcoholic), in which iron accumulates due to the influence of cirrhosis on iron absorption or as a result of increased ingestion of iron, especially from wines or beers; and (2) hemochromatosis is due to an inborn error of metabolism that causes increased intestinal absorption or iron, leading to injury of the liver and other cells in the body.

It is known that cirrhosis of the liver results in increased iron absorption, and this increase may bring about increased iron accumulation in a fibrotic liver. On the other hand, the amount of iron found in the livers of the majority of chronic alcoholics with cirrhosis of the liver, although somewhat increased above that found in normal livers, very rarely shows the massive accumulation found in patients with idiopathic hemochromatosis. Furthermore, in many of their asymptomatic nonalcoholic relatives, the iron content of the serum and the liver is not increased.

Inborn Error of Metabolism

The hypothesis that hemochromatosis represents an inborn error of metabolism was first suggested by Sheldon (1935). Several subsequent studies have added support to the concept of a genetic basis for hemochromatosis (Debré *et al.*, 1952; Dreyfus *et al.*, 1960; Schapira *et al.*, 1962). Most of these studies are consistent with inheritance of a dominant or partially dominant autosomal gene. The genetics of idiopathic hemochromatosis is still not entirely resolved, and the nature of the metabolic error remains in doubt, as does the role of excessive deposition of iron in the genetics of tissue injury (Fairbanks *et al.*, 1971).

Several possible sites for the metabolic lesion have been proposed. An abnormality at the level of the gastrointestinal tract might lead to abnormally high absorption of iron from a diet containing a normal amount of iron. It has been reported that in hemochromatosis, there is a deficiency of gastroferrin, an iron-chelating substance normally present in gastric juice. The role of gastroferrin in hemochromatosis has not yet been fully elucidated. An abnormality in the uptake and release of iron by ferritin or apoferritin is another attractive possibility. Xanthine oxidase has been proposed (Green and Mazur, 1957; Masur *et al.*, 1958) to be a regulator of the mechanism by which iron is released from ferritin, as illustrated here:

1. Storage of iron:
   Apoferritin + Fe^{2+} → ferritin
2. Release of iron:

$$\text{Ferritin} + \text{hypoxanthine} \xrightarrow{\text{xanthine oxidase}} \text{apoferritin} + Fe^{2+} + \text{uric acid}$$

Thus, in the absence of xanthine oxidase, a normal rate of uptake of iron by apoferritin might occur, but the release of iron from ferritin would be decreased. This mechanism would be an attractive explanation of the metabolic lesion in hemachromatosis. However, studies in both man and experimental animals have offered little support for this theory (Fairbanks *et al.*, 1971).

Finally, it might be that one or both of the forms of storage iron, ferritin and hemosiderin, is structurally abnormal in idiopathic hemochromatosis, thus leading to a decrease in the ability of the molecule to release iron. However, Dreyfus and Schapira (1964) were unable to find any differences to distinguish the ferritin and apoferritin of normal liver from those of the livers of patients with idiopathic hemochromatosis. They postulated that the metabolic lesion might represent the abnormal function of a "regulator" gene, leading to excessive biosynthesis of normal apoferritin. This concept was based on the model developed by Jacob and Monod (1961) in their studies of bacterial genetics. This idea is intriguing, but has not been tested and substantiated so far (Fairbanks *et al.*, 1971).

It has been suggested that impairment of the ability of the reticuloendothelial cells to remove iron from the plasma may account for iron accumulation in parenchymal cells (MacDonald *et al.*, 1968a,b; Fairbanks *et al.*, 1971).

Pathogenesis

Another controversy that remains to be settled is whether or not the massive accumulation of iron is responsible for cellular injury and necrosis, followed by fibrotic changes.

Numerous investigators have attempted to produce hemochromatosis in experimental animals by either parenteral or oral administration of iron in large doses over prolonged periods (Andersson, 1950; Brown *et al.*,

1957; Cappell, 1930; Chang *et al.,* 1959; Finch *et al.,* 1950; Goldberg, L., and Smith, 1960; Hegsted *et al.,* 1949; Kinney *et al.,* 1949; Krumbhaar and Chanutin, 1922; MacDonald, 1960; MacDonald and Pechet, 1965; MacDonald *et al.,* 1965; Nissim, 1953; Platzer *et al.,* 1955; Polson, 1929a,b; Rather, 1956; Rous and Oliver, 1918). Although it has been possible to produce hemosiderosis of liver and other viscera, convincing evidence of cellular injury and fibrosis has not been demonstrated. The production of hemosiderosis accompanied by cellular injury and portal fibrosis in experimental animals required two conditions: iron overloading and a choline-deficient diet (MacDonald and Pechet, 1965; MacDonald *et al.,* 1968b). Administration of folic acid to rats receiving a choline-deficient diet (MacDonald *et al.,* 1965) prevented cellular necrosis and fibrosis, thus suggesting that folic acid deficiency may play a role in the genetics of the hepatic lesion in rats (Fairbanks *et al.,* 1971).

The role of iron was particularly challenged by MacDonald and Pechet (MacDonald, 1963, 1964; MacDonald and Pechet, 1965). They pointed out that : (1) alcoholism and malnutrition are frequently associated features in patients with hemochromatosis; (2) patients with Laennec's cirrhosis commonly have increased hepatic deposits of hemosiderin; (3) there is a similarity in many of the clinical manifestations of idiopathic hemochromatosis and Laennec's cirrhosis, and all intermediate forms between the two are seen with respect to iron, liver disease, carbohydrate metabolism, and other conditions; and (4) experimental iron overload alone has failed to evoke the histological changes of hemochromatosis in other species. In the opinion of these workers, the hemosiderin deposits are incidental. The tissue injury and fibrosis in hemochromatosis are evidences primarily of malnutrition, just as in Laennec's cirrhosis (Fairbanks *et al.,* 1971).

On the other hand, neither alcoholic excess nor malnutrition is found universally in patients with well-documented hemochromatosis. In the experience of many investigators, the iron content of livers of patients with Laennec's cirrhosis, while often greater than normal, very rarely approaches the massive amounts found in hemochromatosis. Diabetes mellitus often develops very early and may be severe in hemochromatosis, but is usually only latent or later in onset, and infrequently severe, in Laennec's cirrhosis. In hemochromatosis, liver function is usually normal until very late in the course of the disease, whereas in Laennec's cirrhosis, it is abnormal whenever there is histological evidence of the disease. Portal venous hypertension occurs commonly in Laennec's cirrhosis, leading to esophageal varices, but this complication is infrequent in hemochromatosis (Fairbanks *et al.,* 1971).

The results of studies conducted in other species are not necessarily relevant to human disease, inasmuch as 20–50 years are required in man for hemochromatosis to become clinically manifest. In none of the experimental animal studies of iron overloading has a comparable interval elapsed. Furthermore, in a few cases (Case Records of the Massachusetts General Hospital, 1952; Johnson, 1968; Turnberg, 1965) of iron overloading unintentionally carried out over a course of several years in humans, the classic tissue changes and clinical picture of hemochromatosis have been observed. Finally, the effect of therapeutic phlebotomy in ameliorating the course of hemochromatosis is often so striking as to leave little doubt that large accumulations of hemosiderin contribute in some manner to cellular injury and necrosis. It is possible that one effect of excessive hepatic accumulation of hemosiderin is to reduce the ability of the cells to withstand other injurious processes (such as alcohol or dietary deficiency of lipotropic factors). Supporting this possibility is the observation that the clinical manifestations of hemochromatosis affect only those members of a family who consume alcohol in excess while apparently sparing their more temperate iron-laden siblings and children (Fairbanks *et al.,* 1971).

Pathology

The accumulation of iron pigments in idiopathic hemochromatosis appears to affect nearly all tissues of the body, although the clinical manifestations are predominantly related to hepatic, cardiac, pancreatic, articular, cutaneous, and perhaps pituitary involvement. The total body iron content may be 30–50 g or more. Other elements that have been noted to increase in the livers of patients with hemochromatosis are copper, lead, and molybdenum, whereas aluminum appears to be decreased in comparison to normal livers (Fairbanks *et al.,* 1971).

The deposition of hemosiderin is most intense at the periphery of the liver lobule, which is also where cell necrosis and fibrosis first appear. The peripheral cells become larger and show more prominent nucleoli and chromatin and polar cytoplasm. Clumping of chromatin about nucleoli, combined with the pallor of the cytoplasm, may give the cells a "bull's-eye" appearance. Degenerating cells with pyknotic nuclei may become enmeshed in the proliferating fibrous tissue. As the cells die at the periphery of the lobule, the hemosiderin they release is taken up by fibroblasts at the lobule periphery and in portal space. An increase in small lymphocytes is seen in the interlobular septa, but inflammatory changes are less marked in hemochromatosis as compared with Laennec's cirrhosis. Bile ducts may show marked proliferation. The central portion of the lobule may appear normal except for hemosiderin deposits until later in the course of this disease. Ultimately, the architecture of the lobule may become so distorted, as a result of fibrosis, that the histological picture becomes indistinguishable from that of Laennec's cirrhosis. As in Laennec's cirrhosis, the incidence of carcinoma of the liver is increased in hemochromatosis (Fairbanks *et al.,* 1971).

Pigmentation and fibrosis of the pancreas are very frequent. Gross structural disorganization and infiltration with fibrous connective tissue in addition to the hemosiderin deposits are commonly present in the pancreases of patients with hemochromatosis (Fairbanks *et al.,* 1971).

Splenic involvement varies considerably, and some of the changes may be due to increased portal pressure. Pigmentation is variable, and, when present, is largely confined to the reticuloendothelial cells. Enlargement of the spleen is moderate.

In the absence of hemorrhage or therapeutic phlebotomy, bone marrow iron content is increased in idiopathic hemochromatosis. It is distributed characteristically as small discrete particles of hemosiderin more or less uniformly spread throughout reticulum cells in the bone marrow.

Small deposits of hemosiderin may be found in the entire alimentary tract. Stainable iron is present in the glandular epithelium of the stomach fairly consistently, and may be demonstrated by gastric biopsy in most cases. Brunner's glands in the duodenum are also frequently involved.

The pericardium may be brownish and have some fibrous thickening. As far as one can tell, only one proved case of restrictive (constrictive) pericarditis has been reported (Case Records of the Massachusetts General Hospital, 1960). The ventricular walls are wider and firmer than normal. Iron pigment is demonstrable microscopically in the myocardial fibers. There may be degeneration, fragmentation, and necrosis of cells; myocardial fibrosis; interstitial edema; and fatty infiltration (Blumer and Nesbit, 1938; Horeau *et al.,* 1964; Horns, 1949; Keschner, 1951; Palacio *et al.,* 1960; Petit, 1945; Schreiber, 1957; Ströder, 1942; Swan and Dewar, 1952; Warembourg *et al.,* 1965; Wasserman *et al.,* 1962). The myocardium is commonly infiltrated with inflammatory cells. Endocardial and valvular changes are usually minimal (Fairbanks *et al.,* 1971).

Hemosiderin is deposited in the islets of Langerhans and certain other endocrine organs. The pigment deposition is often marked in the pituitary gland, chiefly in the cells of the anterior pituitary. Iron deposits are also seen in the thyroid, adrenal cortex (zona glomerulosa), and testes. Atrophy of the germinal epithelium of the testes is frequent, and in about 20% of cases, primary hypogonadism may be seen clinically.

Microscopically, two types of pigment changes may be seen in the skin. In the epidermis, increased depotision of melanin is frequently found in the basal layers. Except in rare instances, hemosiderin is not present in the epidermis, but is confined to the sweat glands and the connective tissue of the corneum. Hemosiderin deposition in the central nervous system is usually confined to a few selected areas. The choroid plexus, pineal gland,

and extrapyramidal areas are some of the sites of iron deposition. Gliosis and hemorrhage are not common.

In the kidney, hemosiderin is usually confined to the epithelial cells of the tubules. When present, the iron may be demonstrated in desquamated epithelial cells in the urinary sediment. Intercapillary glomerulosclerosis (Kimmelsteil–Wilson lesion) has been considered rare in the diabetes associated with hemochromatosis, but in one report (Becker and Miller, 1960), one third of 22 patients had diffuse or nodular glomerular lesions (Fairbanks *et al.,* 1971).

In cases of idiopathic hemochromatosis with joint symptoms, the synovial lining cells have been shown to be heavily laden with hemosiderin (Kra *et al.,* 1965; Petit, 1945). Degenerative changes described in articular cartilage include loss of basophilia, flaking, separation of superficial cartilage, and clumping of chondrocytes (Hamilton, E., *et al.,* 1968). The synovial fluid is usually normal. Increased amounts of hemosiderin and ferritin may be found in many other body tissues in patients with idiopathic hemochromatosis without any associated degenerative changes or functional impairment of the involved organs (Fairbanks *et al.,* 1971).

Clinical Features

Symptoms include fatigue, weakness, and lassitude. In about half the patients, the symptoms are accompanied by manifestations of diabetes mellitus, weight loss, polyuria, and polydipsia.

Dyspnea, orthopnea, palpitations, and swelling of the legs, although not usual, may become prominent during the course of the disease in about one third of the patients. These symptoms may be due to necrosis and fibrosis of the myocardium affecting both ventricles.

Arthralgia is very common. The characteristic arthropathy may be seen in 25% of cases. The joint symptoms predominantly affect the small joints of the hands. The knees, ankles, and feet are also frequently involved. In the past, the joint manifestations were attributed to rheumatoid arthritis, "fibrositis," or degenerative arthritis in many cases.

Cutaneous hyperpigmentation, loss of libido, and thinning of hair may be seen in hemochromatosis. Abdominal pain related to liver disease is fairly common. The pain is dull and steady in the upper abdomen without distinct localization. Stretching of the liver capsule and tension on the supporting ligaments due to hepatomegaly may account for this pain. Peripheral neuropathy attributable to diabetes mellitus may be seen.

Brownish discoloration of conjunctivae due to hemosiderin deposition may be seen. Gynecomastia may be present. Cardiac arrhythmias are common. Cardiomegaly may be seen in some patients. Hepatomegaly is almost always present. Splenomegaly is found in about 50% of cases.

Spider telangiectasia and palmar erythema are frequently present. Jaundice is seen infrequently. Ascites is present in one third of patients. Testicular atrophy is found in about 25% of patients with hemochromatosis. Edema of the legs may occur as a result of hepatic dysfunction or congestive heart failure. A characteristic finding in patients with arthritic symptoms is thickening of the soft tissue of the proximal finger joints, knees, and ankles. Some patients may have effusion of the knee (Fairbanks *et al.,* 1971).

Laboratory Data

Although histologically evident liver disease is a constant feature of hemochromatosis, the laboratory tests commonly used as indices of liver function usually give normal results. The rate of sulfobromophthalein (BSP) excretion, generally regarded as a sensitive test of liver function, is usually normal.

Serum iron is increased. Transferrin is usually 70–100% saturated. More than 80% of these patients have diabetes mellitus. There may be a decrease in the plasma concentration of glucocorticoids (Stocks and Martin, 1968). Some investigators have implicated an impairment of pituitary function in hemochromatosis to account for endocrine changes. particularly hypogonadism (Fairbanks *et al.,* 1971).

The rate of absorption of a tracer dose of iron was normal in some studies (Balfour *et al.,* 1942; Chodos *et al.,* 1954) and increased in others (Alper *et al.,* 1951; Bothwell *et al.,* 1953; Deller, 1965; Finch and Bothwell, 1961; Losowsky and Wilson, 1967; Peterson and Ettinger, 1953; Pirzio-Biroli *et al.,* 1958). It is possible that in untreated patients, the massive accumulation of iron results in the diminution of the otherwise enhanced rate of iron absorption. After therapeutic phlebotomies, iron absorption is increased in comparison with that in normal subjects. Ferrokinetic studies reveal a prolongation of plasma iron clearance and an increase in plasma iron turnover rate due to a high serum iron level (Bothwell *et al.,* 1953, 1955, 1957; Brunner, 1966; Clément *et al.,* 1965; Darnis, 1964; Dreyfus and Schapira, 1963; Fairbanks *et al.,* 1971; Hiyeda, 1939; Pollycove and Mortimer, 1961; Rosselin, 1964; Sargent and Winchell, 1967; Scandellari *et al.,* 1967; Schmid *et al.,* 1964a).

The most valuable diagnostic procedure is liver biopsy and assessment of iron store in the liver. Chelating substances have been used as tests for iron overload, particularly diethylenetriaminepentaacetate and desferoxamine (Desferal) (Balcerzak *et al.,* 1968; Barry, M., *et al.,* 1969; Fielding *et al.,* 1966; Hwang and Brown, 1964; Losowsky, 1966; Ploem *et al.,* 1966; Powell and Thomas, 1967; Schmid *et al.,* 1964b; Smith, P. M., *et al.,* 1967; 1969; Walsh, R. J., *et al.,* 1963; Walsh, J. R., *et al.,* 1965; Wöhler, 1964). These tests are performed by injecting specified amounts of the chelating agents, collecting the urine over an interval of 6–24 h, and then measuring the amount of iron excreted. The results indicate that after a parenteral injection of a chelating agent, patients with iron overload, as in hemochromatosis, excrete substantially more iron in the urine than do normal subjects or patients with ordinary Laennec's cirrhosis (Fairbanks *et al.*, 1971).

Treatment

The treatment of idiopathic hemochromatosis can be separated into two aspects. First, there is the management of the failure or dysfunction of whatever organ systems may be involved, primarily the liver, pancreas, and heart. There is nothing unique about these problems in hemochromatosis, and usual management for these conditions is indicated. Infections, most frequently pneumonia, were the cause of death in nearly half the cases in one series (Dillingham, 1960; Fairbanks *et al.*, 1971).

The second aspect of treatment of idiopathic hemochromatosis is removal of the excess iron stores. Two phlebotomies weekly (500 ml each time) may be needed in most patients. This program should be monitored by regular determination of hemoglobin, serum iron, and iron-binding capacity. Another possibility is to use desferoxamine, an iron-chelating agent that is an effective agent for therapy of hemochromatosis. The daily injection of 800 mg desferoxamine might result in removal of 7.3 g iron from the body in 1 year. This is much less than what one might achieve by a program of twice-weekly phlebotomy (Fairbanks *et al.*, 1971).

R. Williams *et al.* (1969) compared survival rates of 40 patients treated by phlebotomy with those of 18 patients who were not so treated. The median survival from the time of admission was 2 years in the nonphlebotomized group and more than 7 years for the phlebotomized group. R. Williams *et al.* (1969) found apparent regression even of perilobular fibrosis in several liver biopsy samples obtained over a period of years in patients undergoing therapeutic phlebotomy (Fairbanks *et al.*, 1971).

JUVENILE IDIOPATHIC HEMOCHROMATOSIS

The onset of the clinical manifestations of idiopathic hemochromatosis before the age of 20 years has been repeatedly reported (Althausen and Kerr, 1933; Bezançon *et al.*, 1932; Bothwell *et al.*, 1959; Boulin and Uhry, 1949; Mielke, 1953; Palacio *et al.*, 1960; Perkins *et al.*, 1965; Portella *et al.*, 1957; Ströder, 1942). Such cases appear to differ from adult cases of idiopathic hemochromatosis only in age at onset and in severity and rapidity of evolution of the disease. Since this variant of idiopathic hemochromatosis has occurred among siblings, a careful study of other members of the family should be made to detect latent disease and arrest its evolution. Treatment should be by therapeutic phlebotomy (Fairbanks *et al.,* 1971).

SECONDARY HEMOCHROMATOSIS

The clinical and pathological picture of hemochromatosis complicates the course in a small group of patients with long-standing anemia (Aufderheide *et al.,* 1953; Chesner, 1946; Gelpi and Ende, 1958; Houston, 1951; Morningstar, 1955; Wallerstein and Robbins, 1953). In general, these patients have had a severe chronic hemolytic anemia such as thalassemia major, sideroblastic anemia, or other anemias with hyperplastic bone marrows. A few cases of hemochromatosis have been reported in patients with congenital spherocytosis or congenital nonspherocytic hemolytic anemia (Barry, M., *et al.,* 1968; Fairbanks *et al.,* 1971; Pletcher *et al.,* 1963; Reeves *et al.,* 1963; Wilson, J. D., *et al.,* 1967).

Many patients who have developed this form of hemochromatosis have received frequent blood transfusions, sometimes totaling several hundred. Because of the association of viral hepatitis with blood transfusion, it is possible that in some patients, the hepatic fibrosis represents the aftereffects of hepatitis. On the other hand, some patients with chronic anemia have developed the clinical picture of hemochromatosis without having ever received transfusion and without any known exposure to hepatotoxic substances. An additional factor in patients with chronic anemias is the indiscriminate use of iron for therapeutic purposes. The continuous oral administration of iron salts over a period of many years can in itself be associated with the clinical syndrome of hemochromatosis (Morningstar, 1955; Fairbanks *et al.,* 1971).

The symptoms and physical findings are usually those of the primary disorder. Probably all the manifestations of idiopathic hemochromatosis may be reproduced in secondary hemochromatosis (Fairbanks *et al.,* 1971).

When there is no anemia or the anemia is mild, a program of therapeutic phlebotomy should be instituted as described for idiopathic hemochromatosis. Unfortunately, this is often not possible because of the severity of the anemia. It is in these patients that the administration of an iron-chelating agent might be useful (Fairbanks *et al.,* 1971).

HEMOSIDEROSIS

Some authors distinguish hemosiderosis from hemochromatosis on the basis of distribution as well as concentration of iron. Thus, in hemosiderosis, the iron deposits are thought to be more prominent in the spleen, lymph nodes, and bone marrow, with relatively less iron found in the liver, pancreas, and other organs (Popper and Schaffner, 1957). Finch *et al.* (1950) stated that irrespective of the route of administration, ferric iron will eventually be distributed largely in the liver after an adequate time interval. Therefore, it may be that the ratio of liver iron to spleen iron depends on the length of time the iron overload has been present. Within the liver itself, the ultimate distribution of iron varies with the preparation used and the species studied. Chronically anemic patients given multiple blood transfusions eventually develop extensive iron deposition in the Kupffer cells and the liver parenchyma. One detailed study of patients with iron overload failed to demonstrate significant differences in iron distribution between patients with hemosiderosis and those with hemochromatosis (Fairbanks *et al.*, 1971; MacDonald and Mallory, 1960).

SHUNT HEMOCHROMATOSIS

In 1959, Tuttle *et al.* (1959) described the unusual course of a patient with Laennec's cirrhosis who had undergone end-to-side portacaval anastomosis because of bleeding esophageal varices. Liver biopsy at the time of operation disclosed extensive cirrhosis, but there was no stainable iron. Three years later, at autopsy, the typical histological picture of hemochromatosis was observed. Others have observed similar cases (Brodanová and Hoenig, 1966; Da Silva *et al.*, 1963; Ecker *et al.*, 1968; Fairbanks *et al.*, 1971; Gardiol *et al.*, 1967; Grace and Balint, 1966; Hoffbauer, 1960; Nixon, 1966; Schaefer *et al.*, 1962; Williams, R., *et al.*, 1969).

The pathogenesis of shunt hemochromatosis is not understood. The clinical manifestations and laboratory findings appear to be similar to those of idiopathic hemochromatosis. Treatment is directed at the complication of the disorder. Although it is reasonable to use phlebotomy in the management of shunt hemochromatosis, such treatment has not been utilized. Survival appears to be only a few years from the time of portosystemic anastomosis, although some patients have lived longer (Ecker *et al.*, 1968; Fairbanks *et al.*, 1971; Tisdale, 1961).

PORPHYRIA CUTANEA TARDA

An interrelationship between porphyria cutanea tarda (PCT) and iron overloading was suggested by several investigators (Brugsch, 1958; Langhof and Mildschlag, 1954). Increased porphyrin excretion in hemochromatosis has been observed. Bolgert *et al.* (1953) reported that of nine patients with PCT, six had hepatomegaly and eight had serum iron concentration of 170 μg/100 ml or higher. Langhof and Mildschlag (1954) in 1954 reported a case of PCT in which there was cutaneous bronzing, increased serum iron, abnormal GTT, and abnormal liver function. According to them, their patient had incipient hemochromatosis in addition to PCT. It was noted that after 2 days of treatment with BAL (British anti-lewisite), cutaneous lesions did not occur even after exposure to sunlight. Similar cases were soon reported (Boulet *et al.,* 1959; Tuffanelli, 1960). It would now appear that the frequent association of PCT with iron overload should permit one to predict with some confidence the existence of excessive iron stores in patients with PCT (Fairbanks *et al.,* 1971).

Etiology and Pathogenesis

The etiology and pathogenesis of PCT have not been established. It is believed that this is not a genetic disorder, although some instances of familial occurrence of PCT have been described (Saltzer *et al.,* 1968). The majority of patients with PCT have had histories of prolonged excessive consumption of alcoholic beverages (Berlin and Brante, 1962; Boulet *et al.,* 1959; Lamont and Hathorn, 1960; Prato *et al.,* 1964; Saltzer *et al.,* 1968; Sauer and Funk, 1969; Saunders, 1963; Tuffanelli, 1960), although this is not true for all patients. The primary cause of the excessive accumulation of iron is not known. Possibly it is secondary to chronic hepatic injury, which is known to increase iron absorption. The increased iron absorption may be due in part to the effect of alcohol on iron absorption, and to the high iron content of some alcoholic beverages. However, the possibility that the increased iron absorption is due to a primary inherent defect at the gastrointestinal level cannot be excluded.

It has been proposed that the excessive accumulation of iron interferes in some manner with the enzymatic synthesis of heme, and that this metabolic inhibition results in the excessive accumulation of heme precursors in plasma and liver. The observation that a decrease in the total body iron content by phlebotomies commonly leads to a marked decrease in porphyrin excretion would support this point of view.

Pathology

The histological changes in the skin are melanosis, fragmentation of elastic tissue, and disorganization of collagen and elastic fibers (Saltzer *et al.,* 1968). The result of this degenerative process if the appearance of relatively homogenous colloid like material in the dermis. These changes, however, are nonspecific. The histopathology of the liver is not distinguishable from that described for idiopathic hemocromatosis. Biopsy specimens exhibit a red fluorescence in ultraviolet light (Fairbanks *et al.,* 1971; Sauer and Funk, 1969).

Clinical Features

The clinical manifestations of PCT have been described in detail by many authors (Bolgert *et al.,* 1953; Boulet *et al.,* 1959; Saltzer *et al.,* 1968;

Sauer and Funk, 1969). Males predominate in a ratio of about 3 : 1, and the disorder is not usually seen prior to the age of 35.

Recurrent formation of bullae followed by ulceration and the formation of atrophic scars on skin in areas exposed to sunlight or trauma is the most characteristic cutaneous manifestation. Cutaneous hyperpigmentation, hypertrichosis, and sclerodermalike dermal thickening are commonly seen. The cutaneous lesions fluoresce in ultraviolet light. Abdominal colic, nausea, vomiting, fever, hypertension, and mental aberrations have been reported to occur. Physical examination may reveal bullae, ulcerations, sometimes pigmented atrophic scars in exposed areas, and hypopigmentation of the skin, and hepatomegaly. Some diminution in vibratory and positional sense in the lower extremities has been described (Fairbanks *et al.,* 1971; Sauer and Funk, 1969).

Laboratory Data

Hemoglobin, leukocyte total and differential counts, platelet count, serum bilirubin, and blood urea nitrogen are usually normal. BSP retention is commonly abnormal, as may be other tests of liver function. Serum iron is increased, and transferrin is usually 60–95% saturated. The serum may exhibit a reddish fluorescence in ultraviolet light (Saltzer *et al.,* 1968). About 20–30% of patients with PCT have abnormal GTTs.

The urine contains a mixture of uroporphyrin I and III and coproporphyrin. Porphobilinogen in urine is not increased. The urine may appear reddish-brown and fluoresce in ultraviolet light (Fairbanks *et al.,* 1971).

Ferrokinetic studies reveal the plasma iron turnover rate to be either normal or slightly increased. Iron utilization has been reported to be either normal or decreased (Prate *et al.,* 1964; Price *et al.,* 1968; Sauer and Funk, 1969). Patients with PCT have been shown to absorb more of an oral dose of ^{59}Fe than normal subjects (Saunders, 1963). After intravenous injection of ^{59}Fe, there is a greater than normal accumulation of the label in the livers of patients with PCT (Berlin and Brante, 1962; Fairbanks *et al.,* 1971; Price *et al.,* 1968; Sauer and Funk, 1969).

Treatment

The treatment of choice, at present, is repeated phlebotomies. The relief of clinical symptoms seems to begin after removal of only about 3–5 g iron (equivalent to removal of 12–20 units of blood), not enough to deplete the iron stores. It is accompanied by a marked decrease in urinary porphyrin excretion. Chloroquine in small doses (0.5 g orally twice weekly) has resulted in decreased urinary uroporphyrin excretion and concomitant remission of the cutaneous phenomenon of PCT. Larger doses of chloroquine, however, appear to cause hepatocellular injury in this condition (Fairbanks *et al.,* 1971).

Alcohol is likely to cause exacerbation in patients with PCT. These patients should be instructed to abstain from use of alcohol and to avoid other hepatotoxins.

BANTU SIDEROSIS (AFRICAN NUTRITIONAL HEMOSIDEROSIS)

Hemosiderosis of dietary origin has been recognized as an endemic disease of the negroid peoples of South Africa since 1929 (Sheldon, 1935). The disorder is commonly known as "Bantu siderosis." It appears that at least 50% of African males in South Africa have moderately to severely increased iron content in their livers, and about 5% have some degree of cirrhosis. The prevalence of hepatic hemosiderosis in African women is much less (Fairbanks *et al.,* 1971).

Etiology

In many areas of Africa, it is customary to prepare food in iron pots. By this process, the iron content of cooked food is increased as much as fourfold above the content of the uncooked food. An alcoholic beverage ("Kaffir beer") is also brewed in iron containers, and the beer contains as much as 15 mg iron/100 ml. The daily dietary intake of iron may be as high as 215 mg (Fairbanks *et al.,* 1971).

Pathology

With minimal hemosiderosis, hemosiderin is deposited predominantly in the liver cord cells, especially in the perilobular areas. As iron accumulation progresses, hemosiderin also appears in the Kupffer cells, cells of the portal tract, and reticuloendothelial cells of the spleen and bone marrow. With massive iron accumulation, there is an associated portal fibrosis, and the hepatic architecture may be indistinguishable from that of idiopathic hemochromatosis. In such cases, hemosiderin is found in the pancreas, adrenal, thyroid, pituitary and myocardium (Fairbanks *et al.,* 1971).

Clinical Features

In patients with hemosiderosis, there may be no signs or symptoms. In patients with hemochromatosis, the clinical features are the same as those described for idiopathic hemochromatosis (Fairbanks *et al.,* 1971).

Tests of glucose metabolism were abnormal in 20% of patients with hemochromatosis. The serum iron is increased, and transferrin saturation has been reported as infrequently being greater than 50% (Fairbanks *et al.,* 1971).

Treatment

It would seem reasonable to treat these patients by phlebotomy and restriction of use of alcoholic beverages. Preventive measures to decrease the iron content of diet seem warranted (Fairbanks *et al.,* 1971).

REFERENCES

Aasa, R., Malmström, B. G., Saltman, P., and Vänngård, T. 1963. The specific binding of iron (III) and copper (II) to transferrin and conalbumin, *Biochim. Biophys. Acta* **75,** 203–222.

Addison, G. M., Beamish, M. R., Hales, C. N., Hodgkins, M., Jacobs, A., and Llewellin, P. 1972. An immunoradiometric assay for ferritin in the serum of normal subjects and patients with iron deficiency and iron overload. *J. Clin. Pathol.* **25,** 326–329.

Allen, D. W., and Jandl, J. H. 1960. Kinetics of intracellular iron in rabbit reticulocytes. *Blood* **15,** 71–81.

Allgood, J. W., and Brown, E. B. 1967. The relationship between duodenal mucosal iron concentration and iron absorption in human subjects. *Scand. J. Haematol.* **4,** 217–229.

Alper, T., Savage, D. V., and Bothwell, T. H. 1951. Radioiron studies in a case of hemochromatosis. *J. Lab. Clin. Med.* **37,** 665–675.

Althausen, T. L., and Kerr, W. J. 1933. Hemochromatosis. II. A report of three cases with endocrine disturbances and notes on a previously reported case: Discussion of etiology. *Endocrinology* **17,** 621–646.

Andersson, N. S. E. 1950. Experimental and clinical investigations into the effect of parenterally administered iron. *Acta Med. Scand.* **138** (Suppl. 241), 1–71.

Aufderheide, A. C., Horns, H. L., and Goldish, R. J. 1953. Secondary hemochromatosis. I. Transfusion (exogenous) hemochromatosis. *Blood* **8,** 824–836.

Aisen, P., and Brown, E. B. 1977 The iron-binding function of transferrin in iron metabolism. *Semin. Hematol.* **14,** 31–53.

Bainton, D. F., and Finch, C. A. 1964. The diagnosis of iron deficiency anemia. *Amer. J. Med.* **37,** 62–70.

Balcerzak, S. P., Westerman, M. P., Heinle, E. W., and Taylor, F. H. 1968. Measurement of iron stores using desferrioxamine. *Ann. Inter. Med.* **68,** 518–525.

Balfour, W. M., Hahn, P. F., Bale, W. F., Pommerenke, W. T., and Whipple, G. H. 1942. Radioactive iron absorption in clinical conditions: Normal pregnancy, anemia, and hemochromatosis. *J. Exp. Med.* **76,** 15–30.

Barkan, G. 1933. Die unterscheidung des "leicht abspaltbaren" Bluteisens vom Hämoglobineisen und vom anorganischem Eise. *Hoppe-Seyler's Z. Physiol. Chem.* **221,** 241–251.

Barry, M., Scheuer, P. J., Sherlock, S., Ross, C. F., and Williams, R. 1968. Hereditary spherocytosis with secondary haemochromatosis. *Lancet* **2,** 481–485.

Barry, M., Cartei, G., and Sherlock, S. 1969. Differential ferrioxamine test in haemochromatosis and liver diseases. *Gut* **10,** 697–704.

Barry. W. E., and Day, H. J. 1964. Refractory sideroblastic anemia: Clinical and hematologic study of ten cases. *Ann. Intern. Med.* **61,** 1029–1044.

Bässler, R. 1961. Elektronenmikroskopische Befunde bei essentieller Lungenhämosiderose. *Z. Pathol.* **71,** 259–282.

Beal, V. A., Meyers, A. J., and McCammon, R. W. 1962. Iron intake, hemoglobin, and physical growth during the first two years of life. *Pediatrics* **30,** 518–539.

Becker, D., and Miller, M. 1960. Presence of diabetic glomerulosclerosis in patients with hemochromatosis. *N. Engl. J. Med.* **263,** 367–373.

Beirne, G. J., Octaviano, G. N., Kopp, W. L., and Burns, R. O. 1968. Immunohistology of the lung in Goodpasture's syndrome. *Ann. Intern. Med.* **69,** 1207–1212.

Berlin, S. O., and Brante, G. 1962. Iron metabolism in porphyria and haemochromatosis (letter to the editor). *Lancet* **2,** 729.

Bessis, M. C., and Breton-Gorius, J. 1957. Iron particles in normal erythroblasts and normal and pathological erthrocytes. *J. Biophys. Biochem. Cytol.* **3,** 503–504.

Bessis, M. C., and Breton-Gorius, J. 1959. Ferritin and ferruginous micelles in normal erythroblasts and hypochromic hypersideremic anemias. *Blood* **14,** 423–432.

Bessis, M. C., and Breton-Gorius, J. 1962. Iron metabolism in the bone marrow as seen by electronmicroscopy. *Blood* **19,** 635–663.

Beutler, E. 1957. Iron enzymes in iron deficiency. *Amer. J. Med. Sci.* **234,** 517–527.

Beutler, E. 1959a. Iron enzymes in iron deficiency. IV. Cytochrome oxidase in rat kidney and heart. *Acta Haematol.* **21,** 371–377.

Beutler, E. 1959b. Iron enzymes in iron deficiency. VI. Aconitase activity and citrate metabolism. *J. Clin. Invest.* **38,** 1605–1616.

Beutler, E. 1961. Hematology: Iron metabolism. *Annu. Rev. Med.* **12,** 195–210.

Beutler, E., and Blaisdell, R. K. 1958. Iron enzymes in iron deficiency. III. Catalase in rat red cells and liver with some further observations in cytochrome *c. J. Lab. Clin. Med.* **52,** 694–699.

Beutler, E., and Blaisdell, R. K. 1960. Iron enzymes in iron deficiency. V. Succinic dehydrogenase in rat liver, kidney, and heart. *Blood* **15,** 30–35.

Beutler, E. Robson, M. J., and Buttenwiëser, E. 1958. A comparison of the plasma iron, iron-binding capacity, sternal marrow iron and other methods in the clinical evaluation of iron stores. *Ann. Inter. Med.* **48,** 60–82.

Bezancon, F., de Gennes, L., Delarue, and Oumansky, 1932. Cirrhose pigmentaire avec infantilisme, insuffisance cardiaque et aplasies endocriniennes multiples. *Bull. Soc. Med. Paris* **48,** 967–974.

Bickers, N. J., Brown, C. L., and Sprague, C. C. 1962. Pyridoxine responsive anemia. *Blood* **19,** 304–312.

Biggs, J. C., and Davis, A. E. 1963. Relationship of diminished pancreatic secretion to haemochromatosis. *Lancet* **2,** 814.

Biggs, J. C., and Davis, A. E. 1966. The exocrine pancreas and iron absorption. *Aust. Ann. Med.* **15,** 36–39.

Bishop, R. C., and Bethell, F. H. 1959. Hereditary hypochromic anemia with transfusion hemosiderosis treated with pyridoxine: Report of a case. *N. Engl. J. Med.* **261,** 486–489.

Björkman, S. E. 1956. Chronic refractory anemia with sideroblastic bone marrow: A study of four cases. *Blood* **11,** 250–259.

Blomstrom, D. C., Knight, E., Jr., Phillips, W. D., and Weiler, J. F. 1964. The nature of iron in ferredoxin. *Proc. Natl. Acad. Sci. U.S.A.* **51,** 1085–1092.

Bloom, V. R., Wayne, D. J., and Wrong, O. M. 1965. Lung purpura and nephritis (Goodpasture's syndrome) complicated by the nephrotic syndrome. *Ann. Intern. Med.* **63,** 752–759.

Blumer, G., and Nesbit, R. R. 1938. A case of hemochromatosis with degeneration of the heart muscle an death from congestive heart failure. *N. Engl. J. Med.* **218,** 295–298.

Bolgert, M., Canivet, J., and Le Sourd, M. 1953. La porphyrie cutanée de l'adulte étude de neuf cas et description. *Sem. Hop. Paris* **29,** 1587–1608.

Bond, C. F. 1948. The nature of the anemia of pregnancy in the rat. *Endocrinology* **43,** 180–191.

Bothwell, T. H., and Finch, C. A. 1962. In: *Iron Metabolism.* Little, Brown, Boston, pp. 1–440.

Bothwell, T. H., van Doorn-Wittkampf, H. van W., Du Preez, M. L., and Alper, T. 1953. The absorption of iron: Radioiron studies in idiopathic hemochromatosis, malnutritional cytosiderosis, and transfusional hemosiderosis. *J. Lab. Clin. Med.* **41,** 836–848.

Bothwell, T. H., Ellis, B. C., van Doorn-Wittkampf, H. van W., and Abrahams, O. L. 1955. Radioiron studies in hemochromatosis: The effects of repeated phlebotomies. *J. Lab. Clin. Med.* **45,** 167–178.

Bothwell, T. H., Hurtado, A. V., Donohue, D. M., and Finch, C. A. 1957. Erythrokinetics. IV. The plasma iron turnover as a measure of erythropoiesis. *Blood* **12,** 409–427.

Bothwell, T. H., Pirzio-Biroli, G., and Finch, C. A. 1958. Iron absorption. I. Factors influencing absorption. *J. Lab. Clin. Med.* **51,** 24–36.

Bothwell, T. H., Cohen, I., Abrahams, O. L., and Perold, S. M. 1959. A familial study in idiopathic hemochromatosis. *Amer. J. Med.* **27,** 730–738.

Bottomley, S. S. 1977. Porphyrin and iron metabolism in sideroblastic anemia. *Semin. Hematol.* **14,** 169–185.

Boulet, P., Mirouze, J., Barjon, P., Mandin, A., Corbiére, J.-Cl., and Duntze, F. 1959. Porphyrie cutanée de l'adulte et diabéte sucré évolutif. *Bull. Mem. Soc. Med. Hop. Paris* **1,** 653–656.

Boulin, R., and Uhry, P. 1949. Le diabéte bronzé. *Acta Gastroenterol. Belg.* **12,** 540–541.

Bourne, M. S., Elves, M. W., and Israëls, M. C. G. 1965. Familial pyridoxine-responsive anaemia. *Brit. J. Haematol.* **11,** 1–10.

Bousser, J., Gajdos, A., Gajdos-Török, M., Bilski-Pasquier, G., and Zittoun, R. 1967. Anémie sidéroblastique idiopathique acquise: Incorporation de la glycine-2-C-14 dans l'héme et la globine des érythroblastes médullaires *in vitro. Nouv. Rev. Fr. Hematol.* **7,** 847–854.

Braude, R., Chamberlain, A. G., Kotarbinski, M., and Mitchell, K. G. 1962. The metabolism of iron in piglets given labelled iron either orally or by injection. *Brit. J. Nutr.* **16,** 427–449.

Britton, G. M. Stohlman, F., Jr., and Tanaka, Y. 1968. A primary sideroblastic anemia terminating in bone marrow aplasia. *Amer. J. Clin. Pathol.* **50,** 467–477.

Brock, J. F., and Diamond, L. K. 1934. Rickets in rats by iron feeding. *J. Pediatr.* **4,** 442–453.

Brodanová, M., and Hoenig, V. 1966. Iron metabolism in patients with portacaval shunts. *Scand. J. Gastroenterol. 1,* 167–172.

Brown, E. B., and Justus, B. W. 1958. *In vitro* absorption of radioiron by everted pouches of rat intestine. *Amer. J. Physiol.* **194,** 319–326.

Brown, E. B., and Rother, M. 1961. Studies of the process of intestinal iron absorption in rats. *Blood* **18,** 780 (abstract).

Brown, E. B., and Rother, M. L. 1963. Studies of the mechanism of iron absorption. I. Iron uptake by the normal rat. *J. Lab. Clin. Med.* **62,** 357–373.

Brown, E. B., Jr., Dubach, R., Smith, D. E., Reynafarje, C., and Moore, C. V. 1957. Studies in iron transportation and metabolism. X. Long-term iron overload in dogs. *J. Lab. Clin. Med.* **50,** 862–893.

Brugsch, J. 1958. Hämochromatose und Melanodermieporphyrie als verschiedene Formen der Hämsynthesestörung bei Pigmentzirrhose und Bronzediabetes. *A. Gesamte Inn. Med.* **13,** 411–415.

Brunner, H. E. 1966. Idiopathische Hämochromatose und Lebercirrhose mit Siderose: Differentialdiagnose durch Untersuchunge der Ferro- und Erythrocytenkinetik mit radioaktiven Eisen (Fe-59) und Chrom (cr-51). *Klin. Wochenschr.* **44,** 1235–1243.

Byrd, R. B., and Cooper, T. 1961. Hereditary iron-loading anemia with secondary hemochromatosis. *Ann. Intern. Med.* **55,** 103–123.

Callender, S. T. 1973. Fortification of food with iron—is it necessary or effective? In: *Nutritional Problems in a Changing World* (D. Hollingsworth and M. Russell, eds.), John Wiley and Sons, New York, pp. 205–210.

Cáp, J. Lehotská, V., and Mayerová, A. 1968. Kongenitálna atransferinémia u 11-mesaěného dietata. *Cesk. Pediatr.* **23,** 1020–1025.

Cappell, D. F. 1930. The late results of intravenous injection of colloidal iron. *J. Pathol.* **33,** 175–196.

Cartwright, G. E., and Wintrobe, M. M. 1954. The anemia of infection. XIX. Studies on free erythrocyte coproporphyrin and protoporphyrin. In: *Modern Trends in Blood Diseases* (J. F. Wilkinson, ed.). Butterworth, London and Washington, D.C., pp. 183–188.

Case Records of the Massachusetts General Hospital. 1952. Case 38512. *N. Engl. J. Med. 247,* 992–995.

Case Records of the Massachusetts General Hospital. 1960. Case 46281. *N. Engl. J. Med.* **263,** 88–94.

Cavell, P. A., and Widdowson, E. M. 1964. Intakes and excretions of iron, copper and zinc in the neonatal period. *Arch. Dis. Chid.* **39,** 496–501.

Chang, H. Y., Robbins, S. L., and Mallory, G. K. 1959. Prolonged intravenous administration of iron to normal and anemic rabbits. *Lab. Invest.* **8,** 1–18.

Charlton, R. W., Jacobs, P., Torrance, J. D., and Bothwell, T. H. 1965. The role of the intestinal mucosa in iron absorption. *J. Clin. Invest.* **44,** 543–554.

Chesner, C. 1946. Hemochromatosis: Review of the literature and presentation of a case without pigmentation or diabetes. *J. Lab. Clin. Med.* **31,** 1029–1036.

Chillar, R. K., Johnson, C. S., and Beutler, E. 1976. Erythrocyte pyridoxine kinase levels in patients with sideroblastic anemia. *N. Engl. J. Med.* **295,** 881–883.

Chodos, R. B., Ross, J. F., Apt, L., Halkett, J., and Pollycove, M. 1954. The absorption of food iron and inorganic iron by normal, iron-deficient, and hemochromatotic subjects. *Clin. Res. Proc.* **2,** 53 (abstract).

Clément, F., Delaloye, B., and Vannotti, A. 1965. L'exploration isotopique du metabolisme du fer: Anciens et nouveaux modeles. *Acta Haematol. (Basel)* **33,** 65–85.

Coltman, C. A., Jr. 1969. Pagophagia and iron lack. *J. Amer. Med. Assoc.* **207,** 513–516.

Conrad, M. E., Jr., and Crosby, W. H. 1963. Intestinal mucosal mechanisms controlling iron absorption. *Blood* **22,** 406–415.

Conrad, M. E., Weintraub, L. R., and Crosby, W. H. 1964. The role of the intestine in iron kinetics. *J. Clin. Invest.* **43,** 963–974.

Conrad, M. E., Weintraub, L. R., Sears, D. A., and Crosby, W. H. 1966. Absorption of hemoglobin iron. *Amer. J. Physiol.* **211,** 1123–1130.

Cooley, T. B. 1945. A severe type of hereditary anemia with elliptocytosis: Interesting sequence of splenectomy. *Amer. J. Med. Sci.* **209,** 561–568.

Cotton, H. B., and Harris, J. W. 1962. Familial pyridoxine-responsive anemia. *J. Clin. Invest.* **41,** 1352 (abstract).

Crosby, W. H. 1970. Iron enrichment: One's food, another's poison (editorial). *Arch. Int. Med.* **126,** 911–913.

Crosby, W. H. 1977. Current concepts in nutrition: Who needs iron? *New Engl. J. Med.* **297,** 543–545.

Crosby, W. H., and Sheehy, T. W. 1960. Hypochromic iron-loading anaemia: Studies of iron and haemoglobin metabolism by means of vigorous phlebotomy. *Brit. J. Haematol.* **6,** 56–65.

Cusack, R. P., and Brown, W. D. 1965. Iron deficiency in rats: Changes in body and organ weights, plasma proteins, hemoglobins, myoglobins, and catalase. *J. Nutr.* **86,** 383–393.

Czerniejewski, C. P., Shank, C. W., Bechtel, W. G., and Bradley, W. B. 1964. The minerals of wheat, flour, and bread. *Cereal Chem.* **41,** 67–72.

Dacie, J. V., and Mollin, D. L. 1966. Siderocytes, sideroblasts and sideroblastic anaemia. *Acta Med. Scand. Suppl.* **445,** 237–248.

Dacie, J. V., Smith, M. D., White, J. C., and Mollin, D. L. 1959. Refractory normoblastic anaemia: A clinical and haematological study of seven cases. *Brit. J. Haematol.* **5,** 56–82.

Dallman, P. R. 1969. Iron restriction in the nursing rat: Early effects upon tissue heme proteins, hemoglobin and liver iron. *J. Nutr.* **97,** 475–480.

Dallman, P. R., and Schwartz, H. C. 1965a. Distribution of cytochrome *c* and myoglobin in rats with dietary deficiency. *Pediatrics* **35,** 677–686.

Dallman, P. R., and Schwartz, H. C. 1965b. Myoglobin and cytochrome response during repair of iron deficiency in the rat. *J. Clin. Invest.* **44,** 1631–1638.

Dameshek, W. 1965. Sideroblastic anaemia: Is this a malignancy? *Brit. J. Haematol.* **11,** 52–58.

Darby, W. J. 1951. Iron and copper. In: *Handbook of Nutrition,* 2nd ed. McGraw-Hill (Blakiston), New York, pp. 89–110.

Darnis, F. 1964. Exploration de l'érythropoïèse par le radio-fer 59 dans les hémochromatoses idiopathiques non traitées, et traitées par la méthode des saignées repetées. *Med. Monde* **40,** 159–164.

Da Silve, L. C., Jamra, M. A., Maspes, V., Pontes, J. F., Pieroni, R. R., and de Ulhóa Cintra, A. B. 1963. Pathogenesis of indirect reacting hyperbilirubinemia after portacaval anastomosis. *Gastroenterology* **44,** 117–124.

Davis, A. E., and Biggs, J. C. 1964. Iron absorption in haemochromatosis and cirrhosis of the liver. *Aust. Ann. Med.* **13,** 201–203.

Davis, A. E., and Biggs, J. C. 1965. The pancreas and iron absorption. *Gut* **6,** 140–142.

Davis, P. N., Norris, L. C., and Kratzer, F. H. 1968. Iron utilization and metabolism in the chick. *J. Nutr.* **94,** 407–417.

Davis, P. S., Luke, C. G., and Deller, D. J. 1966. Reduction of gastric iron-binding protein in haemochromatosis: A previously unrecognized metabolic defect. *Lancet* **2,** 1431–1433.

Debrè, R., Schapira, G., Dreyfus, J. C., and Schapira, F. 1952. Métabolisme du fer chez les descendants de malades atteints de cirrhose bronzée. *Bull. Soc. Med. Paris* **1,** 665–669.

DeGowin, R. L., Sorensen, L. B., Charleston, D. B., Gottschalk, A., and Greenwald, J. H. 1968. Retention of radioiron in the lungs of a woman with idiopathic pulmonary hemosiderosis. *Ann. Intern. Med.* **69,** 1213–1220.

Deiss, A., and Cartwright, G. E. 1970. Ferritin metabolism in reticulated siderocytes. *J. Clin. Invest.* **49,** 517–523.

de Leeuw, N. K. M., Lowenstein, L., and Hsieh, Y. S. 1966. Iron deficiency in hydremia in normal pregnancy. *Medicine (Baltimore)* **45,** 291–315.

Deller, D. J. 1965. $Iron^{59}$ absorption measurements by whole-body counting: Studies in alcoholic cirrhosis, hemochromatosis, and pancreatitis. *Amer. J. Dig. Dis.* **10,** 249–258.

Derechin, S. S., and Johnson, P. 1962. Red proteins from bovine milk. *Nature (London)* **194,** 473–474.

Dieckmann, W. J., and Wegner, C. R. 1934. The blood in normal pregnancy. I. Blood in plasma volumes. *Arch. Intern. Med.* **53,** 71–86.

Dillingham, C. H. 1960. Familial occurrence of hemochromatosis: Report of four cases in siblings. *N. Engl. J. Med.* **262,** 1128–1130.

Donati, R. M., Warnecke, M. A., and Gallagher, N. I. 1966. *In vivo* reticulocyte radioiron assimilation. *J. Nucl. Med.* **7,** 928–934.

Douglas, A. S., and Dacie, J. V. 1953. Incidence and significance of iron-containing granules in human erythrocytes and their precursors. *J. Clin. Pathol.* **6,** 307–313.

Dowdle, E. B., Schachter, D., and Schenker, H. 1960. Active transport of Fe^{59} by everted segments of rat duodenum. *Amer. J. Physiol.* **198,** 609–613.

Drabkin, D. L. 1951. Metabolism of the hemin chromoproteins. *Physiol. Rev.* **31,** 345–431.

Dressel, E. I. B., and Falk, J. E. 1956. Studies on the biosynthesis of blood pigments. 3. Haeme and porphyrin formation from δ-aminolaevulic acid and from porphobilinogen in haemolysed chicken erythrocytes. *Biochem. J.* **63,** 80–87.

Dreyfus, J. C., and Schapira, G. 1963. Metabolisme du fer dans l'hemochromatose. *Congr. Franc. Med. (Les Hemochromatoses)* **34,** 11–34.

Dreyfus, J. C., and Schapira, G. 1964. The metabolism of iron in haemochromatosis. In; *Iron Metabolism: An International Symposium* (F. Gross, ed.). Springer-Verlag, Berlin, pp. 296–325.

Dreyfus, J. C., Schapira, G., Schwarzmann, V., and Abbou, R. 1960. Surcharge ferrique hépatique: Forme inapparente chez un fils d'hémochromatosique. *Presse Med.* **68,** 577–578.

Dubach, R., Callender, S. T., and Moore, C. V. 1948. Studies in iron transportation and metabolism: Absorption of radioactive iron in patients with fever and with anemias of varied etiology. *Blood* **3,** 526–540.

Ecker, J. A., Gray, P. A., McKittrick, J. E., and Dickson, D. R. 1968. The development of postshunt hemochromatosis–parenchymal siderosis in patients with cirrhosis occurring after portasystemic shunt surgery: A review of the literature and report of two additional cases. *Amer. J. Gastroenterol.* **50,** 13–29.

Ehrenberg, A., and Laurell, C.-B. 1955. Magnetic measurements on crystallized iron-transferrin isolated from the blood plasma of swine. *Acta Chem. Scand.* **9,** 68–72.

Ehrenberg, A., and Theorell, H. 1955. Stereochemical structure of cytochrome *c*. *Acta. Chem. Scand.* **9,** 1193–1205.

Elves, M. W., Bourne, M. S., and Israeëls, M. C. G. 1966. Pyridoxine-responsive anaemia determined by an X-linked gene. *J. Med. Genet.* **3,** 1–4.

Elwood, P. C. 1963. A clinical trial of iron-fortified bread. *Brit. Med. J.* **1,** 224–227.

Evans, G. W., and Grace, C. I. 1974. Interaction of transferrin with iron-binding sites on rat intestinal epithelial cell plasma membranes. *Proc. Soc. Exp. Biol. Med.* **147,** 687–689.

Fairbanks, V. F., Fahey, J. L., and Beutler, E. 1971. *Clinical Disorders of Iron Metabolism* 2nd ed. Grune and Stratton, New York, pp. 1–486.

Farquhar, J. D. 1963. Iron supplementation during first year of life. *Amer. J. Dis. Child.* **106,** 201–206.

Feigelson, P., and Greengard, O. 1961. The activation and induction of trypotophan pyrrolase during experimental porphyria and by amino-triazole. *Biochim. Biophys. Acta* **52,** 509–516.

Feuillen, Y. M., and Plumier, M. 1952. Iron metabolism in infants. I. The intake of iron in breastfeedings and artificial feeding (milk and milk foods). *Acta Pediatr.* (Stockholm) **41,** 138–144.

Fielding, J. 1967. Desferrioxamine chelatable body iron. *J. Clin. Pathol.* **20,** 668–670.

Fielding, J., O'Shaughnessy, M. C., and Brunström, G. M. 1965. Iron deficiency without anaemia. *Lancet* **2,** 9–12.

Fielding, J., O'Shaughnessy, M. C., and Brunström, G. M. 1966. Differential ferrioxamine test in idiopathic haemochromatosis and transfusional haemosiderosis. *J. Clin. Pathol.* **19,** 159–164.

Finch, C. A., and Bothwell, T. H. 1961. The syndrome of hemochromatosis (editorial). *Arch. Intern. Med. (Chicago)* **107,** 807–810.

Finch, C. A., Hegsted, M., Kinney, T. D., Thomas, E. D., Rath, C. E., Hoskins, D., Finch, S., and Fluharty, R. G. 1950. Iron metabolism: The pathophysiology of iron storage. *Blood* **5,** 983–1008.

Fischer, H., and Zeile, K. 1929. Syntheses of hematoporphyrin,protoporphyrin, and hemin. *Ann.* **468,** 98–116.

Fitch, W. M., and Margoliash, E. 1967. Construction of phylogenetic trees. *Science* **155,** 279–284.

Fletcher, J., and Huehns, E. R. 1967. Significance of the binding of iron by transferrin. *Nature (London)* **215,** 584–586.

Fontès, G., and Thivolle, L. 1925. Sur la teneur du serum en fer non hemoglobinique et sur sa diminution au cours de l'anemie experimentale. *C. R. Soc. Bio. (Paris)* **93,** 687–689.

Foy, H., and Kondi, A. 1957. Anaemias of the tropics: Relation to iron intake, absorption and losses during growth, pregnancy and lactation. *J. Trop. Med. Hyg.* **60,** 105–118.

Freeman, R. M., Vertel, R. M., and Esterling, R. E. 1966. Goodpasture's syndrome: Prolonged survival with chronic hemodialysis. *Arch. Intern. Med. (Chicago)* **117,** 643–647.

Fritz, J. C., Pla, G. W., Roberts, T., Baehne, J. W., and Have, E. L. 1970. Biological availability in animals of iron from common dietary sources. *Agric. Food Chem* **18,** 647–651.

Gabrio, B. W., and Salomon, K. 1950. Distribution of total ferritin in intestine and mesenteric lymph nodes of horses after iron feeding. *Proc. Soc. Exp. Biol. Med.* **75,** 124–127.

Gabrio, B. W., Shoden, A., and Finch, C. A. 1953. A quantitative fractionation of tissue ferritin and hemosiderin. *J. Biol. Chem.* **204,** 815–821.

Gajdos, A. 1966. Les enzymes de la biosynthèse de l'hème et leurs anomalies au cours de la thalassémie, l'anémie sidéroachrestique héréditaire et l'anémie sidéroblastique idiopathique acquise. *Nouv. Rev. Franc. Hematol.* **6,** 845–857.

Garby, L., Irnell, L., and Werner, I. 1969a. Iron deficiency in women of fertile age in a Swedish community. II. Efficiency of several laboratory tests to predict the response to iron supplementation. *Acta Med. Scand.* **185,** 107–111.

Garby, L., Irnell, L., and Werner, I. 1969b. Iron deficiency in women of fertile age in a Swedish community, III. Estimation of prevalence based on response to iron supplementation. *Acta Med. Scand.* **185,** 113–117.

Gardiol, D., Corbat, F., and Magnenat, P. 1967. Un cas d'hémochromatose secondaire aprés anastomose porto-cave. *Schweiz. Med. Wochenschr.* **97,** 1404–1498.

Garretson, F. D., and Conrad, M. E. 1967. Starch and iron absorption. *Proc. Soc. Exp. Biol. Med.* **126,** 304–308.

Gelpi, A. P., and Ende, N. 1958. An hereidtary anemia with hemochromatosis: Studies on an unusual hemopathic syndrome resembling thalassemia. *Amer. J. Med.* **25,** 303–314.

Gemzell, C. A., Robbe, H., and Sjöstrand, T. 1954. Blood volume and total amount of haemoglobin in normal pregnancy and the puerperium. *Acta Obstet. Gynecol. Scand.* **33,** 289–302.

Gidari, A. S., and Levere, R. D. 1977. Enzymatic formation and cellular regulation of heme synthesis. *Semin. Hematol.* **14,** 145–168.

Gitlin, D., Kumate, J., Urrusti, J., and Morales, C. 1964. The selectivity of the human placenta in the transfer of plasma proteins from mother to fetus. *J. Clin. Invest.* **43,** 1938–1951.

Goldberg, A. 1959. The enzymic formation of haem by the incorporation of iron into protoporphyrin: Importance of ascorbic acid, ergothioneine and glutathione. *Brit. J. Haematol.* **5,** 150–157.

Goldberg, A., Ashenbrucker, H., Cartwright, G. E., and Wintrobe, M. M. 1956. Studies on the biosynthesis of heme *in vitro* by avian eryhrocytes. *Blood* **11,** 821–833.

Goldberg, L., and Smith, J. P. 1960. Iron overloading and hepatic vulnerability. *Amer. J. Pathol.* **36,** 125–149.

Goodpasture, E. W. 1919. The significance of certain pulmonary lesions in relation to the etiology of influenza. *Amer. J. Med. Sci.* **158,** 863–870.

Gordon, W. G., Ziegler, J., and Basch, J. J. 1962. Isolation of an iron-binding protein from cow's milk. *Biochim. Biophys. Acta* **60,** 410–411.

Grace, N. D., and Balint, J. A. 1966. Hemochromatosis associated with end-to-side portacaval anastomosis. *Amer. J. Dig. Dis. N. Ser.* **11,** 351–358.

Granick, S. 1946. Ferritin. IX. Increase of the protein apoferritin in the gastrointestinal mucosa as a direct response to iron feeding. The function of ferritin in the regulation of iron absorption. *J. Biol. Chem.* **164,** 737–746.

Granick, S. 1951. Structure and physiological functions of ferritin. *Physiol. Rev.* **31,** 489–511.

Granick, S., and Michaelis, L. 1942. Ferritin and apoferritin. *Science* **95,** 439–440.

Green, S., and Mazur, A. 1957. Relation of uric acid metabolism to release of iron from hepatic ferritin. *J. Biol. Chem.* **227,** 653–668.

Green, S., Saha, A. K., Carleton, A. W., and Mazur, A. 1958. Release of storage iron to the plasma by xanthine oxidase after purine administration. *Fed. Proc. Fed. Amer. Soc. Exp. Biol.* **17,** 233.

Groves, M. L. 1960. The isolation of a red protein from milk. *J. Amer. Chem. Soc.* **82,** 3345–3350.

Gutelius, M. F., Millican, F. K., Layman, E. M., Cohen, G. J., and Dublin, C. C. 1962. Nutritional studies of children with pica. II. Treatment of pica with iron given intramuscularly. *Pediatrics* **29,** 1018–1023.

Haden, R. L. 1932. Simple achlorhydric anemia. *J. Amer. Med. Assoc.* **99,** 1398–1404.

Hahn, P. F., Bale, W. F., Lawrence, E. O., and Whipple, G. H. 1939. Radioactive iron and its metabolism in anemia: Its absorption, transportation, and utilization. *J. Exp. Med.* **69,** 739–753.

Hahn, P. F., Bale, W. F., Ross, J. F., Balfour, W. M., and Whipple, G. H. 1943. Radioactive iron absorption in gastro-intestinal tract: Influence of anemia, anoxia, and antecedent feeding distribution in growing dogs. *J. Exp. Med.* **78,** 169–188.

Hallberg, L., and Sölvell, L. 1967. Absorption of hemoglobin iron in man. *Acta Med. Scand.* **181,** 335–354.

Hallgren, B. 1954. Haemoglobin formation and storage of iron in protein deficiency. *Acta Soc. Med. Ups.* **59,** 79–208.

Halsted, J. A., Prasad, A. S., and Nadimi, M. 1965. Gastrointestinal function in iron deficiency anemia. *AMA Arch. Intern. Med.* **66,** 508–516.

Hamilton, E., Williams, R., Barlow, K. A., and Smith, P. M. 1968. The arthropathy of idiopathic haemochromatosis. *Q. J. Med.* **37,** 171–182.

Handler, P., Rajogopalan, K. V., and Aleman, V. 1964. Structure and function of iron flavoproteins. *Fed. Proc. Fed. Amer. Soc. Exp. Biol.* **23,** 30–38.

Hansen, H. A., and Weinfeld, A. 1959. Hemosiderin estimations and sideroblast counts in the differential diagnosis of iron deficiency and other anemias. *Acta Med. Scand.* **165,** 333–356.

Harris, C. 1957. The vicious circle of anaemia and menorrhagia. *Canad. Med. Assoc. J.* **77,** 98–100.

Harris, E. B., MacGibbon, B. H., and Mollin, D. L. 1965. Experimental sideroblastic anaemia. *Brit. J. Haematol.* **11,** 99–106.

Harris, J. W., Whittington, R. M., Weisman, R., Jr., and Horrigan, D. L. 1956. Pyridoxine responsive anemia in the human adult. *Proc. Soc. Exp. Biol. Med.* **91,** 427–432.

Harrison, P. M. 1977. Ferritin: An iron-storage molecule. *Semin. Hematol.* **14,** 55–70.

Hartman, R. S., Conrad, M. E., Jr., Hartman, R. E., Joy, R. J. T., and Crosby, W. H. 1963. Ferritin-containing bodies in human small intestinal epithelium. *Blood* **22,** 397–405.

Hawksley, J. C., Lightwood, R., and Bailey, U. M. 1934. Iron deficiency anaemia in children: Its association with gastrointestinal disease, achlorhydria and haemorrhage. *Arch. Dis. Child.* **9,** 359–372.

Hayhoe, F. G., and Quaglino, D. 1960. Refractory sideroblastic anaemia and erythaemic myelosis: Possible reltionship and cytochemical observations. *Brit. J. Haematol.* **6,** 381–387.

Heath, C. W., and Patek, A. J., Jr. 1937. Anemia of iron deficiency. *Medicine (Baltimore)* **16,** 267–350.

Heath, C. W., Strauss, M. B., and Castle, W. B. 1932. Quantitative aspects of iron deficiency in hypochromic anemia (the parenteral administration of iron). *J. Clin. Invest.* **11,** 1293–1312.

Hegsted, D. M., Finch, C. A., and Kinney, T. D. 1949. The influence of diet on iron absorption. II. The interrelation of iron and phosphorus. *J. Exp. Med.* **90,** 147–156.

Heilmeyer, L. 1966. *Disturbances in Heme Synthesis: Special Considerations of the Sideroachrestic Anemias and Erythropoietc Porphyrias.* Charles C. Thomas, Springfield, Illinois, pp. 103–178.

Heilmeyer, L., and Plötner, K. 1937. Das Serumeisen und die Eisenmangelkrankheit (Pathogenese, Symptomatologie und Therapie). G. Fischer, Jena, Germany, pp. 1–92.

Heilmeyer, L., Emmrich, J., Hennenann, H. H., Schubothe, H., Keiderling, W., Lee, M. H., Bilger, R., and Bernauer, W. 1957. Über eine neuartige hypochrome Anämie bei zwei Geschwistern auf der Grundlage einer Eisenverwertungsstörung: Anaemia sideroachrestica hereditaria. *Schweiz. Med. Wochenschr.* **87,** 1237–1238.

Heilmeyer, L., Keller, W., Vivell, O., Betke, K., Wöehler, F., and Keiderling, W. 1961. Die kongenitale Atransferrinämie. *Schweiz. Med. Wochenschr.* **91,** 1203–1205.

Heiner, D. C., Sears, J. W., and Kniker, W. T. 1962. Multiple precipitins to cow's milk in chronic respiratory disease: A syndrome including poor growth, gastrointestinal symptoms, evidence of allergy, iron deficiency anemia, and pulmonary hemosiderosis. *Amer. J. Dis. Child.* **103,** 634–654.

Heinrich, H. C. 1968. Iron deficiency without anaemia. *Lancet* **2,** 460.

Hines, J. D. 1969. Reversible megaloblastic and sideroblastic marrow abnormalities in alcoholic patients. *Brit. J. Haematol.* **16,** 87–101.

Hines, J. D. 1975. Hematologic abnormalities involving vitamin B_6 and folate metabolism in alcoholic subjects. *Ann. N. Y. Acad. Sci.* **252,** 316–327.

Hines, J. D., and Grasso, J. A. 1970. The sideroblastic anemias. *Semin. Hematol.* **7,** 86–106.

Hines, J. D., and Harris, J. M. 1964. Pyridoxine-responsive anemia: Description of three patients with megaloblastic erythropoiesis. *Amer. J. Clin. Nutr.* **14,** 137–146.

Hiyeda, K. 1939. The cause of Kaschin–Beck's disease. *Jpn. J. Med. Sci. Biol.* **4,** 91–106.

Hoffbauer, F. W. 1960. Primary biliary cirrhosis: Observations on the natural course of the disease in 25 women. *Amer. J. Dig. Dis.* **5,** 348–383.

Holmberg, C. G., and Laurell, C.-B. 1947. Investigations in serum copper. I. Nature of serum copper and its relation to the iron-binding protein in human serum. *Acta Chem. Scand.* **1,** 944–950.

Horeau, J., Nicolas, G., Lerous, M.-J., Babin-Chevaye, L., and Robin, C. 1964. Étude anatomo-clinique du coeur dans l'hémochromatose idiopathique. *Med. Monde* **40,** 132–136.

Horns, H. L. 1949. Hemochromatosis: Cardiac failure associated with extensive hemosiderosis of the myocardium. *Amer. J. Med.* **6,** 272–274.

Horrigan, D. L., and Harris, J. W. 1964. Pyridoxine-responsive anemia: Analysis of 62 cases. *Adv. Intern. Med.* **12,** 103–174.

Houston, J. C. 1951. Haemochromatosis and refractory anemia. *Guy Hosp. Rep.* **100,** 355–361.

Hwang, Y.-F., and Brown, E. B. 1964. Evaluation of deferoxamine in iron overload. *Arch. Intern. Med.* (Chicago) **114,** 741–753.

Ingram, D. J. E., Gibson, J. F., and Perutz, M. F. 1956. Orientation of the four haem groups in haemoglobin. *Nature (London)* **178,** 906–908.

Jacob, F., and Monod, J. 1961. Genetic regulatory mechanisms in the synthesis of proteins. *J. Mol. Biol.* **3,** 318–356.

Jacobs, A., and Butler, E. B. 1965. Menstrual blood-loss in iron-deficiency anaemia. *Lancet* **2,** 407–409.

Jacobs, A., Kilpatrick, G. S., and Withey, J. L. 1965. Iron deficiency anaemia in adults: Prevalence and prevention. *Postgrad. Med. J.* **41,** 418–424.

Jacobs, P., Bothwell, T. H., and Charlton, R. W. 1966. Intestinal iron transport: Studies using a loop of gut with an artificial circulation. *Amer. J. Physiol.* **210,** 694–700.

Jandl, J. H., and Katz, J. H. 1963. The plasma-to-cell cycle of transferrin. *J. Clin. Invest.* **42,** 314–326.

Jandl, J. H., Inman, J. K., Simmons, R. L., and Allen, D. W. 1959. Transfer of iron from serum iron-binding protein to human reticulocytes. *J. Clin. Invest.* **38,** 161–185.

Johannson, B. 1960. Isolation of iron-containing red protein from human milk. *Acta Chem. Scand.* **14,** 510–512.

Johnson, B. F. 1968. Hemochromatosis resulting from prolonged oral iron therapy. *N. Engl. J. Med.* **278,** 1100–1101.

Josephs, H. W. 1959. The iron of the newborn baby. *Acta Paediatr. (Stockholm)* **48,** 403–418.

Kaldor, I. 1958. Studies on intermediary iron metabolism. XII. Measurement of the iron derived from water soluble and water insoluble non-haem compounds (ferritin and haemosiderin iron) in liver and spleen. *Austral. J. Exp. Biol.* **36,** 173–182.

Kaplan, E., Zuelzer, W. W., and Mouriquand, C. 1954. Sideroblasts: Study of stainable non-hemoglobin iron in marrow normoblasts. *Blood* **9,** 203–213.

Katz, J. H. 1965. The delivery of iron to the immature red cell: A critical review. *Ser. Haematol.* **6,** 15–29.

Kelly, A. B. 1919. Spasm at the entrance to the esophagus. *J. Laryngol.* **34,** 285–289.

Kennedy, W. P. U., Shearman, D. J. C., Delamore, I. W., Simpson, J. D., Black, J. W., and Grant, I. W. B. 1966. Idiopathic pulmonary haemosiderosis with myocarditis: Radioisotope studies in a patient treated with prednisone. *Thorax* **21,** 220–229.

Keschner, H. W. 1951. The heart in hemochromatosis. *South. Med. J.* **44,** 927–930.

Kinney, T. D., Hegsted, D. M., and Finch, C. A. 1949. The influence of diet on iron absorption. I. The pathology of iron excess. *J. Exp. Med.* **90,** 137–146.

Kra, S. J., Hollingsworth, J. W., and Finch, S. C. 1965. Arthritis with synovial iron deposition in a patient with hemochromatosis. *N. Engl. J. Med.* **272,** 1268–1271.

Kroe, D. J., Kaufman, N., Klavins, J. V., and Kinney, T. D. 1966. Interrelation of amino acids and pH in intestinal iron absorption. *Amer. J. Physiol.* **211,** 414–418.

Krumbhaar, E. B., and Chanutin, A. 1922. Studies on experimental plethora in dogs and rabbits. *J. Exp. Med.* **35,** 847–871.

Kuhn, E., Brodan, V., Brodanova, M., and Friedmann, B. 1967. Influence of sleep deprivation on iron metabolism. *Nature (London)* **213,** 1041–1042.

Kurth, D., Deiss, A., and Cartwright, G. E. 1969. Circulating siderocytes in human subjects. *Blood* **34,** 754–764.

Kushner, J. P., Lee, G. R., Wintrobe, M. M., and Cartwright, G. E. 1971. Idiopathic refractory sideroblastic anemia: Clinical and laboratory investigation of 17 pateints and review of the literature. *Medicine (Baltimore)* **50,** 139–158.

Lamont, N. McE., and Hathorn, M. 1960. Increased plasma iron and liver pathology in Africans with porphyria. *S. Afr. Med. J.* **34,** 279–281.

Langhof, H., and Mildschlag, G. 1954. Aktinisch-traumatisch-bullöse Porphyrin-dermatose kombiniert mit beginnender Hamöchromatose. *Arch. Dermatol.* **199,** 21–32.

Laufberger, V. 1937. Sur la cristallisation de la ferritine. *Bull. Soc. Chim. Biol. (Paris)* **19,** 1575–1582.

Laurell, C.-B. 1952. Plasma iron and the transport of iron in the organism. *Pharmacol. Rev.* **4,** 371–395.

Layrisse, M., Martinex-Torres, C., Valez, F., and Gonzalez, M. 1976. Sugar as a vehicle for iron fortification. *Am. J. Clin. Nutr.* **29,** 8–18.

Leading article: Iron deficiency without anaemia. 1968. *Lancet* **1,** 462–463.

Lee, G. R., Cartwright, C. E., and Wintrobe, M. M. 1966. The response of free erythrocyte protoporphyrin to pyridoxine therapy in a patient with sideroachrestic (sideroblastic) anemia. *Blood* **27,** 557–567.

Lee, G. R., MacDiarmid, W. D., Cartwright, G. E., and Wintrobe, M. M. 1968. Hereditary X-linked sideroachrestic anemia. The isolation of two erythrocyte populations differing in X_ga blood type and porphyrin content. *Blood* **32,** 59–70.

Lee, S. L., Rosner, F., Rivero, I., Feldman, F., and Hurwitz, A. 1965. Refractory anemia with abnormal iron metabolism: Its remission after resection of hyperplastic mediastinal lymph nodes. *N. Engl. J. Med.* **272,** 761–766.

Lees, F., and Rosenthal, F. D. 1958. Gastric mucosal lesions before and after treatment in iron deficiency anemia. *Q. J. Med.* **27,** 19–26.

Lichtman, H. C., and Feldman, F. 1963. *In vitro* pyrrole and porphyrin synthesis in lead poisoning and iron deficiency. *J. Clin. Invest.* **42,** 830–839.

Lipschitz, D. A., Cook, J. D., and Finch, C. A. 1974. A clinical evaluation of serum ferritin as an index of iron stores. *N. Engl. J. Med.* **290,** 1213–1216.

Losowsky, M. S. 1966. Effects of desferrioxamine in patients with iron-loading with a simple method for estimating urinary iron. *J. Clin. Pathol.* **19,** 165–169.

Losowsky, M. S., and Hall, R. 1965. Hereditary sideroblastic anaemia. *Brit. J. Haematol.* **11,** 70–85.

Losowsky, M. S., and Wilson, A. R. 1967. Whole-body counting of the absorption and distribution of iron in haemochromatosis. *Clin. Sci.* **32,** 151–160.

Lukl, P., Wiedermann, B., and Barborik, M. 1958. Hereditäre Leptocytsen-anämie bei Männern mit Hämochromatose. *Folia Haematol.(Leipzig)* **3,** 17–45.

Lumeng, L., and Li, T. K. 1974. Vitamin B_6 metabolism in chronic alcohol abuse: Pyridoxal phosphate levels in plasma and the effects of acetaldehyde on pyridoxal phosphate synthesis and degradation in erythrocytes. *J. Clin. Invest.* **53,** 693–704.

Lüthi, H., Sordat, B., and Bütler, R. 1968. Therapieresistente Anämie und humorale Veränderungen bei plasmacellulärem hämosiderotischem Tumor im Mesenterium: Ein besonderes Syndrom? *Schweiz. Med. Wochenschr.* **98,** 816–821.

MacDonald, R. A. 1960. Experimental pigment cirrhosis: Its production in rats by feeding a choline-deficient diet with excess iron. *Amer. J. Pathol.* **36,** 499–519.

MacDonald, R. A. 1963. Idiopathic hemochromatosis: Genetic or acquired? *Arch. Intern. Med. (Chicago)* **112,** 184–190.

MacDonald, R. A. 1964. *Hemochromatosis and Hemosiderosis.* Charles C. Thomas, Springfield, Illinois, pp. 1–374.

MacDonald, R. A., and Mallory, G. K. 1960. Hemochromatosis and hemosiderosis: Study of 211 autopsied cases. *Arch. Intern. Med. (Chicago)* **105,** 686–700.

MacDonald, R. A., and Pechet, G. S. 1965. Experimental hemochromatosis in rats. *Amer. J. Pathol.* **46,** 85–109.

MacDonald, R. A., Jones, R. S., and Pechet, G. S. 1965. Folic acid deficiency and hemochromatosis. *Arch. Pathol. (Chicago)* **80,** 153–160.

MacDonald, R. A., Endo, H., and Pechet, G. S. 1968a. Pathogenesis of experimental hemochromatosis: Reticuloendothelial system disorder and excess iron. *Gastroenterology* **54,** 161 (abstract).

MacDonald, R. A., Endo, H., and Pechet, G. S. 1968b. Studies of experimental hemochromatosis: Disorder of the reticuloendothelial system and excess iron. *Arch. Pathol. (Chicago)* **85,** 366–387.

MacGibbon, B. H., and Mollin, D. L. 1965. Sideroblastic anaemia in man: Observations on seventy cases. *Brit. J. Haematol.* **11,** 59–69.

MacGregor, C. S., Johnson, R. S., and Turk, K. A. D. 1960. Fatal nephritis complicating idiopathic pulmonary haemosiderosis in young adults. *Thorax* **15,** 198–203.

Maddock, R. K., Jr., Stevens, L. E., Reemtsma, K., and Bloomer, H. A. 1967. Goodpasture's syndrome: Cessation of pulmonary hemorrhage after bilateral nephrectomy. *Ann. Intern. Med.* **67,** 1258–1264.

Mahler, H. R., and Elowe, D. G. 1953. DPNH-cytochrome reductase, a ferro-flavo protein. *J. Amer. Chem. Soc.* **75,** 5769–5770.

Maier, C. 1966. Eisenmangel ohne Anämie: Die Hämatologie des praktischen Arztes. *Praxis* **55,** 54–58.

Margoliash, E., Frohwirt, N., and Wiener, E. 1959. A study of the cytochrome C haemochromogen. *Biochem. J. (London)* **71,** 559–570.

Martinez-Torres, C., and Layrisse, M. 1974. Interest for the study of dietary absorption and iron fortification. *World Rev. Nutr. Dietet.* **19,** 51–70.

Matsaniotis, N., Karpouzas, J., Apostolopoulo, E., and Messaritakis, J. 1968. Idiopathic pulmonary haemosiderosis in children. *Arch. Dis. Child.* **43,** 307–309.

Mazur, A., Green, S., Saha, A., and Carleton, A. 1958. Mechanism of release of ferritin iron *in vivo* by xanthine oxidase. *J. Clin. Invest.* **37,** 1809–1817.

McCance, R. A., and Widdowson, E. M. 1937. Absorption and excretion of iron. *Lancet* **2,** 680–684.

McCance, R. A., and Widdowson, E. M. 1938. The absorption and excretion of iron following oral and intravenous administration. *J. Physiol. (London)* **94,** 148–154.

McCance, R. A., and Widdowson, E. M. 1951. Composition of the body. *Brit. Med. Bull.* **7,** 297–306.

McFarlane, D. B., Pinkerton, P. H., Dagg, J. H., and Goldberg, A. 1967. Incidence of iron deficiency, with and without anaemia, in women in general practice. *Brit. J. Haematol.* **13,** 790–796.

Mendel, G. A. 1961. Studies on iron absorption. I. The relationships between the rate of erythropoiesis, hypoxia and iron absorption. *Blood* **18,** 727–736.

Mendel, G. A., Weiler, R. J., and Mangalik, A. 1963. Studies on iron absorption. II. The absorption of iron in experimental anemias of diverse etiogy. *Blood* **22,** 450–458.

Mengel, C. E., Carter, W. A., and Horton, E. S. 1964. Geophagia with iron deficiency and hypokalemia: Cachexia Afrikana. *Arch. Intern. Med. (Chicago)* **114,** 470–474.

Mielke, H. G. 1953. Hämochromatose—ein seltenes Krakheitsbild bei der Frau. *Arztl. Wochnschr.* **8,** 646–648.

Minnich, V., Okcuoglu, A., Tarcon, Y., Arcasoy, A., Cin, S., Yörükoglu, O., Renda, F. and Demirag, B. 1968. Pica in Turkey. II. Effect of clay upon iron absorption. *Amer. J. Clin. Nutr.* **21,** 78–86.

Mollin, D. L. 1965. Sideroblasts and sideroblastic anemia. *Brit. J. Hematol.* 11, 41–48.

Monsen, E. R., Kuhn, I. N., and Finch, C. A. 1967. Iron status of menstruating women. *Amer. J. Clin. Nutr.* **20,** 842–849.

Moore, C. V. 1955 The importance of nutritional factors in the pathogenesis of iron-deficiency anemia. *Amer. J. Clin. Nutr.* **3,** 3–10.

Moore, C. V., and Dubach, R. 1951. Observations on absorption of iron from foods tagged with radioiron. *Trans. Assoc. Amer. Physicians* **64,** 245–256.

Moore, C. V., and Dubach, R. 1956. Metabolism and requirements of iron in the human. *J. Amer. Med. Assoc.* **162,** 197–204.

Moore, C. V., Doan, C. A., and Arrowsmith, W. R. 1937. Studies in iron transportation and metabolism; mechanism of iron transportation: Its significance in iron utilization in anemic states of varied etiology. *J. Clin. Invest.* **16,** 627–1937.

Morgan, E. H. 1961. Plasma-iron and haemoglobin levels in pregnancy: The effect of oral iron. *Lancet* **1,** 9–12.

Morgan, E. H. 1963. Exchange of iron and transferrin across endothelial surfaces in the rat and rabbit. *J. Physiol. (London)* **169,** 339–352.

Morgan, E. H. 1964a. The interaction between the rabbit, human and rat transferrin and reticulocytes. *Brit. J. Haematol.* **10,** 442–452.

Morgan, E. H. 1964b. Passage of transferrin, albumin, and gamma globulin from maternal plasma to fetus in the rat and rabbit. *J. Physiol. (London)* **171,** 26–41.

Morgan, E. H., and Appleton, T. C. 1969. Autoradiographic localization of 125-I-labelled transferrin in rabbit reticulocytes. *Nature (London)* **223,** 1371–1372.

Morgan, E. H., and Baker, E. 1969. The effect of metabolic inhibitors on transferrin and iron and transferrin release from reticulocytes. *Biochim. Biophys. Acta* **184,** 442–454.

Morgan, E. H., and Laurell, C. B. 1963. Studies on the exchange of iron between transferrin and reticulocytes. *Brit. J. Haematol.* **9,** 471–483.

Morgan, E. H., and Walters, M. N. I. 1963. Iron storage in human disease: Fractionation of hepatic and splenic iron into ferritin and haemosiderin with histochemical correlations. *J. Clin. Pathol.* **16,** 101–107.

Morgan. E. H., Huehns, E. R., and Finch, C. A. 1966. Iron reflux from reticulocytes and bone marrow cells *in vitro. Amer. J. Physiol.* **210,** 579–585.

Morningstar, W. A. 1955. Exogenous hemochromatosis: A report of three cases. *Arch. Pathol. (Chicago)* **59,** 355–358.

Morrison, S. D. 1952. Human milk yield, proximate principles, and inorganic constituents. Tech. communication No. 18 of Commonwealth Bureau of Animal Nutrition, Rowell Research Institute, Backsburn, Aberdeenshire, Scotland, Commonwealth Agricultural Bureau, Farnham Royal Slough, Bucks, England, pp. 1–99.

Morse, W. I., and Read, H. C. 1954. Stainable iron in marrow cells and erythrocytes in anemia. *Canad. Serv. Med. J.* **10,** 244–252.

Muir, A. R. 1960. The molecular structure of isolated and intracellular ferritin. *Quart. J. Exp. Physiol. Cogn. Med. Sci.* **45,** 192–201.

Mukherjee, C., and Mukherjee, S. K. 1953. Studies in iron metabolism in anaemias in pregnancy. *J. Indian Med. Assoc.* **22,** 345–351.

Munro, J. F., Geddes, A. M., and Lamb, W. L. 1967. Goodpasture's syndrome: Survival after acute renal failure. *Brit. Med. J.* **4,** 95.

Murphy, K. J. 1965. Pulmonary haemosiderosis (apparently idiopathic) associated with myocarditis, with bilateral penetrating corneal ulceration, and with diabetes mellitus. *Thorax* **20,** 341–347.

National Health and Medical Research Council Report (Canberra), No. 1. 1945.

Neerhout, R. C., Larson, W., and Mansur, P. 1969. Mesenteric lymphoid hamartoma associated with chronic hypoferremia, anemia, growth failure, and hyperglobulinemia. *N. Engl. J. Med.* **280,** 922–925.

Niccum, W. L., Jackson, R. L., and Stearns, G. 1953. Use of ferric and ferrous iron in the prevention of hypochromic anemia in infants. *Amer. J. Dis. Child.* **96,** 5533–5567.

Nissim, J. A. 1953. Experimental siderosis: A study of the distribution, delayed effects, and metabolism of massive amounts of various iron preparations. *J. Pathol.* **66,** 185–204.

Nixon, D. D. 1966. Spontaneous shunt siderosis. *Amer. J. Dig. Dis.* **11,** 359–366.

Noyes, W. D., Bothwell, T. H., and Finch, C. A. 1960. The role of the reticulo-endothelial cell in iron metabolism. *Brit. J. Haematol.* **6,** 43–55.

Noyes, W. D., Hosain, F., and Finch, C. A. 1964. Incorporation of radioiron into marrow heme. *J. Lab. Clin. Med.* **64,** 574–580.

O'Dell, B. L., Hardwock, B. C., and Reynolds, G. 1961. Mineral deficiencies of milk and congenital malformations in the rat. *J. Nutr.* **73,** 151–157.

Osaki, S., and Sirivech, S. 1971. Identification and partial purification of ferritin reducing enzyme in liver. *Fed. Proc. Fed. Am. Soc. Exp. Biol.* **30,** 1292 (abstract)

Palacio, J., Sanchez, B., Hojman, D., and Perez, A. H. 1960. Hemochromatosis: Forma cardíaca juvenil. *Prensa Med. Argent.* **47,** 2943–2949.

Paléus, S., Ehrenberg, A., and Tuppy, H. 1955. II. Investigation of the linkage between peptide moiety and prosthetic group. *Acta Chem. Scand.* **9,** 365–374.

Paterson, D. R. 1919. A clinical type of dysphagia. *J. Laryngol.* **24,** 289–291.

Patterson, J. C. S., Marrack, D., and Wiggins, H. S. 1953. The diurnal variation of the serum iron level in erythropoietic disorders. *J. Clin. Pathol.* **6,** 105–109.

Perkins, K. W., McInnes, I. W. S., Blackburn, C. R. B., and Beal, R. W. 1965. Idiopathic haemochromatosis in children: Report of a family. *Amer. J. Med.* **39,** 118–126.

Peterson, R. E., and Ettinger, R. H. 1953. Radiactive iron absorption in siderosis (hemochromatosis) of the liver. *Amer. J. Med.* **15,** 518–524.

Petit. D. W. 1945. Hemochromatosis with complete heart block: With a discussion of the cardiac complications. *Amer. Heart J.* **29,** 253–260.

Pirzio-Biroli, G., Bothwell, T. H., and Finch, C. A. 1958. Iron absorption. II. The absorption of radioiron administered with a standard meal in man. *J. Lab. Clin. Med.* **51,** 37–48.

Platzer, R. F., Young, L. E., and Yuile, C. L. 1955. Hemosiderosis resembling hemochromatosis following multiple transfusions. *Acta Haematol. (Basel)* **14,** 185–192.

Pletcher, W. D., Brody, G. L., and Meyers, M. C. 1963. Hemochromatosis following prolonged iron therapy in a patient with hereditary nonspherocytic hemolytic anemia. *Amer. J. Med. Sci.* **246,** 27–34.

Ploem, J. E., Wael, J. de, Verloop, M. C., and Punt, K. 1966. Sideruria following a single dose of desferrioxamine-B as a diagnostic test in iron overload. *Brit. J. Haematol.* **12,** 396–408.

Pollycove, M. 1958. Iron kinetics. In: *Iron in Clinical Medicine* (R. O. Wallerstein and S. R. Mettier, eds.). University of California Press, Berkeley, pp. 43–57.

Pollycove, M., and Mortimer, R. 1961. The quantitative determination of iron kinetics and hemoglobin synthesis in human subjects. *J. Clin. Invest.* **40,** 753–782.

Polson, C. J. 1929a. The storage of iron following its oral and subcutaneous administration. *Q. J. Med.* **23,** 77–84.

Polson, C. J. 1919b. The fate of colloidal iron administered intravenously. II. Long experiments. *J. Pathol.* **32,** 247–260.

Popper, H. P., and Schaffner, F. 1957. *Liver: Structure and Function.* McGraw-Hill, New York, 777 pp.

Portella, A., Guida, V., and Valerio, V. 1957. Su di un caso di emocromatosi giovanile con alterazioni endocrine. *Riforma Med.* **71,** 1246–1254.

Powell, L. W., and Thomas, M. J. 1967. Use of diethylenetriamine penta-acetic acid (D.T.P.A.) in the clinical assessment of total body iron stores. *J. Clin. Pathol.* **20,** 896–904.

Prasad, A. S. 1966. Zinc metabolism and its deficiency in human subjects, In: *Zinc Metabolism* (A. S. Prasad, ed.). Charles C. Thomas, Springfield, Illinois, pp. 250–302.

Prasad, A. S., and Oberleas, D. 1971. Binding of iron to amino acids and serum proteins *in vitro. Proc. Soc. Exp. Biol. Med.* **138,** 932–935.

Prasad, A. S., Halsted, J. A., and Nadimi, M. 1961. Syndrome of iron deficiency anemia, hepatosplenomegaly, hypogonadism, dwarfism, and geophagia. *Amer. J. Med.* **31,** 532–546.

Prasad, A. S., Tranchida, L., Konno, E. T., Berman, L., Albert, S.. Sing, C. F., and Brewer, G. J. 1968. Hereditary sideroblastic anemia and glucose-6-phosphate dehydrogenase deficiency in a Negro family. *J. Clin. Invest.* **47,** 1415–1424.

Prato, V., Chiandussi, L., Massaro, A., Massa, U., and Zina, G. 1964. La porfiria cutanea tarda ereditaria. *Minerva Med.* **55,** 1897–1905.

Price, D. C., Epstein, J. H., Winchell, H. S., Sargent, T. W., Pollycove, M., and Cavalieri, R. R. 1968. Iron kinetics in porphyria cutanea tarda. *Clin. Res.* **16,** 1–124.

Quaglino, D., and Hayhoe, F. G. 1960. Periodic-acid–Schiff positivity in erythroblasts with special reference to Di Guglielmo's disease. *Brit. J. Haematol.* **6,** 26–33.

Raab, S. O., Haut, A., Cartwright, G. E., and Wintrobe, M. M. 1961. Pyridoxine-response anemia. *Blood* **18,** 285–302.

Rather, L. J. 1956. Hemochromatosis and hemosiderosis: Does iron overload cause diffuse fibrosis of the liver? *Amer. J. Med.* **21,** 857–866.

Recommended Dietary Allowances, 8th ed. 1974. National Research Council, National Academy of Sciences, Washington, D. C.

Reeves, G., Rigby, P. G., Rosen, H., Friedell, G. H., and Emerson, C. P. 1963. Hemochromatosis and congenital nonspherocytic hemolytic anemia in siblings. *J. Amer. Med. Assoc.* **186,** 123–126.

Reimann, F., Fritsch, F., and Schick, K. 1937. Eisenbilanzversuche bei Gesunden und bei Anämischen. II. Untersuchungen über das Wesen der eisenempfindlichen Anämien ("Asiderosen") und der therapeutischen Wirkung des Eisens bei diesen Anämien. *Z. Klin. Med.* **131,** 1–50.

Reimann, F., 1955. Wachstumsanomalien und Missbildungen bei Eisenmangelzuständen (Asiderosen). In: *5th Kongress der europäischen Gesellschaft für Hämatologie,* Freiburg, pp. 546–550.

Reynolds, R. D., Binder, H. J., Miller, M. B., Chang, W. W. Y., and Horan, S. 1968. Pagophagia and iron deficiency anemia. *Ann. Intern. Med.* **69,** 435–440.

Richert, D. A., and Westerfeld, W. W. 1954. The relationship of iron to xanthine oxidase. *J. Biol. Chem.* **209,** 179–189.

Rimington, C. 1959. Biosynthesis of haemoglobin. *Brit. Med. Bull.* **15,** 19–29.

Roath, S., Bourne, M. S., and Israëls, M. C. G. 1964. Ferrokinetics in pyridoxine-responsive anaemia. *Acta Haematol. (Basel)* **32,** 1–8.

Rosselin, G. 1964. Ëtude ferrodynamique de l'hémochromatose primitive. *Med. Monde* **40,** 107–115.

Rothen, A. 1944. Ferritin and apoferritin in the ultracentrifuge: Studies on the relationship of ferritin and apoferritin; precision measurements of the rates of sedimentation of apoferritin. *J. Biol. Chem.* **152,** 679–693.

Rothstein, G., Lee, G. R., and Cartwright, G. E. 1969. Sideroblastic anemia with dermal photosensitivity and greatly increased erythrocyte protoporphyrin. *N. Engl. J. Med.* **280,** 587–590.

Rous, P., and Oliver, J. 1918. Experimental hemochromatosis. *J. Exp. Med.* **28,** 629–644.

Rundles, R. W., and Falls, H. F. 1946. Hereditary (?sex-linked)anemia. *Amer. J. Med. Sci. N. Ser.* **211,** 641–658.

Rybo, G. 1966. Clinical and experimental studies on menstrual blood loss. *Acta Obstet. Gynecol. Scand.* **45,** Suppl. 7, pp. 1–23.

Salmon, H. A. 1962. The cytochrome *c* content of the heart, kidney, liver, and skeletal muscle of iron-deficient rats. *J. Physiol. (London)* **164,** 17–30.

Saltzer, E. I., Redeker, A. G., and Wilson, J. W. 1968. Porphyria cutanea tarda: Remission following cloroquine administration without adverse effects. *Arch. Dermatol. (Chicago)* **98,** 496–498.

Sargent, T., and Winchell, H. S. 1967. Iron absorption in hemochromatosis before and after therapy. *Clin. Res.* **15,** 107 (abstract).

Sauer, G. F., and Funk, D. D. 1969. Iron overload in cutaneous porphyria. *Arch. Intern. Med. (Chicago)* **124,** 190–196.

Saunders, S. J. 1963. Iron metabolism in symptomatic porphyria: A preliminary communication. *S. Afr. J. Lab. Clin. Med.* **9,** 277–282.

Scandellari, C., Dobrilla, G., Bosello, O., Cavallini, G., Lo Cascio, V., and Cartei, G. 1967. Sulla validità della ferrocinetica mediante Fe^{59} per la diagnosi differenziale tra siderocromatosi idiopatica e secondaria epatopatica. *Acta Isot. (Padova)* **7,** 117–134.

Schade, A. L., Reinhart, R. W., and Levy, H. 1949. Carbon dioxide and oxygen in complex formation with iron and siderophilin, the iron-binding component of human plasma. *Arch. Biochem.* **20,** 170–172.

Schaefer, J. W., Amick, C. J., Oikawa, Y., and Schiff, L. 1962. The development of hemochromatosis following portacaval anastomosis. *Gastroenterology* **42,** 181–188.

Schapira, G., Dreyfus, J.-C., Schwarzmann, V., and Étévé, J. 1962. Hypersidérémie et surcharge ferrique hépatique chez les decendents d'hémochromatosiques. *Rev. Franc. Etud. Clin. Biol.* **7,** 485–491.

Schmid, J. R., Oechslin, R. J., and Schnider, Th. 1964a. Ferrokinetische Untersuchungen bei primärer Hämochromatose und sideroachrestischer Anämie. *Schweiz. Med. Wochenschr.* **94,** 1158–1164.

Schmid, J. R., Oechslin, R. J., Schnider, Th., and Moeschlin, S. 1964b. Ein einfacher 6 stündiger i.m. Test mit Desferrioxamin-B (Desferal) zur Diagnose der Hämochromatose. *Schweiz. Med. Wochenschr.* **94,** 1652.-1655.

Schreiber, A. W. 1957. Hemochromatosis and the heart. *Ann. Intern. Med.* **47,** 1015–1021.

Schubert, W. K., and Lahey, M. E. 1959. Copper and protein depletion complicating hypoferric anemia of infancy. *Pediatrics* **24,** 710–733.

Settlemire, C. T., and Matrone, G. 1967a. *In vivo* interference of zinc with ferritin iron in the rat. *J. Nutr.* **92,** 153–158.

Settlemire, C. T., and Matrone, G. 1967b. *In vivo* effect of zinc on iron turnover in rats and life span of the erythrocyte. *J. Nutr.* **92,** 159–164.

Shahidi, N. T. 1964. Anémie hypochrome par un trouble du métabolisme du fer. *Schweiz. Med. Wochenschr.* **94,** 1385–1386.

Shahidi, N. T., Nathan, D. G., and Diamond, L. K. 1964. Iron deficiency anemia associated with an error of iron metabolism in two siblings. *J. Clin. Invest.* **43,** 510–521.

Sheldon, J. H. 1935. *Haemochromatosis.* Oxford University Press, London, pp. 1–382.

Sherman, H. C. 1935. *Chemistry of Food and Nutrition.* Macmillan, New York, 640 pp.

Shoden, A., and Sturgeon, P. 1959. Iron storage. II. The influence of the type of compound administered on the distribution of iron between ferritin and hemosiderin. *Acta Haematol.* **22,** 140–145.

Shoden, A., and Sturgeon, P. 1960. Hemosiderin. I. A physico-chemical study. *Acta Haematol.* **23,** 376–392.

Shoden, A., and Sturgeon, P. 1961. Formation of haemosiderin and its relation to ferritin. *Nature (London)* **189,** 846–847.

Shoden, A., and Sturgeon, P. 1962. Iron storage, III. The influence of rates of administration of iron on its distribution between ferritin and hemosiderin. *Acta Haematol.* **27,** 33–46.

Shoden, A., and Sturgeon, P. 1963. On the formation of haemosiderin and its relation to ferritin. II. A radioisotopic study. *Brit. J. Haematol.* **9,** 513–522.

Siimes, M. A., Addiego, J. E., Jr. and Dallman, P. R. 1974. Ferritin in serum: Diagnosis of iron deficiency and iron overload in infants and children. *Blood* **43,** 581–590.

Sirivech, S., Frieden, E., and Osaki, S. 1974. The release of iron from horse spleen ferritin by reduced flavins. *Biochem. J.* **143,** 311–315.

Smith, H. D. 1964. Pediatric lead poisoning. *Arch Environ. Health (Chicago)* **8,** 256–261.

Smith, J. A., Drysdale, J. W., Goldberg, A., and Munroe, H. N. 1968. The effect of enteral and parenteral iron on ferritin syntehsis in the intestinal mucosa of the rat. *Brit. J. Haematol.* **14,** 79–86.

Smith, P. M., Studley, F., and Williams, R. 1967. Assessment of body-iron stores in cirrhosis and haemochromatosis with the differential ferrioxamine test. *Lancet* **1,** 133–136.

Smith, P. M., Lestas, A. N., Miller, J. P., Pitcher, C. S., Dymock, I. W., and Williams, R. 1969. The differential ferrioxamine test in the management of idiopathic haemochromatosis. *Lancet* **2,** 402–405.

Soergel, K. H., and Sommers, S. C. 1962. Idiopathic pulmonary hemosiderosis and related syndromes. *Amer. J. Med.* **32,** 499–511.

Spitzer, N., Newcomb, T. F., and Noyes, W. D. 1966. Pyridoxine-responsive hypolipidemia and hypocholesterolemia in a patient with pyridoxine-responsive anemia. *N. Engl. J. Med.* **274,** 772–775.

Srivastava, S. K., Sanwal, G. G., and Tewari, K. K. 1965. Biochemical alterations in rat tissue in iron deficiency anaemia and repletion with iron. *Indian J. Biochem.* **2,** 257–266.

Steiner, B., and Nabrady, J. 1965. Immunoallergic lung purpura treated with azathioprine. *Lancet* **1,** 140–141.

Stevens, A. R., Jr., Coleman, D. H., and Finch, C. A. 1953. Iron metabolism: Clinical evaluation of iron stores. *Ann. Intern. Med.* **38,** 199–205.

Stewart, W. B., Yuile, C. L., Clairborne, H. A., Snowman, R. T., and Whipple, G. H. 1950. Radioiron absorption in anemic dogs: Fluctuation in mucosal blocks and evidence for gradient of absorption in gastrointestinal tract. *J. Exp. Med.* **921,** 375–382.

Stocks, A. E., and Martin, F. I. R. 1968. Pituitary function in haemochromatosis. *Amer. J. Med.* **45,** 839–845.

Streeter, R. R., Presant, C. A., and Reinhard, E. 1977. Prognostic significance of thrombocytosis in idiopathic sideroblastic anemia. *Blood* **50,** 427–432.

Ströder, U. 1942. Infantilismus und Myokardfibrose bei der Hämochromatose. *Dsch. Arch. Klin. Med.* **189,** 141–166.

Sturgeon, P. 1956a. Studies in iron requirements in infants and children. II. The influence on normal infants of oral iron in therapeutic doses. *Pediatrics* **17,** 341–348.

Sturgeon, P. 1956b. Iron metabolism: A review with special consideration of iron requirements during normal infancy. *Pediatrics* **18,** 267–298.

Sturgeon, P. 1959. Studies of iron requirements in infants. III. Influence of supplemental iron during normal pregnancy on mother and infant. *Brit. J. Haematol.* **5,** 31–44.

Swan, W. G. A., and Dewar, H. A. 1952. The heart in haemochromatosis. *Brit. Heart J.* **14,** 117–124.

Swiss, L. D., and Beaton, G. H. 1974. A prediction of the effects of iron fortification. *Am. J. Clin. Nutr.* **27,** 373–379.

Synderman, S. E., Holt, L. E., Jr., Carretero, R., and Jacobs, K. 1953. Pyridoxine deficiency in the human infant. *J. Clin. Nutr.* **1,** 200–207.

Tisdale, W. A. 1961. Parenchymal siderosis in patients with cirrhosis after portasystemic-shunt surgery. *N. Engl. J. Med.* **265,** 928–932.

Tranchida, L., Palutke, M., Poulik, M. D., and Prasad, A. S. 1973. Primary acquired sideroblastic anemia preceding monoclonal gammopathy and malignant lymphoma. *Amer. J. Med.* **55,** 559–564.

Tuffanelli, D. L. 1960. Porphyria cutanea tarda associated with hemochromatosis. *U.S. Armed Forces Med. J.* **11,** 1210–1216.

Tuppy, H., and Paléus, S. 1955. A peptic degradation product of cytochrome *c*. I. Purification and chemical composition. *Acta Chem. Scand.* **9,** 353–364.

Turnberg, L. A. 1965. Excessive oral iron therapy causing haemochromatosis. *Brit. Med. J.* **1,** 1360.

Tuttle, S. G., Figueroa, W. G., and Grossman, M. I. 1959. Development of hemochromatosis in a patient with Laennec's cirrhosis. *Amer. J. Med.* **26,** 655–658.

Udenfriend, S. 1970. Biosynthesis of hydroxyproline in collagen. In: *Chemistry and Molecular Biology of the Intercellular Matrix,* Vol. (E. A. Balezs, ed.). Academic Press, New York, pp. 371–384.

Ulstrom, R. A., Smith, N. J., and Heinlich, E. M. 1956. Transient dysproteinemia in infants: A new syndrome. I. Clinical studies. *Am. J. Dis. Child.* **92,** 219–253.

Underwood, E. J. 1977. *Trace Elements in Human and Animal Nutrition,* 4th ed. Academic Press, New York, pp. 13–55.

Vahlquist, B. C. 1941. Das Serumeisen-eine pädiatrischklinische und experimentelle Studie. *Acta Paediatr. (Suppl. 5)* **28,** 1–374.

Vahlquist, B. 1950. The cause of the sexual differences in erythrocyte, hemoglobin and serum iron levels in human adults. *Blood* **5,** 874–875.

Van Campen, D. and Gross, E. 1969. Effect of histidine and certain other amino acids on the absorption of iron-59 by rats. *J. Nutr.* **99,** 68–74.

Vavra, J. D., and Poff, S. A. 1967. Heme and porphyrin synthesis in sideroblastic anemia. *J. Lab. Clin. Med.* **69,** 904–918.

Vavra, J. D., Mayer, V. K., and Moore, C. V. 1964. *In vitro* heme synthesis by human blood: Abnormal heme synthesis in thalassemia major. *J. Lab. Clin. Med.* **63,** 736–753.

Velez, H., Restrepo, A., Vitale, J. J., and Hellerstein, E. E. 1966. Folic acid deficiency secondary to iron deficiency in man: Remission with iron therapy and a diet low in folic acid. *Amer. J. Clin. Nutr.* **19,** 27–36.

Verloop, M. C., and Rademaker, W. 1960. Anaemia due to pyridoxine deficiency in man. *Brit. J. Haematol.* **6,** 66–80.

Verloop, M. C., Panders, J. T., Ploem, J. E., and Bos, C. C. 1964. Sideroachrestic anaemias. In: *International Society of Haematology, 10th Congress, Stockholm,* Vol. 5-6. Ejnar Munksgaards Forlag, Copenhagen, pp. 76–87.

Vilter, R. W., Mueller, J. F., Glazer, H. S., Jarrold, T., Abraham, J., Thompson, C., and Hawkins, V. R. 1953. The effect of vitamin B_6 deficiency induced by desoxypyridoxine in human beings. *J. Lab. Clin. Med.* **42,** 335–357.

Vinson, P. P. 1922. Hysterical dysphagia. *Minn. Med.* **5,** 107–108.

Vogler, W. R., and Mingioli, E. S. 1965. Heme synthesis in pyridoxine-responsive anemia. *N. Engl. J. Med.* **273,** 347–353.

Vogler, W. R., and Mingioli, E. S. 1968. Porphyrin synthesis and heme synthetase activity in pyridoxine-responsive anemia. *Blood* **32,** 979–988.

Vuylsteke, J., Verloop, M. C., and Drogendijk, A. C. 1961. Favorable effect of pyridoxine and ascorbic acid in a patient with refractory sideroblastic anaemia and haemochromatosis. *Acta Med. Scand.* **169,** 113–123.

Wallerstein, R. O., and Robbins, S. L. 1953. Hemochromatosis after prolonged oral iron therapy in a patient with chronic hemolytic anemia. *Amer. J. Med.* **14,** 256–260.

Walsh, J. R., Kaldor, I., Brading, I., and George, E. P. 1955. The availability of iron in meat: Some experiments with radioactive iron. *Aust. Ann. Med.* **4,** 272–276.

Walsh, J. R., Perkins, K. W., Blackburn, C. R., Sanford, R., and Cantrill, S. 1963. The use of DTPA in the diagnosis and management of idiopathic haemochromatosis. *Aust. Ann. Med.* **12,** 192–196.

Walsh, J. R., Mass, R. E., Smith, F. W., and Lange, V. 1965. Iron chelation with deferoxamine in hepatic disease. *Gastroenterology* **49,** 134–140.

Warembourg, H., Niquet, G., Ducloux, G., and Théry, C. 1965. Adiastolie par péricardite constrictive et hémochromatose. *Little Med.* **10,** 599–604.

Wasserman, A. J., Richardson, D. W., Baird, C. L., and Wyso, E. M. 1962. Cardiac hemochromatosis simulating constrictive pericarditis. *Amer. J. Med.* **32,** 316–323.

Weatherall, D. J., Pembrey, M. E., Hall, E. G. Sanger, R., Tippett, P., and Glavin, J. 1970. Familial sideroblastic anemia: Problem of X_g and X chromosome inactivation. *Lancet* **2,** 744–748.

Weintraub, L. R., Conrad, M. E., and Crosby, W. H. 1964. The role of hepatic iron stores in the control of iron absorption. *J. Clin. Invest.* **43,** 40–44.

Weintraub, L. R., Conrad, M. E., and Crosby, W. H. 1965. Regulation of the intestinal absorption of iron by the rate of erythropoiesis. *Brit. J. Haematol.* **11,** 432–438.

Weintraub, L. R., Weinstein, M. B., Huser, H., and Rafal, S. 1968. Absorption of hemoglobin iron: The role of a heme-splitting substance in the intestinal mucosa. *J. Clin. Invest.* **47,** 531–539.

Weiss, E. B., Earnest, D. L., and Greally, J. F. 1968. Goodpasture's syndrome: Case report with emphasis on pulmonary physiology. *Amer. Rev. Respir. Dis.* **97,** 444–450.

Wheby, M. S., and Crosby, W. H. 1963. The gastrointestinal tract and iron absorption. *Blood* **22,** 416–428.

Whipple, G. H., and Robscheit-Robbins, F. S. 1925. Blood regeneration in severe anemia. *Amer. J. Physiol.* **72,** 395–435.

W.H.O. Health Bulletin No. 23. 1951. Government of India Press, New Delhi.

Williams, D. M., Loukopoulos, D., Lee, G. R., and Cartwright, G. E. 1976. Role of copper in mitochondrial iron metabolism. *Blood* **48,** 77–85.

Williams, R., Smith, P. M., Spicer, E. J. F., Barry, M., and Sherlock, S. 1969. Venesection therapy in idiopathic haemochromatosis: An analysis of 40 treated and 18 untreated patients. *Q. J. Med.* **38,** 1–16.

Wilson, J. D., Scott, P. J., and North, J. D. K. 1967. Hemochromatosis in association with hereditary spherocytosis. *Arch. Intern. Med. (Chicago)* **120,** 701–707.

Wilson, J. F., Heiner, D. C., and Lahey, M. E. 1962. Studies on iron from metabolism. I. Evidence of gastrointestinal dysfunction in infants with iron deficiency anemia. A preliminary report. *J. Pediatr.* **60,** 787–800.

Wintrobe, M. M., and Beebe, R. T. 1933. Idiopathic hypochromic anemia. *Medicine (Baltimore)* **12,** 187–243.

Wöhler, F. 1964. Diagnosis of iron storage diseases with desferrioxamine (Desferal test). *Acta Haematol. (Basel)* **32,** 321–337.

Worwood, M. 1977. The clinical biochemistry of iron. *Semin. Hematol.* **14,** 3–30.

CHAPTER 6

MAGNESIUM

INTRODUCTION

Magnesium is one of the most plentiful elements on earth, and it is the fourth most abundant cation in the vertebrate. Magnesium is associated with many different biological processes, indicating that it may have a fundamental role in life (Aikawa, 1971, 1976).

BIOCHEMISTRY

ROLE OF MAGNESIUM IN PHOTOSYNTHESIS

Among the greatest triumphs of early evolution was the development of a method of harnessing the energy of the sun, which is transmitted as light, to drive energy-requiring synthetic processes. This process occurs in higher plants in an especially organized subcellular organelle, the chloroplast. The chloroplast is an organized set of membranes crowded with water-insoluble lipid and containing the central pigment chlorophyll, which is the magnesium chelate of porphyrin (Aikawa, 1976).

The light quantum activates the chlorophyll molecule (an electron moves from the π orbitals to the exterior of an atomic shell, and is ejected, leaving behind a chlorophyll free radical). This occurrence terminates the true photochemical event, whereby a light quantum is transmuted into a high-energy electron (Aikawa, 1976).

The energy of electrons is used to produce adenosine triphosphate (ATP), which, along with reduced nicotinamide adenine dinucleotide (NADPH), generates carbohydrates from CO_2. The chloroplast is therefore a transducer that converts the electromagnetic energy from the sun into the chemical energy of ATP. This transduction does not occur in the absence of chelated magnesium (Aikawa, 1976).

Lin and Nobel (1971) observed an increase in the concentration of chloroplast Mg^{2+} *in vivo* caused by illuminating the plant. This was the first direct evidence indicating that changes in magnesium level actually occur in the plant cell. The photophosphorylation rate was enhanced by magnesium in the chloroplasts. The increase of magnesium in chloroplasts may thus be a regulatory mechanism whereby light controls photosynthetic activity.

ROLE OF MAGNESIUM IN OXIDATIVE PHOSPHORYLATION

In the absence of sunlight, plants depend on stored chemical energy to maintain life. This stored energy is released by oxidative phosphorylation, a process that occurs in the mitochondrial membrane of both plant and animal cells. The main function of all mitochondria is to couple phosphorylation to oxidation. ATP, the main fuel of life, is produced in oxidative phosphorylation. All enzyme reactions known to be catalyzed by ATP show an absolute requirement for magnesium. These reactions include a very wide spectrum of synthetic processes (Aikawa, 1976).

A rapid swelling of heart and liver mitochondria can be produced in rats fed a magnesium-deficient diet for 10 days, while no significant decrease in the magnesium content of the mitochondrion results. ATP reverses the swelling of mitochondria from the hearts and livers of magnesium-deficient rats (Aikawa, 1976).

Much of the magnesium in the cell nucleus is combined with those phosphoric groups of DNA that are not occupied by histone. The chemical factors that control the variable activity at the sites along a chromosome are largely unknown. There is a suggestion that the sites along the DNA chain at which the phosphoric acid groups are combined with histone are inactive and, conversely, that those at which they are combined with magnesium are active. The physical integrity of the DNA helix seems to be dependent on magnesium. Evidence suggests that Mg^{2+} is necessary as an intermediate complexing agent during cell duplication and during the formation of RNA on a double-stranded DNA template (Aikawa, 1976).

Both magnesium and ATP are involved in the synthesis of nucleic acids. Because sections of the chromosomes in the nucleus are held together by calcium and magnesium, it appears likely that changes in the concentration of magnesium in the medium might determine the degree of chromosomal aberration. There is evidence indicating that variations in the concentration of magnesium *in vivo* exert control on DNA synthesis (Aikawa, 1976).

The principal and probably the only function of the ribosome, which occurs universally in microorganisms, higher plants, and animals, is the biosynthesis of protein. The rate of protein synthesis is proportional to the number of ribosomes present. Ribosomes require magnesium ions to maintain their physical stability (Hughes, 1972), and they dissociate into smaller particles when the magnesium concentration becomes low (Zitomer and Flaks, 1972). An optimum intracellular concentration of magnesium is needed for the integrity of the macromolecules necessary for RNA synthesis (Clement *et al.,* 1973). The physical size of the RNA aggregates is controlled by the concentration of magnesium, and polypeptide formation cannot proceed without optimal magnesium concentration (Willick and Kay, 1971). Mg^{2+} most likely acts to stabilize a favorable protein conformation (Aikawa, 1976; Case *et al.,* 1973).

PHYSIOLOGY AND METABOLISM IN MAN

NORMAL DISTRIBUTION AND TURNOVER

The magnesium content of the human body ranges between 22.7 and 35.0 meq/kg wet weight of tissue (Widdowson *et al.,* 1951). Extrapolations from tissue analyses performed on victims of accidental death indicate that the body content of magnesium for a man weighing 70 kg would be approximately 2000 meq (24 g) (Aikawa, 1976; Schroeder *et al.,* 1969).

Of the total magnesium in the body, 89% resides in bone and muscle, with bone containing about 60% of the total body content of magnesium at a concentration of about 90 meq/kg wet weight. Most of the remaining magnesium is equally distributed between muscle and nonmuscular soft tissues. Of the nonosseous tissues, liver and striated muscle contain the highest concentration (14–16 meq/kg). About 1% of the total body content of magnesium is extracellular. The levels of magnesium in the serum of healthy people are remarkably constant, remaining on the average at 1.7 meq/liter, and varying less than 15% from this mean value (Wacker and Parisi, 1968). The distribution of normal values for serum magnesium is identical in men and women and remains constant with advancing age (Aikawa 1976; Keating *et al.,* 1969).

The total and ultrafiltrable magnesium in normals are (means ± S.D.) 1.809 ± 0.132 meq/liter and 1.175 ± 0.096 meq/liter, respectively, and the mean percentage of ultrafiltrable magnesium is 64 ± 2.4. An increased percentage of ultrafiltrable magnesium is associated with decreased levels of plasma proteins that bind magnesium. The pK of magnesium protein in normal subjects has been calculated to be 1.927 ± 0.052. Roughly 10–15% of the nonultrafiltrable magnesium in normal subjects appears to be independent of the serum protein. One gram of albumin binds approximately 0.012 meq magnesium. Of the nonultrafiltrable magnesium 60–65% could be accounted for by the serum albumin in normal persons (Prasad *et al.*, 1959, 1961). The ratio of bound to unbound magnesium, as well as to total serum levels, appears remarkably constant. The magnesium content of erythrocytes ranges from 4.4 to 6.0 meq/liter (Baron and Ahmet, 1969).

INTAKE

An average American daily ingests between 20 and 40 meq magnesium. Magnesium intakes of 0.30–0.35 meq/kg per day are considered adequate to maintain magnesium balance in normal adults (Jones *et al.*, 1967). A daily intake of 17 meq (0.25 meq/kg) magnesium may meet nutritive requirements, provided the person remains in positive magnesium balance.

For a child, the estimated daily intake is 12.5 meq (150 mg) (Coussons, 1969). Greater importance of magnesium in childhood is suggested by the relative ease with which deficiency states can be produced experimentally in young animals as compared with adult animals (Coussons, 1969).

The following common foods can be ranked in order of decreasing mean concentrations of magnesium (in meq/kg): nuts, 162; cereals, 66; seafoods, 29; meats, 22; legumes, 20; vegetables, 14; dairy products, 13; fruits, 6; refined sugars, 5; fats, 0.6. This order differs when the concentrations are ranked on the basis of caloric values of the foods, as follows: vegetables, legumes, seafoods, nuts, cereals, dairy products, fruit, meat, refined sugars, and fats. The very small contribution of fats and refined sugars to the total intake of magnesium is worth noting. These two foodstuffs (the major sources of caloric energy) are virtually devoid of magnesium (Schroeder *et al.*, 1969).

ABSORPTION

When a tracer dose of ^{28}Mg was administered orally to 26 subjects, the fecal excretion within 120 hr accounted for 60–88% of the administered dose (Aikawa *et al.*, 1958). At 4 hr, the concentration of radioactivity in the plasma was maximal, but the actual increase in serum magnesium concentration was negligible. When ^{28}Mg was injected intravenously into a normal human subject, only 1.8% of the radioactivity had been recovered in the stool within 72 hr (Aikawa *et al.*, 1960). The fecal magnesium seems to be primarily magnesium from material that is not absorbed by the body, rather than magnesium secreted by the intestine. Ingested magnesium seems to be absorbed mainly by the small intestine (Schroeder *et al.*, 1969). The factors that control the gastrointestinal absorption of magnesium are poorly understood (Aikawa, 1976).

In normal subjects on regular diets, the average daily absorption of magnesium from the gastrointestinal tract is 0.14 meq/kg, an amount that is about 40% of the size of the extracellular pool. The rate of entry of magnesium into the intracellular pool would be about 0.0058 meq/kg per hr if one assumes that absorption occurs continuously throughout the day. This rate of entry is about 1% of the rate of removal of magnesium from the extracellular pool by all routes (Aikawa, 1976; Wallach *et al.*, 1966).

No single factor seems to play a dominant role in the absorption of magnesium, as does vitamin D in the absorption of calcium. Numerous studies using ^{28}Mg suggest that the absorption of magnesium in man is influenced by the load presented to the intestinal mucosa (Aikawa, 1959b; Graham *et al.*, 1960). On a regular diet containing 20 meq magnesium, 44% of the ingested radioactivity was absorbed per day. Whereas on a low-magnesium diet (1.9 meq/day), 76% was absorbed, on ingestion of a high-magnesium diet (47 meq/day), the absorption was decreased to 24% (Aikawa, 1976).

Absorption of magnesium begins within an hour of ingestion and then continues at a steady rate for 2–8 hr; after 12 hr, absorption is minimal. In man, absorption throughout the small intestine is fairly uniform, although little or no magnesium is absorbed from the large bowel (Graham *et al.*, 1960).

Evidence from various species of animals suggests that the small intestine is the main site of magnesium absorption, but that the pattern of absorption varies with the species studied (Graham *et al.*, 1960; Field, 1961). In the rabbit, absorption from the large intestine is negligible (Aikawa, 1959a, 1976). In male albino rats, more than 79% of the total absorption of ^{28}Mg takes place in the colon, and excretion of endogenous magnesium occurs mainly in the proximal gut (Chutkow, 1964). Both magnesium and calcium are bound to phosphate and to nonphosphate binding material of an unknown nature in the ileal contents of ruminating calves (Smith, R. H., and McAllan, 1966) and are therefore rendered nonultrafiltrable.

It has been suggested that there is a common mechanism for transporting calcium and magnesium across the intestinal wall (Aikawa, 1976; Alcock and MacIntyre, 1962; Hendrix *et al.*, 1963; MacIntyre, 1960). There is at present no unequivocal evidence that magnesium is actively transported across the gut wall (Aikawa, 1976). It appears reasonable to assume that the net amount of dietary magnesium absorbed is directly related to the intake and to the time available for absorption from the small intestine. Thus, apart from a small effect from the difference in potential across the wall of the small intestine, the concentration of ionic magnesium in the digest at the absorption site must be the main factor that controls the amount absorbed in a given time (Aikawa, 1976; Smith, R. H., and McAllan, 1966).

SECRETION

Undoubtedly, there is considerable secretion of magnesium into the intestinal tract from the bile and from the pancreatic and intestinal juices; this secretion is followed by almost complete reabsorption. Parotid saliva contains approximately 0.3 meq magnesium (Lear and Grøn, 1968) and pancreatic juice about 0.1 meq/liter. The observation that hypomagnesemia may occur in subjects suffering from large losses of intestinal fluids suggests that intestinal juices contain enough magnesium to deplete the serum when magnesium is not reabsorbed by the colon (Aikawa, 1976).

Studies have just begun on the role played by cells of the intestinal mucosa in the transport of divalent cations (Szelényi, 1973). Further studies might reveal that the cells of the intestinal mucosa, like those in the kidney and elsewhere in the body, may depend in part on metabolic activity for the uptake and release of calcium and magnesium (Aikawa, 1976).

EXCRETION

The majority of the magnesium absorbed into the body is excreted by the kidney; fecal magnesium represents mainly the unabsorbed fraction. In subjects on a normal diet, one third or less of the ingested magnesium (5–17 meq) is excreted by the kidney. Following intravenous injection of a tracer dose of ^{28}Mg in 12–16 meq of stable magnesium, the daily urinary excretion of magnesium in eight normal subjects ranged between 6 and 36 meq (Aikawa *et al.*, 1960). The urinary excretion increased when the parenteral dose was increased. The maximal renal capacity for excretion is unknown, but it probably is quite high, perhaps more than 164 meq/day (Aikawa, 1976; Wacker and Parisi, 1968).

The ultrafiltrable magnesium in the plasma is filtered by the glomeruli and is reabsorbed by the renal tubules, most likely by an active process, although the control mechanisms are not known. There is some evidence that magnesium might be secreted by the renal tubule (Forster and Berglund, 1956). Both the mercurial and thiazide diuretics increase the excretion of magnesium, calcium, potassium, and sodium (Aikawa, 1976).

In subjects on a normal diet, the renal excretion amounts to one third or less of the 5–17 meq magnesium that is ingested daily. In 12 normal men on an unrestricted diet, the mean daily excretion of magnesium in the urine was 13.3 ± 3.5 meq (Aikawa, 1976; Wacker and Vallee, 1958).

The mechanism of magnesium excretion by the mammalian kidney is still unclear. It may involve glomerular filtration and partial reabsorption of the filtered material by the renal tubules, or the filtered material may be completely reabsorbed and the excreted magnesium appear by tubular secretion, as is believed to occur with potassium. Tubular secretion of magnesium undoubtedly occurs in the aglomerular fish (Berglund and Forster, 1958), although stop-flow studies with radioactive magnesium in dogs have produced conflicting evidence regarding secretion of magnesium by the tubules (Ginn *et al.*, 1959; Murdaugh and Robinson, 1960). The renal excretion of magnesium in the rabbit appears to be essentially glomerular; the tubular wall appears to be impermeable by magnesium throughout its length (Aikawa, 1976; Raynaud, 1962).

The amount of magnesium that is filtered at the glomerulus in an adult human is about 9.6 meq/hr, assuming a glomerular filtration rate of 130 ml/min, a total plasma magnesium concentration of 1.6 meq/liter, and an ultrafiltrable fraction that comprises 75% of the total. The mean rate of magnesium excretion in the urine (about 0.33 meq/hr) thus represents only 3.5% of the filtered load. Therefore, the whole range of excretion observed under physiological conditions in man may be explained if the tubular reabsorption of magnesium varies between 91 and 99% of the amount filtered at the glomerulus. In the rat (Averill and Heaton, 1966), sheep (Wilson, 1960), and cattle (Storry and Rook, 1962), evidence exists that there is a renal threshold for excretion of magnesium at a value close to the lower limit of the normal blood level.

The possibility of secretion of magnesium by the renal tubules has been studied under conditions of magnesium loading (Heaton, 1969). When serum concentrations were above 6.2 meq/liter, the amount excreted exceeded twice the filtered load, thereby demonstrating tubular secretion of magnesium beyond any likely experimental error. Response to the administration of 2,4-dinitrophenol suggested that magnesium is also secreted by the tubules under physiological conditions (Aikawa, 1976).

Until recently, all the available evidence in the rat has been consistent with a mechanism for magnesium excretion that involves reabsorption of the filtered material, with the excreted magnesium derived chiefly by tubular secretion. This secretion seems to commence only when the magnesium concentration in serum exceeds a critical value that is close to the lower limit of the normal range. Studies with stop-flow techniques, however, did not find magnesium secretion in acutely magnesium-loaded rats undergoing mannitol or sulfate diuresis (Aikawa, 1976; Alfredson and Walser, 1970).

Magnesium excretion in the dog (Massry *et al.*, 1969), like sodium and calcium excretion, is determined by filtration and reabsorption alone, without evidence for tubular secretion. There is a maximal tubular reabsorption capacity (Tm) for magnesium of about 11.5 μeq/min per kg body weight. Parathyroid hormone might directly enhance tubular reabsorption of magnesium (Aikawa, 1976).

Magnesium is also excreted in sweat (Consolazio *et al.*, 1963). In men exposed to high temperatures for several days, from 10 to 15% of the total output of magnesium is recovered in sweat. Acclimatization does not occur as it does for sodium and potassium. Sweat can account for 25% of the magnesium lost daily under extreme conditions; this factor would be important when the magnesium intake is low.

MAGNESIUM CONSERVATION ON A LOW-MAGNESIUM DIET

It is primarily the ionic fraction of the magnesium in plasma that appears in the glomerular filtrate. Any protein-bound magnesium that is filtered is probably returned to the circulation via lymph. The excretion of magnesium can be greater than normal in renal diseases associated with heavy proteinuria (Aikawa, 1976).

Magnesium clearance (corrected for protein binding) increases as a linear function of serum magnesium concentration and approaches the inulin clearance at high plasma magnesium levels (Aikawa, 1976; Chesley and Tepper, 1958).

Despite the probability of diets being low in magnesium under some circumstances, magnesium deficiency does not occur in human beings with healthy kidneys. The explanation for this clinical observation seems to be that renal mechanisms are efficient enough to conserve all but approximately 1 meq magnesium/day. The fecal losses are minimal (Aikawa, 1976; Barnes *et al.,* 1958).

PLASMA CLEARANCE AND TISSUE UPTAKE OF MAGNESIUM

The introduction of the radioactive isotope of magnesium, ^{28}Mg, for clinical studies in 1957 made determination of the ''exchangeable'' pool in human subjects possible. When nine normal subjects were given intravenous infusions of 12–30 meq magnesium tagged with ^{28}Mg, the material was cleared very rapidly from the extracellular fluid (Aikawa *et al.,* 1960). The concentration of radioactivity in the plasma and urine was too low to follow after 36 hr. After a few hours, the volume of fluid available for the dilution of this ion, as calculated from the plasma concentration of ^{28}Mg, exceeded the volume of total body water (Aikawa, 1976).

In general, the clearance curves showed a rapid phase during the first 4 hr, a subsequent more gradual decline until about 14 hr, and a slow exponential slope thereafter. Tissue biopsies contained concentrations of ^{28}Mg in liver, appendix, fat, skin, and subcutaneous connective tissue that could not be attributed solely to the extracellular components of these tissues. These observations suggested that ^{28}Mg rapidly entered cells of the soft tissues, and that 70% or more of the infused magnesium was retained in the body for at least 24 hr (Aikawa, 1976).

The 24-hr urinary excretion of stable magnesium after the infusion of ^{28}Mg approximated the amount of nonradioactive magnesium infused, while only 20% of the ^{28}Mg infused was recovered. Earlier investigators without the benefit of the radioisotopic data assumed that most of the infused magnesium was rapidly excreted by the kidney. The additional isotopic data indicate that the infusion of fairly large amounts of magnesium results in a compensatory renal excretion of the body store of magnesium, and that the material excreted is most likely not the ions that were administered (Aikawa, 1976).

Serial external surveys of radioactivity over the entire body revealed the maximal distribution of radioactivity at the end of infusion to be over the right upper quadrant of the abdomen. This evidence suggests initial concentration of magnesium in the liver. The specific activity in bile at 18 hr was equal to that of serum. This equilibration of the infused ^{28}Mg occurred earlier in bile than in any other tissue or fluid available for study (Aikawa, 1976; Aikawa *et al.*, 1960).

The specific activities in plasma and urine showed only a slight gradual increase after about 18 hr, suggesting that the infused material had equilibrated with the stable magnesium in a rather labile pool, and that further exchange was occurring very slowly in a less labile pool. In normal subjects, the size of this labile pool ranged between 135 and 397 meq (2.6–5.3 meq/kg body weight). The body content of magnesium is estimated to be 30 meq/kg; therefore, it appears that less than 16% of the total body content of magnesium is measured by the ^{28}Mg exchange technique (Aikawa, 1976).

Results of the external survey and the tissue analyses suggest that the labile pool of magnesium is contained primarily in connective tissue, skin, and the soft tissues of the abdominal cavity (such as the liver and intestine), and that the magnesium in bone, muscle, and red cells exchanges very slowly (Aikawa, 1976).

In another study, Silver *et al.* (1960) followed the magnesium turnover for periods up to 90 hr following intravenous injection of ^{28}Mg into human subjects. Even at 90 hr, only one third of the body's magnesium had reached equilibrium with the isotope. These results confirmed the impression that gastrointestinal absorption of magnesium is very limited. In terms of exponential components, graphic analysis of urinary ^{28}Mg curves yielded a slow component with a half-time of 13–35 hr, accounting for 10–15% of the injected dose, and two more rapid components with a half-time of 1 and 3 hr, respectively, accounting for 15–25% of the injected dose. The large remaining fraction (about 25–50% of the body's total pool) had a turnover rate of less than 2%/day. Since about 25–50% of the total body content exchanges at a turnover rate of less than 2%/day, this isotopic dilution method, used so successfully with sodium and potassium, cannot be employed to quantitate the total body content of magnesium in man. In rabbits, however, the exchangeable magnesium value at 24 hr agrees well with the total carcass content of magnesium (Aikawa *et al.*, 1959).

MAGNESIUM EQUILIBRATION IN BONE

The reactivity of the skeleton, as measured by isotopic exchange, declines with age (Breibart *et al.*, 1960). The exchange of ^{28}Mg, expressed as bone/serum specific activity, occurs more rapidly in younger animals than in older ones. ^{28}Mg accumulates in the bones of young rats approximately twice as fast as in the bones of adult rats (Lengemann, 1959).

Exchange of ^{28}Mg in cortical bone occurs much more rapidly in young rats than in adult rats. The stable magnesium content of bone increases with age, and it varies inversely with the water content of the bone. ^{28}Mg studies in lambs indicate that the magnesium reserve in bone is mobilized during dietary magnesium deficiency (Aikawa, 1976; McAleese *et al.*, 1960).

^{28}Mg COMPARTMENTAL ANALYSIS IN MAN

Avioli and Berman (1966) used a combination of metabolic balance and ^{28}Mg turnover techniques to develop a mathematical model for magnesium metabolism in man. These data were subjected to compartmental analysis using digital-computer techniques.

Following intravenous administration of ^{28}Mg, the decline in the specific activity of plasma or urine can be expressed as the sum of several exponential terms by the method of graphic analysis. On the basis of such analyses, Silver *et al.* (1960) defined in man three exchangeable magnesium compartments with half-times of 38, 3, and 1 hr. In 1961, MacIntyre *et al.* (1961) described three exchangeable magnesium compartments containing 7.3, 24.4, and 98.7 meq magnesium. Similar data were obtained by Zumoff *et al.* (1958).

Multicompartmental analysis indicates that there are at least three exchangeable magnesium pools in man with varied rates of turnover: compartments 1 and 2, exemplifying pools with a relatively fast turnover, together approximating extracellular fluid in distribution; compartment 3, an intracellular pool containing over 80% of the exchanging magnesium having a turnover rate one half that of the most rapid pool; and compartment 4, which probably accounts for most of the whole-body magnesium (Wallach *et al.*, 1966). Only 15% of whole-body magnesium, averaging 3.54 meq/kg body weight, is accounted for by relatively rapid exchange processes (Aikawa, 1976; Avioli and Berman, 1966).

HOMEOSTASIS

The physiological mechanisms responsible for maintaining the plasma magnesium concentration at a constant level are not well understood (MacIntyre, 1967). Both calcitonin (Littledike and Arnaud, 1971) and parathormone might be involved. Nevertheless, animals and human beings on an adequate intake of magnesium do remain in magnesium balance, and the two main regulatory sites appear to be the gastrointestinal tract and the kidney (Aikawa, 1976).

INTERRELATIONSHIP OF PARATHYROID HORMONE AND MAGNESIUM

Considerable evidence exists for the hypothesis that parathyroid hormone might help to control the concentration of plasma magnesium through a negative feedback mechanism (Aikawa, 1976; Heaton, 1965; Gill *et al.*, 1967; MacIntyre *et al.*, 1963).

Magnesium deficiency in the intact rat is accompanied by hypercalcemia and hypophosphatemia, provided the parathyroid glands are intact. The concentration of ionic calcium in plasma is elevated. In the absence of the parathyroid gland, magnesium-deficient rats do not develop hypercalcemia or hypophosphatemia. Also, parathyroidectomized animals with magnesium deficiency develop a concentration of ionized calcium in plasma lower than that observed in parathyroidectomized rats on a normal diet (Aikawa, 1976; Gitelman *et al.*, 1968a; Sallis and DeLuca, 1966).

These observations help in establishing a relationship between an apparent increased function of the parathyroid gland and magnesium deficiency (Sallis and DeLuca, 1966). Data from Anast *et al.* (1972) and Suh *et al.* (1973) suggest that magnesium depletion in man could result in impaired synthesis or release of parathyroid hormone, or both. If parathyroid regulation is influenced by the concentration of magnesium in plasma, its activity should be diminished with hypermagnesemia (Altenähr and Leonhardt, 1972; Aikawa 1976; Gitelman *et al.*, 1968b).

The influence of the plasma magnesium concentration on parathyroid gland function was studied in goats and in sheep by perfusion of the isolated parathyroid gland with whole blood of varying magnesium concentration (Buckle *et al.*, 1968). The parathyroid hormone concentration in venous plasma from the gland was estimated by a specific radioimmunoassay. The concentration of parathyroid hormone in the effluent plasma diminished in each animal when the concentration of magnesium was raised; the concentration of hormone increased when the magnesium concentration was lowered. The response of the parathyroid hormone concentration to changes in plasma magnesium concentration occurred within minutes. Magnesium seemed to have a specific influence on the rate of release of parathyroid hormone (Aikawa, 1976).

Sherwood *et al.* (1970) developed an organ culture system utilizing normal bovine parathyroid tissue. Studies with this system give direct evidence that the release of parathyroid hormone is inversely proportional to both the calcium and the magnesium ion concentrations. These two cations are equipotent in blocking hormone release (Aikawa, 1976).

Parathyroid extract increases the rate of magnesium loss from either fresh or boiled bone *in vitro* in a magnesium-low medium that contains 50% bovine serum. The extract, however, has no effect in a protein-free medium. These data are consistent with the hypothesis that the physiocochemical action of parathyroid preparations may involve the binding of divalent cations by a parathyroid–albumin complex (Martindale and Heaton, 1965; Gordon, 1963). This phenomenon in dead tissue, which could partially explain an important biological function, is definitely not in accord with current concepts of the mechanism of hormonal action (Aikawa, 1976).

RELATIONSHIP BETWEEN BONE AND EXTRACELLULAR MAGNESIUM

In the rat, magnesium deficiency has been shown repeatedly to cause lowering of the magnesium concentration in bone (Martindale and Heaton, 1965). The observation of a direct close relationship between the magnesium concentrations in the plasma and the femurs of magnesium-deficient rats and calves supports the concept that the skeleton provides the magnesium reserve in the body and suggests that an equilibrium exists between the magnesium of the plasma and the bone. This equilibrium is apparently independent of enzymatic activity, and therefore must be physicochemical in nature. That the equilibrium depends on the concentration of magnesium in both the medium and the bone suggests that the relationship between bone and extracellular fluid magnesium is analogous to the ionization of a poorly dissociated salt, with the magnesium in bone corresponding to the undissociated salt (Aikawa, 1976).

MAGNESIUM DEFICIENCY IN MAN

There are many causes of clinical magnesium deficiency (Table IV). Symptomatic deficiency usually depends on severity and duration.

Fraser and Flink (1951) reported an instance of prolonged parenteral magnesium-free fluid administration that resulted in hypomagnesemia and

Table IV. Causes of Magnesium Deficiency and Hypomagnesemia[a]

A. Gastrointestinal and nutritional causes
  1. Prolonged parenteral fluid administration without magnesium (beginning after 3 weeks)
  2. Prolonged severe diarrhea, e.g., ulcerative colitis, regional enteritis, and chronic laxative abuse
  3. Intestinal malabsorption
    a. Idiopathic steatorrhea
    b. Tropical sprue
    c. Short-bowel syndrome from any cause, resection for enteritis or vascular lesion, jejunocolic fistula for weight reduction, gastrojejunocolic fistula
  4. Alcoholism
  5. Acute and recurrent pancreatitis
  6. Starvation with attendant metabolic acidosis
  7. Diabetic ketoacidosis
  8. Protein–calorie malnutrition including kwashiorkor

B. Renal causes
  1. Prolonged use of the diuretics (especially furosemide and ethacrynic acid)
  2. Renal diseases
    a. Renal tubular acidosis
    b. Recovery from acute tubular necrosis (diuretic phase)
    c. Chronic glomerulonephritis and pyelonephritis (rarely)
    d. Familial renal magnesium wastage
    e. Gentamycin-induced renal injury

C. Endocrine and metabolic causes
  1. Hyperthyroidism
  2. Hyperparathyroidism with osteitis fibrosa cystica
  3. Malacic bone disease with hypercalcemia
  4. Primary and secondary aldosteronism (mineralocorticoid excess)
  5. Excessive lactation
  6. Congenital hypoparathyroidism
  7. Infant born of mother with hyperparathyroidism

D. Neonatal and childhood causes
  1. Infantile convulsions with hypomagnesemia and hypocalcemia
  2. Newborns of diabetic mothers
  3. Genetic (male) hypomagnesemia
  4. Exchange transfusions

[a]From Flink (1976).

clincal manifestations that are now considered by many to be characteristic of magnesium deficiency (Fraser and Flink, 1951). High-calorie amino acid hyperalimentation fluid without adequate magnesium enhances the rate at which deficiency develops. In a previously well-nourished subject, administration of magnesium-free fluid for 3 weeks or longer is needed to produce depletion. In animals, experimental magnesium depletion is enhanced by high protein and high calcium intake (Bunce *et al.*, 1963; Colby and Frye, 1951). Large volume losses of gastrointestinal fluids simultaneously enhance deficiency, in part because of the associated interruption of food intake, but also because of significant loss of magnesium in the fluid when the volume is large (Barnes, 1969; Thoren, 1963). Burn patients are particularly vulnerable to depletion due to the large volumes of exudate formed and also because of the prolonged need for parenteral therapy (Broughton *et al.,* 1968). Complicated surgical problems that result from trauma or mishap and require long maintenance on parenteral nutrition predispose the patient to magnesium depletion unless adequate supplementation of magnesium is used as a preventive measure during the entire illness (Baron, 1960; Broughton *et al.,* 1968; Flink, 1976; Flink *et al.,* 1954, 1957; Fletcher *et al.,* 1960; Kallas, 1970; Randall *et al.,* 1959; Smith, W. D., 1963; Thoren, 1963).

Prolonged severe diarrhea from any cause may result in magnesium depletion. Therefore, chronic ulcerative colitis and regional enteritis in an active phase, amebic colitis, or chronic laxative abuse could result in magnesium depletion. Some of these questions were studied in detail by Thoren (1963), but there have been many reports of series of patients with magnesium depletion resulting from severe chronic diarrhea (Flink, 1976; Gerlach *et al.,* 1970; Hammarsten and Smith, 1957; Thoren, 1963).

Intestinal malabsorption for various reasons is a common factor in mangesium deficiency (Balint and Hirschowitz, 1961; Booth *et al.,* 1963; Fletcher *et al.,* 1960; Gerlach *et al.,* 1970; Goldman *et al.,* 1962; Heaton and Fourman, 1965; MacIntyre *et al.,* 1961; Muldowney *et al.,* 1970; Nielsen and Thaysen, 1971; Opie *et al.,* 1964). The simplest form is extensive resection of the small bowel, particularly when the ileum is resected for any reason. Malabsorption of many nutrients results. Other causes of malabsorption are spontaneous enterocolonic fistulas and surgically induced fistulas. One complication of enterocolonic fistulas for treatment of obesity is magnesium deficiency. Steatorrhea from any cause, e.g., nontropical sprue (celiac disease), tropical sprue, or chronic pancreatic insufficiency, can result in magnesium deficiency. Steatorrhea may have an enhancing effect in addition to large intestinal fluid loss due to the loss of fats and fatty acids. Magnesium and calcium have the chemical property of combining with fatty acids to produce soaps. Steatorrhea may therefore enhance the loss of magnesium. Some striking examples of hypocalcemia have been reported in patients with steatorrhea. Correction of magnesium depletion is necessary to correct hypocalcemia (Estep *et al.,* 1969; Flink, 1976; Heaton and Fourman, 1965; Muldowney *et al.,* 1970).

Alcoholism was recognized by Flink *et al.* (1954) in 1954 to cause magnesium deficiency. Evidence to support this concept includes the following: (1) hypomagnesemia occurs frequently as a result of alcoholism (Flink *et al.,* 1954; Heaton *et al.,* 1962; Martin *et al.,* 1959; Mendelson *et al.,* 1959; Milner and Johnson, 1965; Nielsen, 1963; Smith, W. D., and Hammarsten, 1959); (2) alcohol induces magnesium diuresis (Heaton *et al.,*

1962; Kalbfleisch *et al.*, 1963; McCollister *et al.*, 1958, 1963); (3) a positive external balance of magnesium amounting to a mean of 1.0 meq/kg during recovery has been demonstrated (Flink *et al.*, 1957; Jones *et al.*, 1969; Lim and Jacob, 1972; McCollister *et al.*, 1960). Low exchangeable magnesium (^{28}Mg) has been found by three groups with similar results (Jones *et al.*, 1969; Martin and Bauer, 1962; Mendelson *et al.*, 1965). Low magnesium concentration in muscles of patients with alcoholism at the beginning of withdrawal has been shown by several investigators (Jones *et al.*, 1969; Lim and Jacob, 1972) to be similar to decreases observed in celiac disease and kwashiorkor (MacIntyre *et al.*, 1961; Metcoff *et al.*, 1960; Montgomery, 1960). A favorable response to therapy has been observed often, but not always. Instances of severe hypomagnesemia associated with cardiac irregularity (Chadda *et al.*, 1973; Kim *et al.*, 1961; Loeb *et al.*, 1968; Ricketts *et al.*, 1969) and hypocalcemia responsive only to magnesium repletion (Estep *et al.*, 1969) have been found during the withdrawal period. The pathogenesis of magnesium depletion in chronic alcololism is related to loss in the urine resulting from alcohol ingestion primarily of magnesium-free calories. The malnutrition probably is the most important factor. As a result of the high incidence of serious alcoholism worldwide, alcohol is probably the most important cause of magnesium deficiency in adults (Flink, 1976).

Although cerebrospinal fluid (CSF) has not been extensively studied, Glickman *et al.* (1962) found mean values of magnesium in CSF to be lower than normal in alcoholic patients with delirium tremens. Although the means were not significantly lower by statistical analysis, some of the magnesium values in alcoholic patients were greater than 3 standard deviations of the mean. Chutkow and Myers (1968) found low CSF magnesium in nonalcoholic patients with magnesium deficiency and in experimental magnesium deficiency (Flink, 1976).

Among the first diseases to be identified as accompanied by hypomagnesemia were acute pancreatitis and recurrent acute pancreatitis (Edmondson *et al.*, 1952). The more severe the episode, the more severe are the hypomagnesemia and hypocalcemia. Prolonged illness due to pancreatitis necessitating total parenteral nutrition may accentuate magnesium depletion. When the cause of the pancreatitis is alcoholism, it can be an important contributing factor to magnesium depletion (Flink, 1976).

Starvation during World War II was the first recognized nutritional cause of magnesium depletion (Mellinghoff, 1949). Symptoms were not noted. The mechanism of magnesium deficiency during starvation was elucidated in a study of patients undergoing voluntary starvation for obesity (Jones *et al.*, 1966a). During total starvation, an average loss of 10 meq magnesium/day was found. It appears that ketoacidosis is the principal pathogenic mechanism. Symptomatic magnesium deficiency has been reported following prolonged starvation for obesity. Butler *et al.* (1947) and Nabarro *et al.* (1952) reported significant magnesium depletion during diabetic ketoacidosis, although no symptoms related to this depletion were reported. A high incidence of hypomagnesemia in diabetic ketoacidosis was reported by Martin and Wertman (1947). Occasionally, symptoms do occur from this cause, especially when there has been a prolonged period of acidosis (Flink, 1976).

Since 1960, protein–calorie malnutrition and kwashiorkor have been recognized as causes of serious depletion (Caddell, 1969; Metcoff *et al.*, 1960). Evidence of this is low muscle magnesium concentration, retention of a large quantity of infused magnesium, and favorable response to magnesium therapy (Caddell, 1969; Caddell *et al.*, 1973; Montgomery, 1960, 1961). There is no universal agreement, however, about the therapeutic benefits of magnesium in this condition (Rosen *et al.*, 1970). Both early (Caddell, 1969) and later serial studies (Caddell *et al.*, 1973) showed slow repletion of magnesium in the muscles of this patient group. By means of an infusion test, Caddell *et al.* (1973) were able to document a prolonged period before there is return to a normal response, which suggests a prolonged recovery period before homeostasis is reestablished (Flink, 1976).

The diuretic agents furosemide and ethacrynic acid cause a twofold or greater increase in magnesium excretion (Hänze and Seyberth, 1967). Thiazide diuretics increase magnesium excretion less than furosemide and ethacrynic acid (McCollister *et al.*, 1958). Ammonium chloride and mercury diuretics also cause increased excretion of magnesium in some patients. Depletion of magnesium and potassium can occur simultaneously and cause serious cardiac arrhythmia or enhanced digitalis toxicity (Flink, 1976).

Renal causes of hypomagnesemia include renal tubular acidosis, recovery from acute tubular necrosis, chronic glomerulonephritis and pyelonephritis, gentamycin-induced renal injury (Holmes *et al.*, 1969), and familial renal magnesium wastage (Glickman *et al.*, 1962). Clinical symptoms of hypomagnesemia were first reported by Hirschfelder and Haury (1934) in patients with chronic renal diseases. Severe chronic renal failure (as defined by a glomerular clearance rate of less than 10 ml/min) is often associated with hypermagnesemia, but above this clearance, hypomagnesemia may also occur. Randall (1969) was able to produce a sharp decrease in magnesium level from high values to normal or low levels by correction of acidosis with sodium bicarbonate in patients with serious renal failure. This study demonstrates the importance of knowing the condition of patients at the time of blood sampling. Familial magnesium wastage is often, but not always, associated with hypokalemic metabolic alkalosis (Gitelman *et al.*, 1969). The critical evidence to support this diagnosis is a lack of renal conservation of magnesium despite hypomagnesemia. The syndrome can be asymptomatic, but usually has one or more of the manifestations of magnesium or potassium deficiency or both. This is particularly true in young children. No other renal lesion is demonstrable other than renal wastage (Flink, 1976).

Several endocrine disturbances are associated with hypomagnesemia. Hyperthyroidism is associated with hypomagnesemia, whereas hypothyroidism is associated with hypermagnesemia (Jones *et al.,* 1966b; Tapley, 1955). By means of balance studies, it has been possible to demonstrate retention of magnesium during therapy of hyperthyroidism and a negative balance during thyroid replacement. It is possible that some of the manifestations of thyroid crises are due to this deficiency, but this is not clearly established. When ^{28}Mg is used as a tracer, exchangeable magnesium is actually decreased in hypothyroidism (Dimich *et al.,* 1966). The paradoxically diminished exchangeable magnesium in the face of demonstrated increase of body magnesium makes interpretation of ^{28}Mg studies difficult (Flink, 1976).

In isolated instances, hyperparathyroidism has resulted in symptomatic magnesium deficiency (Agna and Goldsmith, 1958; Harman, 1956; Heaton and Pyrah, 1963; Potts and Roberts, 1958). It appears that the patients who develop hypomagnesemia with or without symptoms postoperatively are mainly those with osteitis fibrosa cystica or marked hypercalcemia. Hypercalcemia from other causes can also be associated with hypomagnesemia, with or without symptoms (Eliel *et al.,* 1969), probably because hypercalcemia promotes magnesium excretion. Parathyroid extract administration to hypoparathyroid patients initially produces increased renal conservation, followed by increased magnesium excretion, but many variations in response to parathyroid extract occur. Hypomagnesemia may be associated with congenital hypoparathyroidism, and is either transient due to maternal hyperparathyroidism or permanent due to a rare instance of familial hypoparathyroidism. Of course, in such instances, hypocalcemia is a prominent or dominant feature (Flink, 1976).

Primary and secondary aldosteronism causes loss of magnesium (Cohen *et al.,* 1970; Gitelman *et al.,* 1969; Mader and Iseri, 1955). Many patients with aldosteronism have had tetany. Secondary aldosteronism in cirrhosis accounts for the hypomagnesemia found in children and adults with cirrhosis and ascites and edema. The hypomagnesemia responds to an aldosterone antagonist. Deoxycorticosterone also causes magnesium loss. Lactation has resulted in hypomagnesemia and tetany in a "wet nurse" producing a very large volume of milk (Flink, 1976; Greenwald *et al.,* 1963).

There are several instances of infantile hypomagnesemia, which is often associated with hypocalcemia (Bajpai *et al.,* 1967; Black *et al.,* 1962; Flink, 1976; Friedman *et al.,* 1967; Haijamae and MacDowall, 1972; Keipert, 1969; Nordia *et al.,* 1971; Paunier *et al.,* 1965; Skyberg *et al.,* 1967; Strømme *et al.,* 1969; Tsang, 1972; Wong and Teh, 1968). The pathogenesis is varied and complex, as outlined by Tsang (1972). Among those most easily explained are infants born to diabetic mothers or mothers with sprue who have low serum magnesium levels (Clarke and Carré, 1967).

A syndrome in male infants, characterized by hypomagnesemia and hypocalcemia, is due to malabsorption of magnesium from the gut (Friedman *et al.,* 1967; Haijamae and MacDowall, 1972; Keipert, 1969; Nordia *et al.,* 1971; Paunier *et al.,* 1965, 1968; Skyberg *et al.,* 1967; Strømme *et al.,* 1969). Therapy with parenteral magnesium salts initially followed by oral supplementation of magnesium corrects the symptoms. In addition to this fairly specific syndrome, which is dependent on intestinal malabsorption, there are numerous infants and young children of both sexes who develop hypomagnesemia and hypocalcemia with symptoms responding only to magnesium therapy. These patients usually recover completely without the need for continued therapy.

A diagnosis of a magnesium-deficiency state in human subjects is not easily established. Hypomagnesemia (more than 2 standard deviations below the mean) is not conclusive evidence *per se,* and a large deficit may occur without hypomagnesemia (Caddell and Olson, 1973; Caddell *et al.,* 1973; Jones *et al.,* 1969; Opie *et al.,* 1964). In man, erythrocyte magnesium concentration has been used by many to diagnose magnesium deficiency, although red cells are not quickly responsive to a deficit (Smith, W. D., and Hammarsten, 1959). Total external balance studies are the most convincing evidence, but often such a study is not feasible. Magnesium infusion tests afford fairly good evidence and are often feasible. The amount of magnesium in the urine in either 24 or 48 hr, depending on the test, is subtracted from the amount of magnesium given intravenously over a 6-hr period (Caddell *et al.,* 1973; Thoren, 1963). Unequivocal response of patients' symptoms that have failed to respond to other measures is also good evidence. Chemical analysis for magnesium in muscle biopsy may be useful, but is not practical. Clinical and chemical evidence together is necessary to establish a diagnosis of magnesium-deficiency syndrome (Flink, 1976).

There is no doubt that even severe hypomagnesemia associated with a significant deficit can be completely asymptomatic and remain clinically undetected (Flink *et al.,* 1957; Hanna *et al.,* 1960; Martin *et al.,* 1952). Considerable controversy has existed regarding characteristic manifestations of magnesium deficiency, although many investigators during the past 20-years have supported the concept of a multifaceted and varied syndrome.

The following manifestations may be noted due to magnesium-deficiency syndrome: muscular twitching and tremor of any or all muscles, including the tongue; athetoid and choreiform movements (rare); vertigo, ataxia, and nystagmus (rare); muscle wasting and muscle weakness; positive Chvostek sign (fairly common); numbness and tingling (fairly common); positive Trousseau sign (rare); spontaneous carpopedal spasm or tetany (rare); convulsions; sweating and tachycardia; apathy, depression, and poor memory; mild to severe delirium (confusion, disorientation, hallucinations, and paranoia); premature ventricular beats, ventricular tachycardia, and ventricular fibrillation; coma; and death. The emphasis should be placed on the neuromuscular and psychiatric aspects of this list, rather than on the more restrictive idea of tetany (Flink, 1976).

The frequent association of hypocalcemia with hypomagnesemia of infancy or in alcoholism, steatorrhea, and malabsorption from any cause has become apparent during the past decade. Noteworthy are the failure of intravenous calcium infusion to influence symptoms and signs, the failure to correct the hypocalcemia, and the correction of hypocalcemic symptoms and signs and of hypomagnesemia by parenteral magnesium (Flink, 1976).

Tetany in the sense of carpal and pedal spasm, muscle rigidity, and even opisthotonus particularly occurs in infants and young children, although it can also occur in adults, as a result of magnesium deficiency. It is usually associated with hypocalcemia, as noted above, but can occur with normal or near-normal calcium (Flink, 1976).

Special mention should be made of cardiac symptoms and signs. Cardiac arrhythmia, which may include frequent premature ventricular contractions, ventricular tachycardia, and ventricular fibrillation, has been reported (Chadda *et al.*, 1973; Kim *et al.*, 1961; Loeb *et al.*, 1968; Ricketts *et al.*, 1969; Seller *et al.*, 1970). In animals and man, digitalis toxicity is enhanced by magnesium deficiency. Sudden death (Milner and Johnson, 1965) in alcoholism, especially during withdrawal, may be related to tachyarrhythmia associated with hypomagnesemia. The danger is enhanced by hypokalemia. The role of magnesium depletion in alcoholic cardiomyopathy remains unclear at present (Alexander, 1966; Flink, 1976; Sullivan *et al.*, 1968).

Magnesium depletion is of importance in the early manifestations of the alcohol withdrawal syndrome. Wolfe and Victor (1969) showed that there was a greatly exaggerated photic sensitivity, as measured by photomyoclonus, and the sensitivity was directly proportionate to the severity of hypomagnesemia. This sensitivity could be abolished by an intravenous infusion of magnesium sulfate. These workers also clearly documented the occurrence of hyperventilation alkalosis during the first 48 hr following withdrawal from alcohol (Flink, 1976).

The role of magnesium deficiency in pathogenesis of the alcohol withdrawal syndrome is still surrounded by controversy. Delirium (confusion, hallucinations, delusions, violent behavior), tremor, and convulsions can occur in alcoholism as well as in non-alcohol-induced magnesium deficiency. Due to the dramatic improvement of neuromuscular symptoms in several patients treated with magnesium salts and symptomatology in common with magnesium deficiency from other causes, manifestations of alcohol withdrawal have been ascribed to magnesium depletion (Flink *et al.,* 1954, 1957, 1973). The apparent complete failure to alter the course in some subjects has created the controversy regarding the role of magnesium in delirium (Flink, 1976).

THERAPY

Therapy of patients with magnesium salts can safely be carried out by following the guidelines listed below. The program, which has been used with many hundreds of patients, is safe and effective (Flink, 1969). It should be noted that this schedule of treatment calls for approximately one fourth the dose given in the treatment of eclampsia (Flink, 1976; Flowers *et al.,* 1962).

The following are suggested guidelines for the treatment of magnesium deficiency regardless of etiology:

1. It is important to know that the kidneys are producing urine and the blood urea nitrogen or creatinine, or both, are normal. Magnesium may be needed and can be administered even in the instance of renal insufficiency, although the treatment must be frequently monitored by serum or plasma levels.
2. At least 1 meq Mg/kg per day should be given parenterally on the first day of therapy. Subsequently, at least 0.5 meq Mg/kg per day should be administered for 3–5 days. If parenteral fluid therapy continues, then at least 0.2 meq/kg per day should be given. This dose may be either administered intramuscularly or added to the intravenous infusion.
3. Intramuscularly, for an average adult, 2.0 g $MgSO_4 \cdot 7\ H_2O$ in 50% solution could be administered every 4 hr for six doses the first day. On days 2–5, the dose can be reduced to 1 g every 6 hr. Intravenously, 5 g $MgSO_4 \cdot 7\ H_2O$/liter may be given the first day up to a total of 2 liters. On subsequent days, a total of 6 g should be given, distributed equally in total fluids of the day (Flink, 1976).

If the patient's condition requires continued intravenous infusions, 2 g $MgSO_4$ should be given daily in the infusion as long as infusions are needed. When a patient with magnesium deficiency is convulsing, 2.0 g $MgSO_4$ solution should be administered intravenously during a 10-min period. For infants and children, this dose should be 0.025 g $MgSO_4$/kg in a 10-min period (Flink, 1976).

Magnesium repletion can occur slowly, particularly in malnourished children (Caddell and Olson, 1973; Caddell *et al.*, 1973; Montgomery, 1961), in malabsorption syndromes (Goldman *et al.*, 1962; Heaton and Fourman, 1965; Opie *et al.*, 1964), and in alcoholism (Flink *et al.*, 1957; Jones *et al.*, 1969). The time lag, or slow response, to injection of magnesium for the correction of sensitivity to audiogenic seizures in magnesium-deficient rats demonstrated by Chutkow (1974) confirms clinical impressions. The response is very different from the immediate response of hypocalcemic tetany to calcium injection. Magnesium therapy must be continued intensively for 4 days and subsequently at a lower dose, as noted above, if interference with normal oral feedings continues. Relapses are likely to occur in the most severely depleted patients unless therapy is continued (Flink, 1976).

EXPERIMENTAL PRODUCTION OF A PURE MAGNESIUM DEFICIENCY

A significant magnesium depletion is difficult to achieve in normal subjects by simple dietary restriction due to the exceedingly efficient renal and gastrointestinal mechanisms for conservation. In normal subjects, the urinary magnesium excretion decreases significantly within 4–6 days of magnesium restriction (Fitzgerald and Fourman, 1956; Barnes *et al.*, 1960). Despite these conservatory mechanisms, Dunn and Walser (1966) did induce in two normal subjects deficits approaching 10% of the total body content of magnesium by infusing sodium sulfate and adding calcium supplements to the magnesium-deficient diet. The magnesium concentration in plasma and erythrocytes decreased moderately. Because the muscle magnesium content remained normal, it was believed that magnesium was lost primarily from the bone. No adverse clinical effects were noted (Aikawa, 1976).

Randall *et al.* (1959) reported data that suggested that total body depletion of magnesium could result in psychiatric and neuromuscular symptoms. Administration of magnesium parenterally or in the diet was associated with clinical improvement that was occasionally dramatic (Aikawa, 1976).

The best study to date of magnesium deficiency in man was reported by Shils (1964, 1969a,b). In this study, seven subjects were placed on a magnesium-deficient diet containing 0.7 meq magnesium/day. The magnesium concentration in plasma decreased perceptibly in all subjects within 7–10 days. Urinary and fecal magnesium and urinary calcium declined markedly. At the height of the deficiency, the plasma magnesium concentration declined to a range of 10–30% of the control values, whereas the red cell magnesium declined more slowly and to a smaller degree. All male subjects developed hypocalcemia, but the one female patient did not. Marked and persistent symptoms developed only when hypocalcemia was present. The serum potassium concentration declined, and in four of the five subjects in whom this measurement was made, the ^{42}K space was decreased. The serum sodium concentration was significantly altered. Three of the four subjects exhibiting the severest symptoms also had metabolic alkalosis (Aikawa, 1976).

A positive Trousseau sign, noted in five of the seven subjects, was the most commonly observed neurological sign. Electromyographic changes, characterized by the development of myopathic potentials, were observed in all five of the patients tested. Anorexia, nausea, and vomiting were often experienced. All clinical and biochemical abnormalities were corrected when magnesium was added to the experimental diet (Aikawa, 1976).

MAGNESIUM TOXICITY

Intoxication and hypermagnesemia occur mainly in patients with serious renal insufficiency and in eclampsia when large doses of magnesium salts are administered. It appears that excess magnesium blocks neuromuscular transmission owing to diminution in end-plate potential (Engbaek, 1952; Goodman and Gilman, 1970). When levels start to exceed 4 meq/liter, the deep-tendon reflexes are decreased and at levels approaching 10 meq/liter may be absent. Respiratory paralysis is a hazard at this point. Cardiac consequences might be observed in the form of heart block at levels below 10 meq/liter. As long as deep-tendon reflexes remain active, it is likely that the patient will not develop respiratory paralysis. The central depression and peripheral nerve transmission defects produced by the magnesium ion may be antagonized by calcium injection. For instance, calcium salt solution for intravenous use must be immediately available whenever large doses of magnesium salts are used in therapy for eclampsia (Flink, 1976).

Infants born to mothers having received $MgSO_4$ treatment for eclampsia are at risk of developing intoxication manifested as depression and hypotonia. Lipsitz and English (1967) reported a study of 16 infants of mothers treated with doses of 16–60 g $MgSO_4$ in 8–33 hr. Within this group, cord blood magnesium was 3.0–11.5 meq/liter. Three of the infants exhibited severe depression and died. If $MgSO_4$ is going to be used in treatment of eclampsia, the dosage must be determined by carefully monitoring the blood levels and by avoiding levels sufficient to abolish tendon reflexes. Marked hypermagnesemia in man and animals has been associated with hypocalcemia (Flink, 1976; Monif and Savory, 1972).

In infants, hypermagnesemia induces hypothermia. Hypermagnesemia induced in the infants of mothers with eclampsia can also develop meconium plug syndrome (Flink, 1976; Sokal *et al.,* 1972).

The use of magnesium-containing antacids, such as magnesium oxide or magnesium trisilicate, as described by Randall in patients with renal failure (Randall, 1969; Randall *et al.,* 1964), is an important cause of magnesium intoxication. An interesting facet of these studies is the relatively low concentrations that contribute to intoxication. This phenomenon may be due to the observation by Fishman and Raskin (1967) that a high urea concentration results in transcellular transfer of cations. The caution about the hazards of magnesium toxicity in patients with renal failure who use magnesium-containing antacids is important (Flink, 1976).

Magnesium has been utilized in anesthesia. Belsche *et al.* (1964) used different calcium and magnesium salts in dogs and rabbits and noted that calcium gluconate and magnesium gluconate produced clinically satisfactory spinal anesthesia lasting 2 hr; there were no neurological sequelae. Aldrete *et al.* (1968) produced muscle relaxation in dogs with magnesium intravenously at about 12 meq/liter, but no real anesthesia at even higher levels. Muscle paralysis resulted in respiratory insufficiency with hypoxia and a sleeplike state. Also, Somjen *et al.* (1966) failed to produce anesthesia with infusions given to humans (Flink, 1976).

REFERENCES

Agna, J. W., and Goldsmith, R. E. 1958. Primary hyperparathyroidism associated with hypomagnesemia. *N. Engl. J. Med.* **258,** 222–225.

Aikawa, J. K. 1959a. Gastrointestinal absorption of Mg^{28} in rabbits. *Proc. Soc. Exp. Biol. Med.* **100,** 293–295.

Aikawa, J. K. 1959b. The role of magnesium in biologic processes: A review of recent developments. In: *Electrolytes and Cardiovascular Diseases* (E. Bajusz, ed.). Karger, Basel, pp. 9–27.

Aikawa, J. K., 1971. *The Relationship of Magnesium to Disease in Domestic Animals and in Humans.* Charles C. Thomas, Springfield, Illinois, pp. 1–145.

Aikawa, J. K. 1976. Biochemistry and physiology of magnesium. In: *Trace Elements in Humans: Health and Disease,* Vol. II (A. S. Prasad, ed.). Academic Press, New York, pp. 47–78.

Aikawa, J. K., Rhoades, E. L., and Gordon, G. S. 1958. Urinary and fecal excretion of orally administered Mg^{28}. *Proc. Soc. Exp. Biol. Med.* **98,** 29–31.

Aikawa, J. K., Rhoades, E. L., Harms, D. R., and Reardon, J. Z. 1959. Magnesium metabolism in rabbits using Mg^{28} as a tracer. *Amer. J. Physiol.* **197,** 99–101.

Aikawa, J. K., Gordon, G. S., and Rhoades, E. L. 1960. Magnesium metabolism in human beings: Studies with Mg^{28}. *J. Appl. Physiol.* **15,** 503–507.

Alcock, N. W., and MacIntyre, I. 1962. Inter-relation of calcium and magnesium absorption. *Clin. Sci.* **22,** 185–193.

Aldrete, J. A., Barnes, D. R., and Aikawa, J. K. 1968. Does magnesium produce anesthesia? *Anesth. Analg. (Cleveland)* **47,** 428–433.

Alexander, C. 1966. Idiopathic heart disease: Electron microscopic examination of myocardial biopsy in alcoholic heart disease. *Amer. J. Med.* **41,** 229–234.

Alfredson, K. S., and Walser, M. 1970. Is magnesium secreted by the rat renal tubule? *Nephron* **7,** 241–247.

Altenähr, E., and Leonhardt, F. 1972. Suppression of parathyroid gland activity by magnesium: Morphometric ultrastructural study. *Virchows Arch. A:* **355,** 297–308.

Anast, C. S., Mohs, J. M., Kaplan, S. L., and Burns, T. W. 1972. Evidence for parathyroid failure in magnesium deficiency. *Science* **177,** 606–608.

Averill, C. M., and Heaton, F. W. 1966. The renal handling of magnesium. *Clin. Sci.* **31,** 353–360.

Avioli, L. V., and Berman, M. 1966. Mg^{28} kinetics in man. *J. Appl. Physiol.* **21,** 1688–1694.

Bajpai, P. C., Sugden, D., Stern, L., and Denton, R. L. 1967. Serum ionic magnesium in exchange transfusion. *J. Pediatr.* **70,** 193–199.

Balint, J. A., and Hirschowitz, B. I. 1961. Hypomagnesemia with tetany in nontropical sprue. *N. Engl. J. Med.* **265,** 631–633.

Barnes, B. A. 1969. Magnesium conservation: A study of surgical patients. *Ann. N. Y. Acad. Sci.* **162,** 786–802.

Barnes, B. A., Cope, O., and Harrison, T. 1958. Magnesium conservation in the human being on low magnesium diet. *J. Clin. Invest.* **37,** 430–440.

Barnes, B. A., Cope, O., and Gordon, E. B. 1960. Magnesium requirements and deficits: An evaluation of two surgical patients. *Ann. Surg.* **152,** 518–533.

Baron, D. N. 1960. Magnesium deficiency after gastrointestinal surgery and loss of excretions. *Brit. J. Surg.* **48,** 344–346.

Baron, D. N., and Ahmet, S. A. 1969. Intracellular concentrations of water and of the principal electrolytes determined by analysis of isolated human leucocytes. *Clin. Sci.* **37,** 205–219.

Belsche, J. D., Buckley, J. J., and VanBergen, F. H. 1964. Use of calcium and magnesium cations as spinal anesthetics. *Univ. Minn. Med. Bull.* **35,** 369–370.

Berglund, F., and Forster, R. P. 1958. Renal tubular transport of inorganic divalent ions by the aglomerular teleost, *Lophius americanus. J. Gen. Physiol.* **31,** 429–440.

Black, E. H., Montgomery, R. D., and Ward, E. E. 1962. Neurological manifestations in infantile gastroenteritis and malnutrition. *Arch. Dis. Child.* **37,** 106–109.

Booth, C. C., Babouris, N., Hanna, S., and MacIntyre, I. 1963. Incidence of hypomagnesemia in intestinal malabsorption. *Brit. Med. J.* **2,** 141–144.

Breibart, S., Lee, J. S., McCoord, A., and Forbes, G. 1960. Relation of age to radiomagnesium in bone. *Proc. Soc. Exp. Biol. Med.* **105,** 361–363.

Broughton, A., Anderson, I. R. M., and Bowden, C. H. 1968. Magnesium deficiency syndrome in burns. *Lancet* **2,** 1156–1158.

Buckle, R. M., Care, A. D., Cooper, C. W., and Gitelman, H. J. 1968. The influence of plasma magnesium concentration on parathyroid hormone secretion. *J. Endocrinol.* **42,** 529–534.

Bunce, G. E., Reeves, P. G., Oba, T. S., and Sauberlich, H. E. 1963. Influence of the dietary protein level on the magnesium requirement. *J. Nutr.* **79,** 2220–226.

Butler, A. M., Talbot, N. B., Burnett, C. H., Stanbury, J. B., and MacLachlan, E. A. 1947. Metabolic studies in diabetic coma. *Trans. Assoc. Amer. Physicians* **60,** 102–109.

Caddell, J. L. 1969. Magnesium deficiency in protein–calorie malnutrition: A follow-up study. *Ann. N.Y. Acad. Sci.* **162,** 874–890.

Caddell, J. L., and Olson, R. E. 1973. An evaluation of the electrolyte status of malnourished Thai children. *J. Pediatr.* **83,** 124–128.

Caddell, J. L., Suskind, R., Sillup, H., and Olson, R. E. 1973. Parenteral magnesium load evaluation of malnourished Thai children. *J. Pediatr.* **83,** 129–135.

Case, G. S., Sinnott, M. L., and Tenu, J. P. 1973. The role of magnesium ions in beta-galactosidase hydrolyses: Studies on charge and shape of the beta-galactopyranosyl binding site. *Biochem. J.* **133,** 99–104.

Chadda, H. D., Lichstein, E., and Gupta, P. 1973. Hypomagnesemia and refractory cardiac arrhythmias in a nondigitalized patient. *Amer. J. Cardiol.* **31,** 98–100.

Chesley, L. C., and Tepper, I. 1958. Some effects of magnesium loading upon renal excretion of magnesium and certain other electrolytes. *J. Clin. Invest.* **37,** 1362–1372.

Chutkow, J. G. 1964. Sites of magnesium absorption and excretion in the intestinal tract of the rat. *J. Lab. Clin. Med.* **63,** 71–79.

Chutkow, J. G. 1974. Clincal–chemical correlations in the encephalopathy of magnesium deficiency. *Mayo Clin. Proc.* **49,** 244–247.

Chutkow, J. G., and Myers, S. B. 1968. Chemical changes in cerebrospinal fluid and brain in magnesium deficiency. *Neurology* **18,** 963–974.

Clarke, P. C. N., and Carré, I. J. 1967. Hypocalcemic, hypomagnesemic convulsions. *J. Pediatr.* **70,** 806–809.

Clement, R. M., Sturm, J., and Daune, M. D. 1973. Interaction of metallic cations with DNA. VI. Specific binding of Mg^{++} and Mn^{++}. *Biopolymers* **12,** 405–421.

Cohen, M. I., McNamera, H., and Finberg, L. 1970. Serum magnesium in children with cirrhosis. *J. Pediatr.* **76,** 453–455.

Colby, R. W., and Frye, C. M. 1951. Effect of feeding high levels of protein and calcium in rat rations on magnesium deficiency syndrome. *Amer. J. Physiol.* **166,** 408–412.

Consolazio, C. F., Matoush, L. O., Nelson, R. A., Harding, R. S., and Canham, J. E. 1963. Excretion of sodium, potassium, magnesium, and iron in human sweat and the relation of each to balance and requirements. *J. Nutr.* **79,** 407–415.

Coussons, H. 1969. Magnesium metabolism in infants and children. *Postgrad. Med.* **46,** 135–139.

Dimich, A., Rizek, J. E., Wallach, S., and Silver, W. 1966. Magnesium transport in patients with thyroid disease. *J. Clin. Endocrinol. Metab.* **26,** 1081–1092.

Dunn, M. J., and Walser, M. 1966. Magnesium depletion in normal man. *Metab. Clin. Exp.* **15,** 884–895.

Edmondson, H. A., Berne, C. J., Homann, R. E., and Wertman, M. 1952. Calcium, potassium, magnesium and amylase disturbances in acute pancreatitis. *Amer. J. Med.* **12,** 34–42.

Eliel, L. P., Smith, W. O., Chanes, R., and Howrylko, J. 1969. Magnesium metabolism in hyperparathyroidism and osteolytic disease. *Ann. N. Y. Acad. Sci.* **162,** 810–830.

Engbaek, L. 1952. Pharmacological actions of magnesium ions with particular reference to neuromuscular and cardiovascular system. *Pharmacol. Rev.* **4,** 396–414.

Estep, H., Shaw, W. A., Waltington, C., Hobe, R., Holland, W., and Tucker, S. G. 1969. Hypocalcemia due to hypomagnesemia and reversible parathyroid hormone unresponsiveness. *J. Clin. Endocrinol. Metab.* **29,** 842–848.

Field, A. C. 1961. Magnesium in ruminant nutrition. III. Distribution of Mg^{28} in the gastrointestinal tract and tissues of sheep. *Brit. J. Nutr.* **15,** 349–359.

Fishman, R. A., and Raskin, N. H. 1967. Experimental uremic encephalopathy: Permeability and electrolyte metabolism of brain and other tissues. *Arch. Neurol. (Chicago)* **17,** 10–21.

Fitzgerald, M. G., and Fourman, P. 1956. An experimental study of magnesium deficiency in man. *Clin. Sci.* **15,** 635–647.

Fletcher, R. F., Henly, A. A., Sammons, H. G., and Squire, J. R. 1960. A case of magnesium deficiency following massive intestinal resection. *Lancet* **1,** 522–525.

Flink, E. B. 1969. Therapy of magnesium deficiency. *Ann. N. Y. Acad. Sci.* **162,** 901–905.

Flink, E. B. 1976. Magnesium deficiency and magnesium toxicity in man. In: *Trace Elements in Human Health and Disease,* Vol. 2 (A. S. Prasad, ed.). Academic Press, New York, pp. 1–21.

Flink, E. B., Stutzman, F. L., Anderson, A. R., Konig, T., and Fraser, R. 1954. Magnesium deficiency after prolonged parenteral fluid administration and after chronic alcoholism, complicated by delirium tremens. *J. Lab. Clin. Med.* **43,** 169–183; *J. Clin. Invest.* **32,** 568, 1953 (abstract).

Flink, E. B., McCollister, R., Prasad, A. S., Melby, J. D., and Doe, R. P. 1957. Evidences for clinical magnesium deficiency. *Ann. Intern. Med.* **47,** 956–968.

Flink, E. B., Flink, P. F., Shane, S. R., Jones, J. E., and Steffes, P. E. 1973. Magnesium and free fatty acids in alcoholism. *Clin. Res.* **21,** 884.

Flowers, C. E., Jr., Easterling, W. E., Jr., White, F. D., Jung, J. M., and Fox, J. T., Jr. 1962. Magnesium sulfate in toxemia of pregnancy. *Obstet. Gynecol.* **19,** 315–327.

Forster, R. P., and Berglund, F. 1956. Osmotic diuresis and its effect on total electrolyte distribution in plasma and urine of the aglomerular teleost, *Lophius americanus. J. Gen. Physiol.* **39,** 349–359.

Fraser, R., and Flink, E. B. 1951. Magnesium, potassium, phosphorus, chloride and vitamin deficiency as a result of prolonged use of parenteral fluids. *J. Lab. Clin. Med.* **38,** 809.

Friedman, M., Hatcher, G., and Watson, L. 1967. Primary hypomagnesemia with secondary hypocalcemia in an infant. *Lancet* **1,** 703–705.

Gerlach, K., Morowitz, D. A., and Kirsner, J. B. 1970. Symptomatic hypomagnesemia complicating regional enteritis. *Gastroenterology* **59,** 567–574.

Gill, J. R., Jr., Bell, N. H., and Bartter, F. C. 1967. Effect of parathyroid extract on magnesium excretion in man. *J. Appl. Physiol.* **22,** 136–138.

Ginn, H. E., Smith, W. O., Hammarsten, J. F., and Snyder, D. 1959. Renal tubular secretion of magnesium in dogs. *Proc. Soc. Exp. Biol. Med.* **101,** 691–692.

Gitelman, H. J., Kukolj, S., and Welt, L. G. 1968a. The influence of the parathyroid glands on the hypercalcemia of experimental magnesium depletion in the rat. *J. Clin. Invest.* **47,** 118–126.

Gitelman, H. J., Kukolj, S., and Welt, L. G. 1968b. Inhibition of parathyroid gland activity by hypermagnesemia. *Amer. J. Physiol.* **215,** 483–485.

Gitelman, H. J., Graham, J. B., and Welt, L. G. 1969. A familial disorder characterized by hypokalemia and hypomagnesemia. *N.Y. Acad. Sci. Annu.* **162,** (Art. 2), 856–864.

Glickman, L. S., Schenker, V., Gronick, S., Green, A., and Schenker, A. 1962. Cerebrospinal fluid cation levels in delirium tremens with special reference to magnesium. *J. Nerv. Ment. Dis.* **134,** 410–414.

Goldman, L. A., Fossan, D. D. V., and Baird, E. E. 1962. Magnesium deficiency in celiac disease. *Pediatrics* **29,** 948–952.

Goodman, L. S., and Gilman, A. (eds.). 1970. *Pharmacological Basis of Therapeutics,* 4th ed. MacMillan, New York, pp. 811–814.

Gordon, G. S. 1963. A direct action of parathyroid hormone on dead bone *in vitro. Acta Endocrol. (Copenhagen)* **44,** 481–489.

Graham, L. A., Caesar, J. J., and Burgen, A. S. V. 1960. Gastrointestinal absorption and excretion of Mg^{28} in man. *Metab. Clin. Exp.* **9,** 646–659.

Greenwald, J. H., Dubin, A., and Cardon, L. 1963. Hypomagnesemic tetany due to excessive lactation. *Amer. J. Med.* **35,** 854–860.

Haijamae, H., and MacDowall, I. G. 1972. Distribution of divalent cations at the cellular level during primary hypomagnesemia in infancy. *Acta Paediatr. Scand.* **61,** 591–596.

Hammarsten, J. F., and Smith, W. O. 1957. Symptomatic magnesium deficiency in man. *N. Engl. J. Med.* **256,** 897–899.

Hanna, S., MacIntyre, I., Harrison, M., and Fraser, R. 1960. The syndrome of magnesium deficiency in man. *Lancet* **2,** 172–175.

Hänze, S., and Seyberth, H. 1967. Untersuchungen zur Wirkung der Diuretica Furosemide, Ethacrynsäure and Triamiteren auf die renale Magnesium und Calcium-ausscheidung. *Klin. Wochenschr.* **45,** 313–314.

Harman, M. 1956. Parathyroid adenoma in a child. *Amer. J. Dis. Child.* **91,** 313–325.

Heaton, F. W. 1965. The parathyroid and magnesium metabolism in the rat. *Clin. Sci.* **28,** 543–553.

Heaton, F. W. 1969. The kidney and magnesium homeostasis. *Ann. N. Y. Acad. Sci.* **162,** 775–785.

Heaton, F. W., and Fourman, P. 1965. Magnesium deficiency and hypocalcemia in intestinal malabsorption. *Lancet* **2,** 50–52.

Heaton, F. W., and Pyrah, L. N. 1963. Magnesium metabolism in patients with parathyroid disorders. *Clin. Sci.* **25,** 475–485.

Heaton, F. W., Pyrah, L. N., Beresford, C. C., Bryson, R. W., and Martin, D. F. 1962. Hypomagnesemia in chronic alcoholism. *Lancet* **2,** 802–805.

Hendrix, J. Z., Alcock, N. W., and Archibald, R. M. 1963. Competition between calcium, strontium, and magnesium for absorption in the isolated rat intestine. *Clin. Chem.* **9,** 734–744.

Hirschfelder, A. D., and Haury, V. G. 1934. Clinical manifestations of high and low plasma magnesium: Dangers of epsom salt purgation in nephritis. *J. Amer. Med. Assoc.* **102,** 1138–1141.

Holmes, A. M., Hesling, C. M., and Wilson, T. M. 1969. Drug induced secondary aldosteronism in patients with pulmonary tuberculosis. *Q. J. Med.* **39,** 299–315.

Hughes, M. N. 1972. *The Inorganic Chemistry of Biological Processes.* Wiley, New York, 304 pp.

Jones, J. E., Albrink, M. J., Davidson, P. D., and Flink, E. B. 1966a. Fasting and refeeding of various suboptimal isocaloric diets. *Amer. J. Clin. Nutr.* **19,** 320–328.

Jones, J. E., Desper, P. C., Shane, S. R., and Flink, E. B. 1966b. Magnesium metabolism in hyperthyroidism and hypothyroidism. *J. Clin. Invest.* **45,** 891–900.

Jones, J. E., Manalo, R., and Flink, E. B. 1967. Magnesium requirements in adults. *Amer. J. Clin. Nutr.* **20,** 632–635.

Jones, J. E., Shane, S. R., Jacobs, W. H., and Flink, E. B. 1969. Magnesium balance studies in chronic alcoholism. *Ann. N.Y. Acad. Sci.* **162,** 934–946.

Kalbfleisch, J. M., Lindeman, R. D., Ginn, H. E., and Smith, W. O. 1963. Effects of ethanol administration on urinary excretion of magnesium and other electrolytes in alcoholic and normal subjects. *J. Clin. Invest.* **42,** 1471–1475.

Kallas, T. 1970. Symptomatic magnesium deficiency in urological patients. *J. Urol.* **104,** 325–327.

Keating, F. R., Jones, J. D., Elveback, L. R., and Randall, R. V. 1969. The relation of age and sex to distribution of values in healthy adults of serum calcium, inorganic phosphorus, magnesium alkaline phosphatase, total proteins, albumin, and blood urea. *J. Lab. Clin. Med.* **73,** 825–834.

Keipert, J. A. 1969. Primary hypomagnesemia with secondary hypocalcemia in an infant. *Med. J. Aust.* **2,** 242–244.

Kim, Y. W., Andrews, C. E., and Ruth, W. E. 1961. Serum magnesium and cardiac arrhythmias with special reference to digitalis intoxication. *Amer. J. Med. Sci.* **242,** 87–92.

Lear, R. D., and Grøn, P. 1968. Magnesium in human saliva. *Arch. Oral Biol.* **13,** 1311–1319.

Lengemann, F. W. 1959. The metabolism of magnesium and calcium by the rat. *Arch. Biochem.* **84,** 278–285.

Lim, P. and Jacob, E. 1972. Magnesium status of alcoholic patients. *Metab. Clin. Exp.* **21,** 1045–1051.

Lin, D. C., and Nobel, P. S. 1971. Control of photosynthesis by Mg^{2+}. *Arch. Biochem. Biophys.* **145,** 622–632.

Lipsitz, P. J., and English, I. C. 1967. Hypermagnesemia in the newborn infant. *Pediatrics* **40,** 856–862.

Littledike, E. T., and Arnaud, C. D. 1971. The influence of plasma magnesium concentrations on calcitonin secretion in the pig. *Proc. Soc. Exp. Biol. Med.* **136,** 1000–1006.

Loeb, H. S., Pietras, R. P., Gunnar, R. M., and Tobin, J. R. 1968. Paroxysmal ventricular fibrillation in two patients with hypomagnesemia. *Circulation* **37,** 210–215.

MacIntyre, I. 1960. Discussion on magnesium metabolism in man and animals. *Proc. R. Soc. Med.* **53,** 1037–1039.

MacIntyre, I. 1967. Magnesium metabolism. *Adv. Intern. Med.* **13,** 143–154.

MacIntyre, I., Hanna, S., Booth, C. C., and Read, A. E. 1961. Intracellular magnesium deficiency in man. *Clin. Sci.* **20,** 297–305.

MacIntyre, I., Boss, S., and Troughton, V. A. 1963. Parathyroid hormone and magnesium homeostasis. *Nature (London)* **198,** 1058–1060.

Mader, I. J., and Iseri, L. T. 1955. Spontaneous hypopotassemia, hypomagnesemia, alkalosis and tetany due to hypersecretion of corticosterone-like mineralocorticoid. *Amer. J. Med.* **19,** 976–988.

Martin, H. E., and Bauer, F. K. 1962. $Magnesium^{28}$ studies in the cirrhotic and alcoholic. *Proc. R. Soc. Med.* **55,** 912–914.

Martin, H. E., and Wertman, M. 1947. Serum potassium, magnesium and calcium levels in diabetic acidosis. *J. Clin. Invest.* **26,** 217–228.

Martin, H. E., Mehl, J., and Wertman, M. 1952. Clinical studies of magnesium metabolism. *Med. Clin. North Amer.* **36,** 1157–1171.

Martin, H. E., McCuskey, C., Jr., and Tupikova, N. 1959. Electrolyte disturbance in acute alcoholism with particular reference to magnesium. *Amer. J. Clin. Nutr.* **7,** 191–196.

Martindale, L., and Heaton, F. W. 1965. The relation between skeletal and extracellular fluid *in vitro. Biochem. J.* **97,** 440–443.

Massry, S. G., Coburn, J. W., and Kleeman, C. R. 1969. Renal handling of magnesium in the dog. *Amer. J. Physiol.* **216,** 1460–1467.

McAleese, E. M., Bell, M. C., and Forbes, R. M. 1960. Mg^{28} studies in lambs. *J. Nutr.* **74,** 505–514.

McCollister, R., Prasad, A. S., Doe, R. P., and Flink, E. B. 1958. Normal renal magnesium clearance and the effect of water loading, chlorothiazide and ethanol on magnesium excretion. *J. Lab. Clin. Med.* **52,** 928.

McCollister, R. J., Flink, E. B., and Doe, R. P. 1960. Magnesium balance studies in chronic alcoholism. *J. Lab. Clin. Med.* **55,** 98–104.

McCollister, R. J., Flink, E. B., and Lewis, M. 1963. Urinary excretion of magnesium in man following ingestion of ethanol. *Amer. J. Clin. Nutr.* **12,** 415–420.

Mellinghoff, K. 1949. Magnesium Stoffwechselstörungen bei Inanition. *Dtsch. Arch. Klin. Med.* **195,** 475.

Mendelson, J., Wexler, D., Kubzansky, P., Leiderman, H., and Solomon, P. 1959. Serum magnesium in delirium tremens and alcoholic hallucinosis. *J. Nerv. Ment. Dis.* **128,** 352–357.

Mendelson, J. H., Barnes, B., Mayman, C., and Victor, M. 1965. The determination of exchangeable magnesium in alcoholic patients. *Metab. Clin. Exp.* **14,** 88–98.

Metcoff, J., Frenk, S., Antonowicz, I., Gordillo, G., and Lopez, E. 1960. Relations of intracellular ions to metabolite sequences in muscle in kwashiorkor. *Pediatrics* **26,** 960–972.

Miller, J. F. 1944. Tetany due to deficiency in magnesium: Its occurrence in a child of six years with associated osteochondrosis of capital epiphysis of femurs. *Amer. J. Dis. Child.* **67,** 117–119.

Milner, G., and Johnson, J. 1965. Hypomagnesemia and delirium tremens: Report of case with fatal outcome. *Amer. J. Psychiatry.* **122,** 701–702.

Monif, G. R. G., and Savory, J. 1972. Iatrogenic maternal hypocalcemia following magnesium sulfate therapy. *J. Amer. Med. Assoc.* **219,** 1469–1470.

Montgomery, R. D. 1960. Magnesium deficiency and tetany in kwashiorkor. *Lancet* **2,** 74–76.

Montgomery, R. D. 1961. Magnesium balance studies in marasmic kwashiorkor. *J. Pediatr.* **59,** 119–123.

Muldowney, F. P., McKenna, T. J., Kyle, L. H., Freaney, R., and Swan, M. 1970. Parathormone-like effect of magnesium replenishment in steatorrhea. *N. Engl. J. Med.* **281,** 61–68.

Murdaugh, H. V., and Robinson, R. R. 1960. Magnesium excretion in the dog studied by stop-flow analysis. *Amer. J. Physiol.* **198,** 571–574.

Nabarro, J. D. N., Spencer, A. G. D., and Stowers, J. M. 1952. Metabolic studies in severe diabetic ketosis. *Q. J. Med.* **21,** 225–248.

Nielsen, J. 1963. Magnesium metabolism in an acute alcoholic. *Dan. Med. Bull.* **10,** 225–233.

Nielsen, J. A., and Thaysen, E. H. 1971. Acute and chronic magnesium deficiency following extensive small gut resection. *Scand. J. Gastroenterol.* **6,** 663–666.

Nordia, S., Donath, F., Macagno, R., and Gatti, T. 1971. Chronic hypomagnesemia with magnesium dependent hypocalcemia. *Acta Paediatr. Scand.* **60,** 441–448.

Opie, L. H., Hurst, B. J., and Finlay, J. M. 1964. Massive small bowel resection with malabsorption and negative magnesium balance. *Gastroenterology* **47,** 415–420.

Paunier, L., Radde, I. C., Kooh, S. W., and Fraser, D. 1965. Primary hypomagnesemia with secondary hypocalcemia. *J. Pediatr.* **67,** 945 (abstract).

Paunier, L., Radde, I. C., Kooh, S. W., Conen, P. E., and Fraser, D. 1968. Primary hypomagnesemia with secondary hypocalcemia in an infant. *Pediatrics* **41,** 385–402.

Potts, J. T., Jr., and Roberst, B. 1958. Clinical significance of magnesium deficiency and its relation to parathyroid disease. *Amer. J. Med. Sci.* **235,** 206–219.

Prasad, A. S., Flink, E. B., and Zinnemann, H. H. 1959. The base binding property of serum proteins with respect to magnesium. *J. Lab. Clin. Med.* **54,** 357–364.

Prasad, A. S., Flink, E. B., and McCollister, R. 1961. Ultrafiltration studies on serum magnesium in normal and diseased states. *J. Lab. Clin. Med.* **58,** 531–541.

Randall, R. E., Jr. 1969. Magnesium metabolism in chronic renal disease. *Ann. N. Y. Acad. Sci.* **162,** 831–842.

Randall, R. E., Rossmeisl, E. C., and Bleifer, K. H. 1959. Magnesium depletion in man. *Ann. Intern. Med.* **50,** 257–287.

Randall, R. E., Jr., Chen, M. D., Spray, C. C., and Rossmeisl, E. C. 1964. Hypermagnesemia in renal failure. *Ann. Intern. Med.* **61,** 73–88.

Raynaud, C. 1962. Renal excretion of magnesium in the rabbit. *Amer. J. Physiol.* **203,** 649–654.

Ricketts, H. H., Denton, E. K., and Haywood, L. J. 1969. Unusual T-wave abnormality: Repolarization alternans associated with hypomagnesemia, acute alcoholism, and cardiomyopathy. *J. Amer. Med. Assoc.* **207,** 365–366.

Rosen, E. A., Campbell, P. G., and Moosa, G. M. 1970. Hypomagnesemia and magnesium therapy in protein–calorie malnutrition. *J. Pediatr.* **77,** 709–714.

Sallis, J. D., and DeLuca, H. F. 1966. Action of parathyroid hormone on mitochondria: Magnesium- and phosphate-independent respiration. *J. Biol. Chem.* **241,** 1122–1127.

Schroeder, H. A., Nason, A. P., and Tipton, I. H. 1969. Essential metals in man: Magnesium. *J. Chronic Dis.* **21,** 815–841.

Seller, R. H., Cangiano, J., Kim, K. E., Mendelssohn, S., Brest, A. N., and Swartz, C. 1970. Digitalis toxicity and hypomagnesemia. *Amer. Heart J.* **79,** 57–68.

Sherwood, L. M., Herrman, I., and Bassett, C. A. 1970. Parathyroid hormone secretion *in vitro:* Regulation by calcium and magnesium ions. *Nature (London)* **225,** 1056–1057.

Shils, M. E. 1964. Experimental human magnesium depletion. I. Clinical observations and blood chemistry alternations. *Amer. J. Clin. Nutr.* **15,** 133–143.

Shils, M. E. 1969a. Experimental production of magnesium deficiency in man. *Ann. N. Y. Acad. Sci.* **162,** 847–855.

Shils, M. E. 1969b. Experimental human magnesium depletion. *Medicine (Baltimore)* **48,** 61–85.

Silver, L., Robertson, J. S., and Dahl, L. K. 1960. Magnesium turnover in the human studied with Mg^{28}. *J. Clin. Invest.* **39,** 420–425.

Skyberg, D., Strømme, J. H., Nesbakken, R., and Harnas, K. 1967. Congenital primary hypomagnesemia, an inborn error of metabolism. *Acta Paediatr. Scand. Suppl.* **177,** 26–27.

Smith, R. H., and McAllan, A. B. 1966. Binding of magnesium and calcium in the contents of the small intestine of the calf. *Brit. J. Nutr.* **20,** 703–718.

Smith, W. O. 1963. Magnesium deficiency in the surgical patient. *Amer. J. Cardiol.* **12,** 667–670.

Smith, W. O., and Hammarsten, J. F. 1959. Intracellular magnesium in delirium tremens and uremia. *Amer. J. Med. Sci.* **237,** 413–417.

Sokal, M. M., Koenigsberger, M. R., Rose, J. S., Berdon, W. E., and Santulli, T. V. 1972. Neonatal hypermagnesemia and the meconium-plug syndrome. *N. Engl. J. Med.* **286,** 823–825.

Somjen, G. G., Hilmy, M., and Stephen, C. R. 1966. Failure to anesthetize human subjects by intravenous administration of magnesium sulfate. *J. Pharmacol. Exp. Ther.* **154,** 652–659.

Storry, J. E., and Rook, J. A. F. 1962. The magnesium nutrition of the dairy cow in relation to the development of hypomagnesaemia in the grazing animal. *J. Sci. Food Agric.* **13,** 621–627.

Strømme, J. H., Nesbakken, R., Norman, T., Skjrten, F., Skyberg, D., and Johannessen, B. 1969. Familial hypomagnesemia: Biochemical, histological and hereditary aspects studied in two brothers. *Acta Paediatr. Scand.* **58,** 433–444.

Suh, S. M., Trashjian, A. H., Jr., Matsuo, N., Parkinson, D. K., and Fraser, D. 1973. Pathogenesis of hypocalcemia in primary hypomagnesemia: Normal end-organ responsiveness to parathyroid hormone, impaired parathyroid gland function. *J. Clin. Invest.* **52,** 153–160.

Sullivan, J. F., Parker, M., and Carsons, S. B. 1968. Tissue cobalt in beer drinkers myocardiopathy. *J. Lab. Clin. Med.* **71,** 893–911.

Szelényi, I. 1973. Magnesium and its significance in cardiovascular and gastro-intestinal disorders. *World Rev. Nutr. Diet* **17,** 189–224.

Tapley, D. F. 1955. Magnesium balance in myxedematous patients treated with triiodothyronine. *Bull. Johns Hopkins Hosp.* **96,** 274–278.

Thoren, L. 1963. Magnesium deficiency in gastrointestinal fluid loss. *Acta Chir. Scand. Suppl.* **306,** 1–65.

Tsang, R. C. 1972. Neonatal magnesium disturbances. *Amer. J. Dis. Child.* **124,** 282–293.

Wacker, W. E. C., and Parisi, A. F. 1968. Magnesium metabolism. *N. Engl. J. Med.* **278,** 658–662, 712–717, 772–776.

Wacker, W. E. C., and Vallee, B. L. 1958. Magnesium metabolism. *N. Engl. J. Med.* **259,** 431–438.

Wallach, S., Rizek, J. E., Dimich, A., Prasad, N., and Siler, W. 1966. Magnesium transport in normal and uremic patients. *J. Clin. Endocrinol. Metab.* **26,** 1069–1080.

Widdowson, E. M., McCance, R. A., and Spray, C. M. 1951. The chemical composition of the human body. *Clin. Sci.* **10,** 113–125.

Willick, G. E., and Kay, C. M. 1971. Magnesium-induced conformational change in transfer ribonucleic acid as measured by circular dichroism. *Biochemistry* **10,** 2216–2222.

Wilson, A. A. 1960. Magnesium homeostasis and hypomagnesaemia in ruminants. *Vet. Rev.* **6,** 39–52.

Wolfe, S., and Victor, N. 1969. The relationship of hypomagnesemia to alcohol withdrawal symptoms. *Ann. N. Y. Acad. Sci.* **162,** 973–984.

Wong, H. B., and Teh, Y. F. 1968. An association between serum magnesium and convulsions in infants and children. *Lancet* **2,** 18–21.

Zitomer, R. S., and Flaks, J. G. 1972. Magnesium dependence and equilibrium of the *Escherichia coli* ribosomal subunit association. *J. Mol. Biol.* **71,** 263–279.

Zumoff, B., Bernstein, E. H., Imarisio, J. J., and Hellman, L. 1958. Radioactive magnesium (Mg^{28}) metabolism in man. *Clin. Res.* **6,** 260.

CHAPTER 7

MANGANESE

INTRODUCTION

In 1931, manganese was shown to be essential for growth and reproduction in rats and mice (Kemmerer *et al.,* 1931; Orent and McCollum, 1931). Wilgus *et al.* (1936) later demonstrated that manganese prevented a skeletal abnormality in chickens, called "perosis." Even though manganese has been shown to be essential for many species of animals, as yet there are no well-defined occurrences of manganese deficiency in man (Leach, 1976).

BIOCHEMISTRY

The relationship between manganese and enzymes can be classified into two categories: (1) metalloenzymes and (2) metal–enzyme complexes. This kind of categorization is based on affinity of the metal for the enzyme, rather than on function (Leach, 1976).

The number of manganese metalloenzymes is quite limited, unlike the case with other essential transition elements, whereas the enzymes that can be activated (metal–enzyme complexes) are numerous. Included in these enzymes are hydrolases, kinases, decarboxylases, and transferases (Vallee and Coleman, 1964). This type of enzymatic activation generally is relatively nonspecific, which makes it difficult to correlate pathological defects with biochemical function. A group of transferases called "glycosyl transferases," however, offers such a possibility (Leach, 1976).

MANGANESE AND GLYCOSYL TRANSFERASES

Glycosyl transferases are enzymes that are involved in the transfer of sugar from sugar nucleotides to a variety of acceptors. These enzymes are important in the synthesis of polysaccharides and glycoproteins, and a survey of their metal requirements indicated that most of the glycosyl transferases require manganese or some other metal ion for activity (Leach, 1971, 1976).

The need for manganese for the activation of enzymes involved in polysaccharide synthesis can therefore be related to the impairment in mucopolysaccharide metabolism associated with the symptoms of manganese deficiency. In 1971, Leach (1971) presented data that support such a relationship. First of all, the glycosyl transferases involved in mucopolysaccharide synthesis required metal ions for optimum activity, and in most instances, manganese was the ion found to be most effective (Leach, 1976).

The enzymatic activity of tissues from manganese-deficient and control animals was reported by Leach *et al.* (1969). When the enzymes required for chondroitin sulfate synthesis in the 105,000 *g* particulate fraction from deficient and control tissues were compared, the preparations from the deficient tissues incorporated more radioactive substrate. The incorporation of more substrate by the deficient tissues was interpreted as an indication that more acceptor sites were available, reflecting suboptimum *in vivo* synthetic activity of this enzyme. Carbohydrate analysis of this particulate fraction supported such a hypothesis (Leach, 1976).

Manganese is also required for cholesterol synthesis, probably at a step between acetate and mevalonate (Olson, 1965). In addition, manganese is required for the enzyme farnesyl pyrophosphate synthetase. Farnesyl-pyrophosphate is needed for squalene, which is a precursor of cholesterol; thus, a decrease in the activity of farnesyl pyrophosphate synthetase due to manganese deficiency may decrease the serum cholesterol level.

MANGANESE METALLOENZYMES

The number of manganese metalloenzymes that have been isolated and identified is limited (see Table V). Several of these enzymes have been isolated from the mitochondrion, an organelle that is rich in manganese (Leach, 1976).

The most extensively studied manganese metalloenzyme is pyruvate carboxylase, which was isolated from chick liver mitochondria by Scrutton *et al.* (1966). This enzyme contains 4 mol of tightly bound manganese and 4 mol of biotin, and catalyzes the conversion of pyruvate to oxaloacetate. Studies on the tightly bound manganese by Mildvan *et al.* (1966) indicate that the electrophilic character of the bound manganese facilitates the proton departure from the methyl group of pyruvate and the carboxyl transfer from the carboxybiotin residue to pyruvate (Leach, 1976).

Table V. Some Characteristics of Manganese-Containing Metalloproteins

Protein	Molecular weight	Mn/mole	Source	Ref.[a]
Pyruvate carboxylase	500,000	4(II)	Avian liver	1
Superoxide dismutase	39,500	2(III)	*E. coli*	2
Superoxide dismutase	40,000	2(III)	*S. mutans*	3
Avimanganin	89,000	1(III)	Avian liver	4
Manganin	56,000	1	Peanuts	5
Concanavalin A	190,000	1(II)	Jackbean	6

[a]References: (1) Scrutton *et al.* (1966); (2) Keele *et al.* (1970); (3) Vance *et al.* (1972); (4) Scrutton (1971); (5) Dickert and Rozacky (1969); (6) Agrawal and Goldstein (1968).

Scrutton *et al.* (1972) also studied the metal content of pyruvate carboxylase under conditions of manganese deficiency. Magnesium was found to replace manganese as the bound metal in pyruvate carboxylase isolated from manganese-deficient chicks. This substitution caused only minor alterations in the catalytic properties of the enzyme. In contrast to the observation with pyruvate carboxylase described above, manganese deficiency resulted in a depletion of manganese from avimanganin as well as a reduction in the amount of this metalloprotein (Scrutton, 1971). Avimanganin is a protein of unknown function that contains 1 mol of bound manganese(III) per 89,000 mole weight (Leach, 1976).

In view of the competition that exists among manganese, copper, iron, and magnesium at the cellular level, it is conceivable that disorders of manganese metabolism do exist in human subjects, perhaps in association with certain disease states. Further research must be carried out to understand the roles of manganese in human metabolism and in health and disease (Leach, 1976).

METABOLISM

ABSORPTION

Little is known regarding the mechanism of manganese absorption. Thomson *et al.* (1971) reported this element to be well absorbed throughout the length of the small intestine. Several dietary substances interfere with manganese absorption in the intestinal tract. Calcium and phosphorus affect the absorption of manganese adversely. Also, Davis *et al.* (1962) reported that isolated soy protein may interfere with manganese utilization.

Addition of ferric citrate to the diet accentuates the severity of perosis in chickens (Wilgus and Patton, 1939). The reciprocal observation was made by Hartman *et al.* (1955) and Matrone *et al.* (1959). Manganese has been shown to interfere with iron absorption rather than hematopoeisis. A mutual inhibition of absorption could be demonstrated for iron and manganese (Forth and Rummel, 1973; Leach, 1976).

HOMEOSTASIS

The metabolism of manganese has been extensively studied (Maynard and Cotzias, 1955; Cotzias and Greenough, 1958; Borg and Cotzias, 1958a,b; Britton and Cotzias, 1966; Hughes *et al.,* 1966; Papavasiliou *et al.,* 1966; Bertinchamps *et al.,* 1966). It appears that manganese homeostasis is regulated at the excretory level, rather than at the site of absorption. The key tissue in this regulation is the liver, with the bile serving as an important route of excretion. Although biliary excretion is important in adjusting to a manganese load, the bile is not the only route of manganese excretion. Biliary ligation does not halt manganese excretion by the intestinal tract (Leach, 1976).

The pathway of manganese within the body seems to be quite specific. Only manganese would accelerate the exit of radiomanganese from the body. The administration of other elements did not increase excretion, which indicates that there was no interaction between manganese and those elements having similar chemical properties as was observed with various other trace elements (Leach, 1976).

Despite this apparent lack of interaction, several substitutions between manganese and other elements have been reported. Many investigators (Borg and Cotzias, 1958b; Hancock and Fritze, 1973) have observed the isolation of manganese-containing porphyrins. In addition, Scrutton *et al.* (1972) found magnesium to substitute for manganese in pyruvate carboxylase, a manganese metalloprotein.

The body of a normal man contains a total of 12–20 mg manganese (Underwood, 1977). Manganese is distributed widely throughout the tissues and fluids in the body, but tends to be higher in concentration in tissues rich in mitochondria. The retina is rich in its manganese content. The whole blood content (mean $\pm$ S.D.) of manganese ranges from 8.44 $\pm$ 2.73 to 9.84 $\pm$ 0.4 μg/liter (Cotzias *et al.,* 1966; Papavasiliou *et al.,* 1966). The serum concentration (mean $\pm$ S.D.) is 1.42 $\pm$ 0.2 μg/liter, and the level in red cells (mean $\pm$ S.D.) is 23.57 $\pm$ 1.2 μg/liter. Serum manganese is increased following acute coronary occlusion. An increased concentration of manganese in the red cell has been observed in patients with rheumatoid arthritis.

Cotzias and Bertinchamps (1960) proposed the existence of a specific manganese-carrying protein called "transmanganin," although there is no widespread agreement that manganese is associated with a specific protein in blood (Nandedkar *et al.*, 1973; Chapman *et al.*, 1973). Within the cell, much of the manganese is found in the mitochondria.

GENETIC INTERACTION WITH MANGANESE METABOLISM

The relationship between the *pallid* gene in mice and manganese metabolism has been extensively studied (Erway *et al.*, 1966, 1971). A mutant gene affecting coat color in mice, *pallid* also produces a congenital ataxia quite similar to that seen with manganese-deficient normal mice. Supplementing the mutant diet with high levels of manganese during pregnancy prevents the occurrence of the congenital ataxia. The mutant gene itself and the effects of this gene on pigmentation remain unaltered by the manganese treatment. It should be noted that the high levels (1500–2000 ppm) of manganese necessary to prevent this condition in mutant mice greatly exceed the amount of manganese required to prevent congenital ataxia in normal mice. Cotzias *et al.* (1972) reported that mice with the *pallid* gene differed from normal mice in the metabolism of radiomanganese. The manganese concentration of certain tissues, such as bone and brain, was also decreased in the mutant mice (Leach, 1976).

Erway and Mitchell (1973) reported similar findings in pastel mink. The occurrence of screw neck, a postural defect, may be reduced with supplementation of 1000 ppm manganese (Leach, 1976).

In addition to the specific relationship between the aforementioned genes and manganese metabolism, Hurley and Bell (1974) reported substantial individual and strain differences in response to the feeding of low or borderline levels of manganese to mice. These data are similar to those of Gallup and Norris (1939), who observed breed and strain differences in the amount of manganese needed for prevention of perosis in the chick.

MANGANESE METABOLISM AND BIOGENIC AMINES

The similarity between the symptoms of chronic manganese poisoning and Parkinson's disease encouraged the study of a possible relationship between manganese and biogenic amines. Subjects with parkinsonism and chronic manganese poisoning have decreased concentration of striatal dopamine. Mena *et al.* (1970) reported that administration of L-dopa (dihydroxy-phenylalanine), an immediate precursor of dopamine, to patients with chronic manganese toxicity resulted in a disappearance of rigidity and hypokinesia in addition to an improvement of postural reflexes and restitution of balance. This compound (L-dopa) has also been shown to be of great benefit in alleviating some of the symptoms of Parkinson's disease (Cotzias *et al.*, 1971; Leach, 1976).

Papavasiliou *et al.* (1968) proposed that cyclic adenosine monophosphate (cyclic 3′,5′-AMP) is the link between biogenic amines and manganese metabolism. In these reports, the substances that altered cyclic AMP also altered manganese metabolism, as shown by increased liver retention accompanied by decreased biliary excretion. Cotzias *et al.* (1972) extended these studies to mice with the *pallid* gene, where it was revealed that mice with this mutant gene differed from normal mice in the metabolism of L-dopa and tryptophan as well as manganese (Leach, 1976).

MANGANESE DEFICIENCY

The changes associated with manganese deficiency vary according to animal species and the degree of deficiency. There are, however, many symptoms that are common to several species of animals, e.g., skeletal abnormalities and postural defects (ataxia). Manganese has been found to prevent skeletal abnormalities in several species of animals, such as the rat (Amdur *et al.,* 1945), guinea pig (Everson *et al.,* 1959), swine (Plumlee *et al.,* 1956), and cattle (Rojas *et al.,* 1965), in addition to preventing the skeletal defect called perosis in chickens (Leach, 1976; Wilgus *et al.,* 1936).

Manganese is believed to play a role in chondrogenesis rather than osteogenesis (Wolbach and Hegsted, 1953). Data have been obtained in several laboratories that would support such a hypothesis. Leach and Muenster (1962) observed a severe reduction in cartilage mucopolysaccharide content associated with manganese deficiency. This evidence, in addition to subsequent histological studies (Leach, 1968), supports the view that manganese affects skeletal formation through chondrogenesis rather than via osteogenesis (Leach, 1976).

It was shown by Tsai and Everson (1967) that manganese deficiency had similar effects on the mucopolysaccharide content of guinea pig cartilage. Changes in ^{35}S metabolism have been reported in mangnaese-deficient rats (Hurley, 1968). Longstaff and Hill (1972) reported, in addition to the effect on skeletal development, similar compositional changes in eggshell matrix. This evidence helps to explain the effects on eggshell formation described earlier by Leach (1976) and Lyons (1939).

The effect of manganese on mucopolysaccharide metabolism is also responsible for the congenital ataxia observed by several investigators when there is a deficiency of this element (Norris and Caskey, 1939; Hill *et al.,* 1950; Hurley *et al.,* 1958). The postural defects (ataxia) associated with both manganese deficiency and the *pallid* gene in mice seem to be a result of defective development of the otoliths, structures located in the inner ear that are considered to be involved in maintenance of equilibrium (Erway *et al.,* 1966, 1970). It has been demonstrated in extensive studies that there are alterations in mucopolysaccharide metabolism associated with abnormal otolith development (Shrader and Everson, 1967; Hurley, 1968; Shrader *et al.,* 1973). Histochemical and radiosulfate metabolism studies were both used in reaching this conclusion (Leach, 1976).

Even though a defect in mucopolysaccharide metabolism explains several of the symptoms associated with manganese deficiency, other changes exist that cannot be explained in this manner. Liver mitochondria isolated from deficient mice demonstrate a normal phosphate esterified to oxygen consumption ratio (P : O), but show a reduced oxygen uptake (Hurley *et al.,* 1970). Abnormalities, including elongation and reorientation of cristae, are revealed by examination of the ultrastructure, and Bell and Hurley (1973) observed that the ultrastructural changes associated with manganese deficiency occur in other tissues as well. All tissues examined revealed alterations in the integrity of their cell membranes as well as changes in the endoplasmic reticulum. It was therefore proposed that the morphological changes observed in the mitochondria might explain the lowered oxidation rate observed in their previous study (Leach, 1976).

Some other defects in carbohydrate metabolism were observed with manganese deficiency. Several of the guinea pigs with a congenital deficiency have short survival times and exhibit aplasia or hypoplasia of pancreatic tissue. Moreover, these studies revealed that those animals that survive to adult age show abnormal tolerance to intravenously administered glucose (Shrader and Everson, 1968; Everson and Shrader, 1968). Later studies in the same laboratory revealed differences in urinary myoinositol content (Everson, 1968; Leach, 1976).

Recently, a deficiency of manganese was observed in a human subject who was receiving an experimental diet deficient in vitamin K (Doisy, 1974). Inadvertently, manganese was not included in the experimental diet, thus leading to a deficient state for both vitamin K and manganese in the experimental subject. The prothrombin time was prolonged, the prolongation being corrected by vitamin K administration. Dietary supplementation with manganese, however, corrected the prothrombin time. A similar decrease in clotting response from vitamin K was observed in manganese-deficient chicks. A decrease in serum cholesterol, triglyceride, and phospholipids was also noted in the manganese-deficient human subject; the decrease was corrected by manganese supplementation.

Prothrombin is a glycoprotein, and inasmuch as manganese is an activator of the enzyme glycosyl transferases, one may postulate the requirement of manganese for this protein needed for blood clotting. Whereas this observation is very interesting, it is an isolated observation, and one must await more definitive studies in the future confirming the essentiality of manganese for prothrombin synthesis.

MANGANESE TOXICITY

Chronic manganese poisoning occurs among miners working with manganese ores. The manganese enters the lungs as oxide dust from the air and also enters the body via the gastrointestinal tract (Cotzias, 1958). The disease is characterized by a severe psychiatric disorder resembling schizophrenia, followed by a permanently crippling neurological (extrapyramidal) disorder clinically similar to Parkinson's disease.

In general, manganese is among the least toxic of the trace elements to mammals and birds. The growth rate is unaffected by dietary manganese intakes as high as 1000–2000 ppm, although larger amounts interfere with phosphorus retention (Gallup and Norris, 1939). The adverse effects of excess manganese on growth are mainly a reflection of depressed appetite (Underwood, 1971).

A relationship among manganese, iron metabolism, and hemoglobin formation has been observed in lambs, cattle, rabbits, and pigs (Hartman *et al.,* 1955; Matrone *et al.,* 1959; Robinson *et al.,* 1960). A decrease in hemoglobin and serum iron was noted in anemic lambs fed diets containing 1000–2000 ppm manganese. At these levels, manganese appeared to interfere with iron absorption, rather than with hematopoiesis. These findings suggest that the Mn:Fe dietary ratio is of greater significance than commonly appreciated.

TREATMENT

Every attempt must be made to remove the subject from further exposure to manganese. Symptomatic therapy for respiratory symptoms, which include cough, nasopharyngitis, bronchitis, and pneumonia, should be given. Antibiotics and steroids may be useful in cases of pneumonitis (Arenas, 1970).

Early administration of versenate (Ca EDTA) may prevent central nervous system damage. Encouraging results have been obtained by the use of L-dopa for the treatment of parkinsonism associated with manganese toxicity (Arenas, 1970).

REFERENCES

Agrawal, B. B. L., and Goldstein, I. J. 1968. Protein carbohydrate interaction. VII. Physical and chemical studies on concanavalin A, the hemogglutinin of the jackbean. *Arch. Biochem. Biophys.* **124,** 218–229.

Arenas, J. M. 1970. *Poisoning: Toxicology—Symptoms—Treatments,* 2nd ed. Charles C. Thomas, Springfield, Illinois, p. 208.

Amdur, M. O., Norris, L. C., and Heuser, G. F. 1945. The need for manganese in bone development by the rat. *Proc. Soc. Exp. Biol. Med.* **59,** 254–255.

Bell, L. T., and Hurley, L. S. 1973. Ultrastructural effects of manganese deficiency in liver, heart, kidney and pancreas of mice. *Lab. Invest.* **29,** 723–736.

Bertinchamps, A. J., Miller, S. T., and Cotzias, G. C. 1966. Interdependence of routes of excreting manganese. *Amer. J. Physiol.* **211,** 217–224.

Borg, D. C., and Cotzias, G. C. 1958a. Manganese metabolism in man: Rapid exchange of Mn^{56} with tissue as demonstrated by blood clearance and liver uptake. *J. Clin. Invest.* **37,** 1269–1278.

Borg, D. C., and Cotzias, G. C. 1958b. Incorporation of manganese into erythrocytes as evidence for a manganese porphyrin in man. *Nature (London)* **182,** 1677–1678.

Britton, A. A., and Cotzias, G. C. 1966. Dependence of manganese turnover on intake. *Amer. J. Physiol.* **211,** 203–206.

Chapman, B. E., MacDermott, T. E., and O'Sullivan, W. J. 1973. Studies on manganese complexes of human serum albumin. *Bioinorg. Chem.* **3,** 27–38.

Cotzias, G. C. 1958. Manganese in health and disease. *Physiol. Rev.* **38,** 503–532.

Cotzias, G. C., and Bertinchamps, J. 1960. Transmanganin, the specific manganese-carrying protein of human plasma. *J. Clin. Invest.* **39,** 979.

Cotzias, G. C., and Greenough, J. J. 1958. The high specificity of the manganese pathway through the body. *J. Clin. Invest.* **37,** 1298–1305.

Cotzias, G. C., Miller, S. T., and Edwards, J. 1966. Neutron activation analysis: The stability of manganese concentrations in human blood and serum. *J. Lab. Clin. Med.* **67,** 836–849.

Cotzias, G. C., Horiuchi, K., Fuenzalida, S., and Mena, I. 1968. Chronic manganese poisoning: Clearance of tissue manganese concentrations with persistence of a neurological picture. *Neurology* **18,** 376–382.

Cotzias, G. C., Papavasiliou, P. S., Ginos, J., Streck, A., and Düby, S. 1971. Metabolic modification of Parkinson's disease and of chronic manganese poisoning. *Annu. Rev. Med.* **22,** 305–326.

Cotzias, G. C., Tang, L. C., Miller, S. T., Sladic-Simic, D., and Hurley, L. S. 1972. A mutation influencing the transportation of manganese, L-dopa, and L-tryptophan. *Science* **176,** 410–412.

Davis, P. N., Norris, L. C., and Kratzer, F. H. 1962. Interference of soybean meal with the utilization of trace minerals. *J. Nutr.* **77,** 217–223.

Dickert, J. W., and Rozacky, E. 1969. Isolation and partial characterization of manganin, a new manganoprotein from peanut seeds. *Arch. Biochem. Biophys.* **134,** 473–477.

Doisy, E. A., Jr. 1974. Effects of deficiency in manganese upon plasma levels of clotting proteins and cholesterol in man. In: *Trace Element Metabolism in Animals* (W. G. Hoekstra *et al,* eds.). *Proceedings of the 2nd International Symposium,* University Park Press, Baltimore, pp. 668–670.

Erway, L. C., and Mitchell, S. E. 1973. Prevention of otolith defect in pastel mink by manganese supplementation. *J. Hered.* **64,** 111–119.

Erway, L., Hurley, L. S., and Fraser, A. 1966. Neurological defect: Manganese in phenocopy and prevention of a genetic abnormality of inner ear. *Science* **152,** 1766–1768.

Erway, L., Hurley, L. S., and Fraser, A. S. 1970. Congenital ataxia and otolith defects due to manganese deficiency in mice. *J. Nutr.* **100,** 643–654.

Erway, L., Fraser, A., and Hurley, L. S. 1971. Prevention of congenital otolith defect in *pallid* mutant mice by manganese supplementation. *Genetics* **67,** 97–108.

Everson, G. J. 1968. Preliminary study of carbohydrates in the urine of manganese deficient guinea pigs at birth. *J. Nutr.* **96,** 283–288.

Everson, G. J., and Shrader, R. E. 1968. Abnormal glucose tolerance in manganese-deficient guinea pigs. *J. Nutr.* **94,** 89–94.

Everson, G. J., Hurley, L. S., and Geiger, J. F. 1959. Manganese deficiency in the guinea pig. *J. Nutr.* **68,** 49–56.

Forth, W., and Rummel, W. 1973. Iron absorption. *Physiol. Rev.* **53,** 724–792.

Gallup, W. D., and Norris, L. C. 1939. The amount of manganese required to prevent perosis in the chick. *Poultry Sci.* **18,** 76–82.

Hancock, R. G. V., and Fritze, K. 1973. Chromatographic evidence for the existence of a manganese porphryin in erythrocytes. *Bioinorg. Chem.* **3,** 77–87.

Hartman, R. H., Matrone, G., and Wise, G. H. 1955. Effect of high dietary manganese on hemoglobin formation. *J. Nutr.* **57,** 429–439.

Hill, R. M., Holtkamp, D. E., Buchanan, A. R., and Rutledge, E. K. 1950. Manganese deficiency in rats with relation to ataxia and loss of equilibrium. *J. Nutr.* **41,** 359–371.

Hughes, E. R., Miller, S. T., and Cotzias, G. C. 1966. Tissue concentrations of manganese and adrenal function. *Amer. J. Physiol.* **211,** 207–210.

Hurley, L. S. 1968. Genetic–nutritional interactions concerning manganese. In: *Trace Substances in Environmental Health,* Vol. II (D. Hemphill, ed.). University of Missouri, Columbia, pp. 41–51.

Hurley, L. S., and Bell, L. T. 1974. Genetic influence on response to dietary manganese deficiency in mice. *J. Nutr.* **104,** 133–137.

Hurley, L. S., Everson, G. J., and Geiger, J. F. 1958. Manganese deficiency in rats: Congenital nature of ataxia. *J. Nutr.* **66,** 309–319.

Hurley, L. S., Theriault, L. L., and Dreosti, I. E. 1970. Liver mitochondria from manganese-deficient and pallid mice: Function and ultrastructure. *Science* **170,** 1316–1318.

Keele, B. B., McCord, J. M., and Fridovich, I. 1970. Superoxide dismutase from *Escherichia coli* B: A new manganese-containing enzyme. *J. Biol. Chem.* **245,** 6176–6181.

Kemmerer, A. R., Elvehjem, C. A., and Hart, E. B. 1931. Studies on the relation of manganese to the nutrition of the mouse. *J. Biol. Chem.* **92,** 623–630.

Leach, R. M., Jr. 1968. Effect of manganese upon the epiphyseal growth plate in the young chick. *Poultry Sci.* **47,** 828–830.

Leach, R. M., Jr. 1971. Role of manganese in mucopolysaccharide metabolism. *Fed. Proc. Fed. Amer. Soc. Exp. Biol.* **30,** 991–994.

Leach, R. M., Jr. 1976. Metabolism and function of manganese. In: *Trace Elements in Human Health and Disease,* Vol. II (A. S. Prasad, ed.). Academic Press, New York, pp. 235–247.

Leach, R. M., Jr., and Muenster, A. M. 1962. Studies on the role of manganese in bone formation. I. Effect upon mucopolysaccharide content of chick bone. *J. Nutr.* **78,** 51–56.

Leach, R. M., Jr., Muenster, A. M., and Wein, E. M. 1969. Studies on the role of manganese in bone formation. II. Effect upon chondroitin sulfate synthesis in chick epiphyseal cartilage. *Arch. Biochem. Biophys.* **133,** 22–28.

Longstaff, M., and Hill, R. 1972. The hexosamine and uronic acid contents of the matrix of shells of eggs from pullets fed on diets of different manganese content. *Brit. Poult. Sci.* **13,** 377–385.

Lyons, M. 1939. Some effects of manganese on eggshell quality. *Ark. Agric. Exp. Sta. Bull.* **374,** 1.

Matrone, G., Hartman, R. H., and Clawson, A. J. 1959. Manganese–iron antagonism in the nutrition of rabbits and baby pigs. *J. Nutr.* **67,** 309–317.

Maynard, L. S., and Cotzias, G. C. 1955. The partition of manganese among organs and intracellular organelles of the rat. *J. Biol. Chem.* **214,** 489–495.

Mena, I., Marin, O., Fuenzalida, S., and Cotzias, G. C. 1967. Chronic manganese poisoning: Clinical picture and manganese turnover. *Neurology* **17,** 128–136.

Mena, I., Court, J., Fuenzalida, S., Papavasiliou, P. S. and Cotzias, G. C. 1970. Modification of chronic manganese poisoning. *New Engl. J. Med.* **282,** 5.

Mildvan, A. S., Scrutton, M. C., and Utter, M. F. 1966. Pyruvate carboxylase. VII. A possible role for tightly bound manganese. *J. Biol. Chem.* **241,** 3488–3498.

Nandedkar, A. K. N., Nurse, C. E., and Friedberg, F. 1973. Mn^{++} binding by plasma proteins. *Int. J. Peptide Protein Res.* **5,** 279–281.

Norris, L. C., and Caskey, C. D. 1939. A chronic congenital ataxia and osteodystrophy in chicks due to manganese deficiency. *J. Nutr.* **17,** (Suppl.), 16–17.

Olson, J. A. 1965. The biosynthesis of cholesterol. *Ergebn. Physiol.* **56,** 173–215.

Orent, E. R., and McCollum, E. V. 1931. Effects of deprivation of manganese in the rat. *J. Biol. Chem.* **92,** 651–678.

Papavasiliou, P. S., Miller, S. T., and Cotzias, G. C. 1966. Role of liver in regulating distribution and excretion of manganese. *Amer. J. Physiol.* **211,** 211–216.

Papavasiliou, P. S., Miller, S. T., and Cotzias, G. C. 1968. Functional interaction between biogenic amines, 3′-5′-cyclic AMP and manganese. *Nature (London)* **220,** 74–75.

Plumlee, M. P., Thrasher, D. M., Beesen, W. M., Andrews, F. N., and Parker, H. E. 1956. The effects of a manganese deficiency upon the growth, development and reproduction of swine. *J. Anim. Sci.* **15,** 352–367.

Robinson, N. W., Hansard, S. L., Johns, D. M., and Robertson, G. L. 1960. Excess dietary manganese and feed lot performance of beef cattle. *J. Anim. Sci.* **19,** 1290.

Rojas, M. A., Dyer, I. A., and Cassatt, W. A. 1965. Manganese deficiency in the bovine. *J. Anim. Sci.* **24,** 664–667.

Scrutton, M. C. 1971. Purification and some properties of a protein containing bound manganese (avimanganin). *Biochemistry* **10,** 3897–3905.

Scrutton, M. C., Utter, M. F., and Mildvan, A. S. 1966. Pyruvate carboxylase. VI. The presence of tightly bound manganese. *J. Biol. Chem.* **241,** 3480–3487.

Scrutton, M. C., Griminger, P., and Wallace, J. C. 1972. Pyruvate carboxylase: Bound metal content of the vertebrate liver enzyme as a function of diet. *J. Biol. Chem.* **247,** 3305–3313.

Shrader, R. E., and Everson, G. J. 1967. Anomalous development of otoliths associated with postural defects in manganese-deficient guinea pigs. *J. Nutr.* **92,** 453–460.

Shrader, R. E., and Everson, G. J. 1968. Pancreatic pathology in manganese-deficient guinea pigs. *J. Nutr.* **94,** 269–281.

Shrader, R. E., Erway, L. C., and Hurley, L. S. 1973. Mucopolysaccharide synthesis in the developing inner ear of manganese-deficient and pallid mutant mice. *Teratology* **8,** 257–266.

Thomson, A. B. R., Olatunbosun, D., and Valberg, L. S. 1971. Interrelation of intestinal transport system of manganese and iron. *J. Lab. Clin. Med.* **78,** 642–655.

Tsai, H. C. C., and Everson, G. J. 1967. Effect of manganese deficiency on the acid mucopolysaccharides in cartilage of guinea pigs. *J. Nutr.* **91,** 447–452.

Underwood, E. J. 1977. *Trace Elements in Human and Animal Nutrition,* 4th ed. Academic Press, New York, pp. 170–195.

Vallee, B. L., and Coleman, J. E. 1964. Metal coordination and enzyme action. In: *Comprehensive Biochemistry,* Vol. 12 (M. Florkin and E. H. Stotz, eds.). Elsevier, Amsterdam, pp. 165–235.

Vance, P. G., Keele, B. B., Jr., and Rajagopalan, K. V. 1972. Superoxide dismutase from *Streptococcus mutans:* Isolation and characterization of two forms of the enzyme. *J. Biol. Chem.* **247,** 4782–4786.

Wilgus, H. S., and Patton, A. R. 1939. Factors affecting manganese utilization in the chicken. *J. Nutr.* **18,** 35–45.

Wilgus, H. S., Norris, L. C., and Heuser, G. F. 1936. The role of certain inorganic elements in the cause and prevention of perosis. *Science* **84,** 252–253.

Wolbach, S. B., and Hegsted, D. M. 1953. Perosis: Epiphyseal cartilage in choline and manganese deficiencies in the chick. *AMA Arch. Pathol.* **56,** 437–453.

CHAPTER 8

NEWER TRACE ELEMENTS

INTRODUCTION

Less than 20 years ago, trace elements such as zinc, copper, and chromium were considered to be esoteric considerations for human nutrition. The importance of these trace elements in human health and disease has now been established. In recent years, the consumption of highly refined foods, food product analogues, and empty calories that are often lacking in trace elements has increased. The use of fad diets, refined diets, or total parenteral feeding may in the future reveal the importance of some "newer" trace elements. Recently, nickel, vanadium, silicon, fluorine, and tin have been found to be beneficial in the diets of laboratory animals. It seems probable that some of these elements may also be essential or beneficial for man (Nielsen, 1976).

NICKEL

Nickel was found to be present in animal tissues in 1920. It is only recently that nickel has been shown to be essential for animals. Pathological signs that are consistent with nickel deficiency have been produced in chicks, rats, and swine (Nielsen, 1976).

Direct evidence for the essentiality of nickel was first reported in 1970 (Nielsen and Sauberlich, 1970). It should be considered, however, that the findings of that study and of those that followed (Nielsen, 1971, 1974; Nielsen and Higgs, 1971; Nielsen and Ollerich, 1974; Nielsen *et al.,* 1974; Sunderman *et al.,* 1972b) were obtained under conditions that produced suboptimal growth in chicks, and that some of the signs thought to be the result of a nickel deficiency were inconsistent (Nielsen, 1976).

Recently, the methodology for the study of nickel deficiency in animals has been improved considerably. A diet based on dried skim milk, EDTA-extracted soy protein, acid-washed ground corn, and corn oil has been used, and under these conditions, day-old control chicks grew to over 600 g in 4 weeks, which is considered to be optimal. This diet contained 2.2 ng nickel/g on an air-dried basis. The diet of control chicks contained an additional 3 μg nickel/g. The chicks were raised in a trace-element-controlled environment (Nielsen, 1974, 1976).

Grossly, at 3½–4 weeks of age, the legs of deficient chicks differed from those of controls. Deficiency resulted in less pigmentation of the shank skin, and the legs also appeared to be shorter and thicker. Other signs of nickel deficiency in chicks included decreased hematocrits, decreased plasma cholesterol, and increased liver cholesterol (Nielsen, 1976).

Ultrastructural abnormalities in the hepatocytes, consisting of pyknotic nuclei and swollen mitochondria, were also a consistent finding. The swelling of the mitochondria was in the compartment of the matrix and was associated with less clearly defined cristae. Additional ultrastructural changes were ribosomal draping around the mitochondria and dilation of the cisterns of the rough endoplasmic reticulum (Nielsen, 1976).

In rats during the suckling stage, the nickel-deficient pups usually had a less thrifty appearance, characterized by a rougher hair coat, and appeared less active (Nielsen, 1976). They also had a slower growth rate, and some actually appeared malnourished. About 17% of the deficient pups died during the last few days of the suckling period. There was no mortality in the controls at this age. After the deficient animals were weaned, their appearance, growth, and activity improved.

When the nickel-deficient rats were 6–8 weeks of age, they showed some alterations in liver metabolism. Their livers weighed less than those of controls and were a muddy brown color compared with a red-brown color for controls. Homogenates of the deficient livers demonstrated a reduced oxidative ability in the presence of α-glycerophosphate. The nickel-deficient livers also contained significantly lower levels of liver glycogen. Previous studies showed that with nickel deficiency, sucrose density gradients of liver postmitochondrial supernatants were consistent with a decrease in polysomes and an increase in monosomes (Nielsen, 1974, 1976; Nielsen and Ollerich, 1974; Nielsen *et al.*, 1974).

Signs of nickel deficiency have also been produced in swine (Anke *et al.*, 1974). Some of the findings include a sparse, rough hair coat and impaired reproduction. First-generation piglets showed poor growth.

Thus, a substantial amount of direct evidence exists showing nickel to be an essential element. So far, however, no experimental evidence that defines the requirement of nickel for animals has been published. An intake of 50–80 ng nickel/g experimental diet is most likely adequate for chicks and rats (Nielsen, 1976).

BIOLOGICAL FUNCTIONS

The biochemical and physiological functions of nickel are not well known at present. Nickel may play a role in metabolism or in the structure of membranes. The liver ultrastructural changes due to nickel deficiency occur mainly in the membraneous organelles. The level of liver cholesterol, an integral part of membranes, is altered by nickel deficiency.

Recent reports indicate that nickel may be important in the regulation of prolactin (LaBella *et al.,* 1973). Some changes, such as are seen with respect to liver glycogen and cholesterol, shank skin yellow pigments, and plasma cholesterol, due to nickel deficiency may be related to its effect on hormones (Nielsen, 1976).

Nickel may have a role in RNA, DNA, and/or protein structure or function. A nickelmetalloprotein that has been named "nickeloplasmin" has been isolated from human and rabbit serum (Nomoto *et al.,* 1971; Sunderman *et al.,* 1972a); however, the function of this protein is unclear at present. There are significant concentrations of nickel present in DNA and RNA (Wacker and Vallee, 1959; Eichhorn, 1962; Wacker *et al.,* 1963; Sunderman, 1965). It has been suggested that nickel and the other metals that are present may contribute to the stabilization of the structure of the nucleic acids. Nickel can preserve the compact structure of ribosomes against thermal denaturation (Tal, 1968, 1969a,b), and will restore the sedimentation characteristics of *Escherichia coli* ribosomes that have been subjected to EDTA denaturation (Nielsen, 1976).

The possibility that nickel may be an important cofactor in some enzyme system should not be precluded, since nickel can activate numerous enzymes *in vitro,* including deoxyribonuclease (Miyaji and Greenstein, 1951), acetyl CoA synthetase (Webster, 1965), and phosphoglucomutase (Nielsen, 1976; Ray, 1969).

POSSIBLE HUMAN REQUIREMENTS

Since nickel is essential for animals, it is highly probable that it is also essential for man. At present, however, it appears that nickel nutriture is not a practical problem for man. If animal data can be extrapolated to man, the dietary requirement is probably in the range of 50–80 ng/g diet. Most diets will provide this amount because grains and vegetables seem to be good sources of dietary nickel. This statement must be qualified, since knowledge regarding the chemical form of nickel in foods of plant origin is limited. It has been shown that nickel translocates in plants as a stable anionic amino acid complex (Tiffin, 1971). Whether organic nickel complexes are the usual compounds of nickel in plant tissues, and whether they influence the bioavailability of nickel in any way, remains to be determined. Decsy and Sunderman (1974) have evidence suggesting that nickeloplasmin preferentially binds nickel in the form of an organic complex that is not synthesized, or is synthesized poorly, by the rabbit *in vivo*. Grains, which are rich in nickel, are usually also high in phytin. Nickel can form a stable complex with phytic acid (Vohra *et al.,* 1965), and thus it may be possible that the phytate in grains and other vegetables could decrease the availability of dietary nickel for intestinal absorption. Another possibility is that nickel may complex with fiber in these foods, which could thereby decrease the availability of dietary nickel. Foods of animal origin contain relatively little nickel, in contrast to foods of plant origin (Nielsen, 1976).

Diets that are based on foods of animal origin, or fats, or both, can be low in nickel. A human diet that contained 7–22 ng nickel/g was prepared from meat, milk, eggs, refined white bread, butter, and corn oil (Schroeder *et al.,* 1962). Carbohydrate supplied 43.5% of the calories; fat, 39.1%; and protein, 17.4% (Nielsen, 1976).

Nickel nutriture may be of concern in persons with diseases that interfere with intestinal absorption, or who are under extreme physiological stress. The level of nickel in plasma is known to be decreased in patients with cirrhosis of the liver, chronic uremia, or chronic renal insufficiency (McNeely *et al.,* 1971). These findings are perhaps indicative of nickel depletion. The relatively high concentrations of nickel in sweat are another consideration (Hohnadel *et al.,* 1973). Conditions resulting in large losses of sweat may conceivably increase the need for nickel (Nielsen, 1976).

VANADIUM

Evidence for the essentiality of vanadium for animals was reported in 1971 by Hopkins and Mohr (1971a,b), who found significantly reduced growth of wing and tail feathers in chicks fed a diet containing less than 10 ng vanadium/g. Strasia (1971) noted that rats fed less than 100 ng vanadium/g diet showed reduced body growth and a significantly increased blood packed cell volume in comparison with controls receiving at least 0.5 μg vanadium/g. He also found an increase in blood and bone iron in deficient rats. Schwarz and Milne (1971) noted that rats fed a highly purified amino acid diet (containing an unknown quantity of vanadium) demonstrated a growth response to 50–100 ng supplemental vanadium/g diet. In addition to these symptoms, several other deficiency symptoms that are attributable to low levels of dietary vanadium have been reported in rats and chicks (Nielsen, 1976).

In chicks, vanadium deficiency has an effect on plasma lipids. Hopkins and Mohr (1971a,b) noted that vanadium-deficient chicks had decreased plasma levels of cholesterol at 28 days of age, while at 49 days, their plasma cholesterol concentrations were greater than those of control chicks. Nielsen (1976) found increased plasma cholesterol levels in deficient chicks following only 28 days of deficiency. Plasma triglyceride levels are also significantly increased in vanadium-deficient chicks (Hopkins and Mohr, 1974).

Vanadium deficiency has adverse effects on bone development in the chick (Nielsen and Ollerich, 1973). The tibiae in deficient chicks revealed increased epiphyseal plate and decreased primary spongiosa as judged by weight ratios and microscopic examination. Histologically, the vanadium-deficient chick tibiae show disorganization of the cells of the epiphysis. The cells appear compressed and their nuclei flattened.

Reproductive performance in rats is impaired by vanadium deprivation (Hopkins and Mohr, 1974). When five fourth-generation female rats were mated, significantly fewer live births resulted and significantly more deaths of neonatal pups occurred than with vanadium-supplemented controls (Nielsen, 1976).

These data from four different laboratories and on two different species established that vanadium is an essential nutrient for experimental animals. Because of limited data, the level of vanadium required to maintain health in rats and chicks can only be estimated. Schwarz (1974) reported a requirement of 100 ng supplemental vanadium/g diet containing an unknown amount of vanadium for an optimal growth response in rats. An additional increment of growth was noted, however, when 500 ng vanadium was supplemented per gram of diet. It has been suggested that the requirement is between 50 and 500 ng/g when a purified diet is fed (Hopkins and Mohr, 1974). The requirement may be even higher when natural feeds are used. When an experimental diet composed of 26% protein, 6% fat, and 57% carbohydrate (balance minerals, vitamins, and nonnutritive fiber) is used, an intake of approximately 100 ng/g for chicks is probably adequate (Nielsen, 1976).

BIOLOGICAL FUNCTIONS

As with nickel, very little is known concerning the specific biological function or functions of vanadium. Probably vanadium is an important cofactor in controlling one or more enzymatic or catalytic reactions. Schwarz (1974) speculated that vanadium may function as an oxidation–reduction catalyst. It was reported that added vanadium markedly increased the oxidation of phospholipids by washed liver suspensions *in vitro* (Bernheim and Bernheim, 1939). Further evidence that vanadium may act as an oxidation–reduction catalyst in biological systems was obtained from a lower group of organisms known as the ascidians. Schroeder *et al.* (1963) and Underwood (1971) briefly reviewed these data. Ascidians contain green blood cells called vandocytes, which contain hemovanadin, a pigment composed of pyrrole rings and a protein. Hemovanadin is a strong reducing agent (Nielsen, 1976).

Studies involving vanadium and its effect on cholesterol metabolism have shown that pharmacological levels of vanadium may affect tissue cholesterol levels. Curran and Burch (1967) were able to relate these altered cholesterol levels to vanadium inhibition of the microsomal enzyme system known as squalene synthetase, and to the vanadium stimulation of acetoacetyl-CoA deacylase in liver mitochondria. These findings of altered lipid metabolism in vanadium deficiency are consistent with an enzymatic role for vanadium in lipid metabolism (Nielsen, 1976).

Vanadium may also have a catalytic or enzymatic function in bone metabolism or formation. The findings of abnormal bone growth in vanadium deficiency suggests that such a function is a possibility. Further evidence for such a function was found when radiovanadium, injected subcutaneously into young rats, showed the highest uptake to be in areas of rapid mineralization in the dentine and bone (Soremark *et al.,* 1962). Radiovanadium injected intravenously into adult mice was also taken up by the teeth and bones. After 24–48 hr, the tissues having the highest concentration were the bones and teeth, with the zones of mineralization showing an especially high uptake (Nielsen, 1976; Soremark and Ullberg, 1962).

POSSIBLE HUMAN REQUIREMENTS

Information regarding the vanadium content of dietary items is limited, partly because of the difficulty of accurately analyzing low levels of vanadium. Soremark (1967) reported values obtained by activation analysis that ranged from less than 0.1 ng vanadium/g in peas, beets, carrots, and pears to 52 ng/g in radishes. Milk usually contained less than 0.1 ng/g (fresh basis), and liver, fish, and meat contained up to 10 ng/g. Some foods that apparently are good sources of vanadium are bread, some grains and nuts, vegetable oils, and some root vegetables (Schroeder *et al.,* 1963). These limited data indicate, however, that many dietary items contain amounts of vanadium that are below 100 ng/g. Also, information regarding the availability of vanadium from foods is limited. The toxicity of vanadium compounds has been found to be greater when the compounds are fed in a purified diet than when these compounds are given in a natural diet (Berg, 1966; Nielsen, 1976).

Obviously, additional data are necessary before firm conclusions can be drawn. If vanadium is required for man, however, adequate vanadium nutrition should not be taken for granted. A diet that consisted exclusively of milk, meat, and certain vegetables could contain less than 100 ng vanadium/g.

SILICON

One of the newest elements shown to be essential for animals is silicon. Although it was previously reported (Carlisle, 1970, 1971) that silicon may be necessary for an early stage of bone calcification, the first actual evidence for the essentiality of silicon was given in 1972 (Carlisle, 1972a,b; Schwarz and Milne, 1972). In studies with chicks Carlisle (1972a,b) showed that feeding a silicon-deficient diet resulted in depressed growth. Pallor of the legs, comb, skin, and mucous membranes was noted. The subcutaneous tissue was a muddy-yellowish color in comparison with the white-pinkish subcutaneous tissue of the silicon-adequate controls. The deficient chicks had no wattles, their combs were severely attenuated, and feathering was retarded. Leg bones had thinner cortices and were shorter and of smaller circumference than those of the controls. The femurs and tibiae fractured more easily. The cranial bones were noted to be flatter, and beaks were more flexible (Nielsen, 1976).

In rats, 500 μg silicon/g amino acid diet as sodium metasilicate produced a growth response (Schwarz and Milne, 1972; Schwarz, 1974). The unsupplemented animals showed skull deformations and poor incisor pigmentation.

More recently, Carlisle (1973) showed that the skeletal alterations involve the cartilage matrix. There is a significant decrease in hexosomines in the silicon-deficient chick metatarsus and tibial epiphyses, epiphyseal plates, and spongiosae.

The requirement of silicon for the chick as sodium metasilicate has been estimated to be in the range of 100–200 μg/g experimental diet containing 26% amino acids, 5% fat, 62% carbohydrate, and 7% minerals and vitamins. It is likely that other forms of silicon are more available than the silicate for the chick, as they are for the rat. The absolute requirement for the chick, therefore, is probably lower than 100–200 μg/g.

BIOLOGICAL FUNCTIONS

Recent studies have given evidence that silicon is an essential cross-linking agent in connective tissue. Such a role is strongly suggested by both the distribution of silicon and the effect of silicon deficiency on connective tissue form and composition. The data from studies of Schwarz (1973) indicate the presence of 331–554 μg bound silicon/g purified hyaluronic acid from human umbilical cord, chondroitin 4-sulfate, dermatan sulfate, and heparan sulfate. These levels correspond to 1 atom of silicon per 50,000–

85,000 molecular weight, or 130–280 repeating units, and lesser amounts (57–191 μg/g) were found in chondroitin 6-sulfate, heparin, and keratan sulfate-2 from cartilage. Hyaluronic acid from vitreous humor and keratan sulfate-one from cornea were silicon-free. Collagen in connective tissue also contains silicon. According to Schwarz and Chen (1974), 3–6 atoms of silicon per each α-protein chain in the collagen molecule are present. Carlisle (1974a) found lesser amounts of silicon in collagen, although it is still apparent that silicon may have a fundamental role in collagen cross-linking mechanisms (Nielsen, 1976).

Several experiments carried out by Schwarz (1973, 1974) to characterize the form in which silicon may be present demonstrate that the silicon atom is bound over oxygen to the carbon skeleton of mucopolysaccharides: –Si–O-C–. It has been concluded that silicon is present as a silanolate, an etherlike or esterlike derivative of silicic acid. Silicon can link portions of the same polysaccharide to each other, or acid mucopolysaccharides to proteins.

In addition to a structural function, it is possible that silicon may have a matrix, or catalytic, function in bone calcification. Carlisle (1970, 1971, 1974b), using electron-microprobe techniques, observed that as mineralization progresses, the silicon and calcium contents rise congruently in osteoid tissue. In the more advanced stages of mineralization, the silicon concentration falls markedly, while calcium concentrations approach proportions found in bone apatite. Minute sites were found in the metaphysis of young bone that corresponded with the margin of trabeculae and bony spicules during bone formation. Silicon was also found in blood vessels between metaphyseal trabeculae. Carlisle stated that "the fact that silicon occurs both in metaphyseal blood vessels and in the silicon-rich sites, along with the observations by earlier workers that invasion of the metaphysis by blood vessels triggers the sequence of matrix alterations leading to calcification, suggests that silicon takes part in the sequence of events leading to calcification" (Carlisle, 1970; Nielsen, 1976).

POSSIBLE HUMAN REQUIREMENTS

Silicon deficiency in humans has not been described; however, it is apparent from the previous discussion that silicon has important functions in man. Mucopolysaccharides, collagen, and silicon are most likely interrelated in human growth and maintenance of connective tissues. Silicon content in the arterial wall has been found to decrease with the development of atherosclerosis (Loeper and Loeper, 1961), and aging results in diminished silicon concentrations in human skin (dermis) (Brown, 1927; MacCardle *et al.,* 1943) and in normal human aorta (Loeper and Loeper, 1961; Nielsen, 1976).

Silicon is probably not a major dietary problem, since many foods contain high levels of silicon. Such foods include those high in fiber (e.g., some cereal grains) and pectin (e.g., citrus fruits). Dietary items of animal origin, except skin (e.g., chicken), are relatively low in silicon.

TIN

Tin occurs in trace amounts in many tissues and dietary items, but until recently it was considered to be an "environmental contaminant" instead of a possibly essential dietary factor. It was reported in 1970 that tin is essential for the growth of rats maintained on purified amino acid diets in a trace-element-controlled environment (Schwarz *et al.,* 1970). Tin also produced significant improvement in incisor pigmentation (Milne and Schwarz, 1972). These observations, however, have not been confirmed (Nielsen, 1976).

BIOLOGICAL FUNCTIONS

Tin has several chemical properties that offer possibilities for biological function. Tetravalent tin has a strong tendency to form coordination complexes with 4, 5, 6, and possibly 8 ligands, and thus, Schwarz *et al.* (1970) suggested that tin may contribute to the tertiary structure of proteins or other components of biological importance. Also, they speculated that tin may participate in oxidation–reduction reactions in biological systems, since the $Sn^{2+} \rightleftharpoons Sn^{4+}$ potential of 0.13 volt is within the physiological range. It is, in fact, near the oxidation–reduction potential of flavine enzymes (Nielsen, 1976).

POSSIBLE HUMAN REQUIREMENTS

It is impossible to state any possible needs for tin in man, since so little is known about the metabolism. The levels of tin found to promote growth in rats are similar to the quantities found in many foods of plant and animal origin (Schwarz *et al.,* 1970). Tin nutriture, therefore, is not of much concern at present. The increased use of highly refined foods or food product analogues that contain little or no tin could alter this judgment in the future (Nielsen, 1976).

REFERENCES

Anke, M., Grun, M., Dittrich, G., Groppel, B., and Hennig, A. 1974. Low nickel rations for growth and reproduction in pigs. In: *Trace Element Metabolism in Animals—2* (W. G. Hoekstra *et al.,* eds.). University Park Press, Baltimore, pp. 715–718.

Berg, L. R. 1966. Effect of diet composition on vanadium toxicity for the chick. *Poultry Sci.* **45,** 1346–1352.

Bernheim, F., and Bernheim, M. L. C. 1939. The action of vanadium on the oxidation of phospholipids by certain tissues. *J. Biol. Chem.* **127,** 353–360.

Brown, H. 1927. The mineral content of human skin. *J. Biol. Chem.* **75,** 789–794.

Carlisle, E. M. 1970. Silicon: A possible factor in bone calcification. *Science* **167,** 279–280.

Carlisle, E. M. 1971. A relationship between silicon, magnesium, and fluorine in bone formation in the chick. *Fed. Proc. Fed. Amer. Soc. Exp. Biol.* **30,** 462 (abstract).

Carlisle, E. M. 1972a. Silicon: An essential element for the chick. *Fed. Proc. Fed. Amer. Soc. Exp. Biol.* **31,** 700 (abstract).

Carlisle, E. M. 1972b. Silicon: An essential element for the chick. *Science* **178,** 619–621.

Carlisle, E. M. 1973. A skeletal alteration associated with silicon deficiency. *Fed. Proc. Fed. Amer. Soc. Exp. Biol.* **32,** 930 (abstract).

Carlisle, E. M. 1974a. A relationship between silicon, glycosaminoglycan and collagen formation. *Fed. Proc. Fed. Amer. Soc. Exp. Biol.* **33,** 704 (abstract).

Carlisle, E. M. 1974b. Silicon as an essential element. *Fed. Proc. Fed. Amer. Soc. Exp. Biol.* **33,** 1758–1766.

Curran, G. L., and Burch, R. E. 1967. Biological and health effects of vanadium. In: *Trace Substances in Environmental Health,* Vol. I (D. D. Hemphill, ed.). University of Missouri Press, Columbia, pp. 96–102.

Decsy, M. I., and Sunderman, F. W., Jr. 1974. Binding of ^{63}Ni to rabbit serum α_1-macroglobulin *in vivo* and *in vitro*. *Bioinorg. Chem.* **3,** 95–105.

Eichhorn, G. L. 1962. Metal ions as stabilizers or destabilizers of the deoxyribonucleic acid structure. *Nature (London)* **194,** 474–475.

Hohnadel, D. C., Sunderman, F. W., Jr., Nechay, M. W., and McNeely, M. D. 1973. Atomic absorption spectrometry of nickel, copper, zinc, and lead in sweat collected from healthy subjects during sauna bathing. *Clin. Chem.* **19,** 1288–1292.

Hopkins, L. L., Jr., and Mohr, H. E. 1971a. The biological essentiality of vanadium. In: *Newer Trace Elements in Nutrition* (W. Mertz and W. E. Cornatzer, eds.). Marcel Dekker, New York, pp. 195–213.

Hopkins, L. L., Jr., and Mohr, H. E. 1971b. Effects of vanadium deficiency on plasma cholesterol of chicks. *Fed. Proc. Fed. Amer. Soc. Exp. Biol.* **30,** 462 (abstract).

Hopkins, L. L., Jr., and Mohr, H. E. 1974. Vanadium as an essential nutrient. *Fed. Proc. Fed. Amer. Soc. Exp. Biol.* **33,** 1773–1775.

LaBella, F. S., Dular, R., Lemon, P., Vivian, S., and Queen, G. 1973. Prolactin secretion is specifically inhibited by nickel. *Nature (London)* **245,** 330–332.

Loeper, J., and Loeper, J. 1961. Role of silicon in the arterial wall. *C. R. Soc. Biol.* **155,** 468–470.

MacCardle, R. C., Engman, M. F., Jr., and Engman, M. F., Sr. 1943. Mineral changes in neurodermatitis revealed by microincineration. *Arch. Dermatol. Syphilol.* **47,** 335–372.

McNeely, M. D., Sunderman, F. W., Jr., Nechay, M. W., and Levine, H. 1971. Abnormal concentrations of nickel in serum in cases of myocardial infarction, stroke, burns, hepatic cirrhosis, and uremia. *Clin. Chem.* **17,** 1123–1128.

Milne, D. B., and Schwarz, K. 1972. Effect of newer essential trace elements on rat incisor pigmentation. *Fed. Proc. Fed. Amer. Soc. Exp. Biol.* **31,** 700 (abstract).

Miyaji, T., and Greenstein, J. P. 1951. Cation activation of desoxyribonuclease. *Arch. Biochem. Biophys.* **32,** 414–423.

Nielsen, F. H. 1971. Studies on the essentiality of nickel. In: *Newer Trace Elements in Nutrition* (W. Mertz and W. E. Cornatzer, eds.). Dekker, New York, pp. 215–253.

Nielsen F. H. 1974. Essentiality and function of nickel. In: *Trace Element Metabolism in Animals—2* (W. G. Hoekstra *et al.,* eds.). University Park Press, Baltimore, pp. 381–395.

Nielsen, F. H. 1976. Newer trace elements and possible application in man. In: *Trace Elements in Human Health and Disease,* Vol. II (A. S. Prasad, ed.). Academic Press, New York, pp. 379–399.

Nielsen, F. H., and Higgs, D. J. 1971. Further studies involving a nickel deficiency in chicks. In: *Trace Substances in Environmental Health—IV* (D. D. Hemphill, ed.). University of Missouri Press, Columbia, pp. 241–246.

Nielsen, F. H., and Ollerich, D. A. 1973. Studies on a vanadium deficiency in chicks. *Fed. Proc. Fed. Amer. Soc. Exp. Biol.* **32,** 929 (abstract).

Nielsen, F. H., and Ollerich, D. A. 1974. Nickel: A new essential trace element. *Fed. Proc. Fed. Amer. Soc. Exp. Biol.* **33,** 1767–1772.

Nielsen, F. H., and Sauberlich, H. E. 1970. Evidence of a possible requirement for nickel by the chick. *Proc. Soc. Exp. Biol. Med.* **134,** 845–849.

Nielsen, F. H., Ollerich, D. A., Fosmire, G. J., and Sandstead, H. H. 1974. Nickel deficiency in chicks and rats: Effects on liver morphology, function and polysomal integrity. In: *Protein–Metal Interactions, Adv. Exp. Med. Biol.* (M. Friedman, ed.), Vol. 48, Plenum Press, New York, pp. 389–403.

Nomoto, S., McNeely, M. D., and Sunderman, F. W., Jr. 1971. Isolation of a nickel α_2-macroglobulin from rabbit serum. *Biochemistry* **10,** 1647–1651.

Ray, W. J., Jr. 1969. Role of bivalent cations in the phosphoglucomutase system. I. Characterization of enzyme–metal complexes. *J. Biol. Chem.* **244,** 3740–3747.

Schroeder, H. A., Balassa, J. J., and Tipton, I. H. 1962. Abnormal trace metals in man—nickel. *J. Chronic Dis.* **15,** 51–65.

Schroeder, H. A., Balassa, J. J., and Tipton, I. H. 1963. Abnormal trace metals in man—vanadium. *J. Chronic Dis.* **16,** 1047–1071.

Schwarz, K. 1973. A bound form of silicon in glycosaminoglycans and polyuronides. *Proc. Natl. Acad. Sci. U.S.A.* **70,** 1608–1612.

Schwarz, K. 1974. Recent dietary trace element research, exemplified by tin, fluorine, and silicon. *Fed. Proc. Fed. Amer. Soc. Exp. Biol.* **33,** 1748–1757.

Schwarz, K., and Chen, S. C. 1974. A bound form of silicon as a constituent of collagens. *Fed. Proc. Fed. Amer. Soc. Exp. Biol.* **33,** 704 (abstract).

Schwarz, K., and Milne, D. B. 1971. Growth effects of vanadium in the rat. *Science* **174,** 426–428.

Schwarz, K., and Milne, D. B. 1972. Growth promoting effects of silicon in rats. *Nature (London)* **239,** 333–334.

Schwarz, K., Milne, D. B., and Vinyard, E. 1970. Growth effects of tin compounds in rats maintained in a trace element controlled environment. *Biochem. Biophys. Res. Commun.* **40,** 22–29.

Soremark, R. 1967. Vanadium in some biological specimens. *J. Nutr.* **92,** 183–190.

Soremark, R., and Ullberg, S. 1962. Distribution and kinetics of $^{48}V_2O_5$ in mice. In: *Use of Radioisotopes in Animal Biology and the Medical Sciences—2* (M. Fried, ed.). Academic Press, New York, pp. 103–114.

Soremark, R., Ullberg, S., and Appelgren, L. E. 1962. Autoradiographic localization of vanadium pentoxide ($V_2{}^{48}O_5$) in developing teeth and bones of rats. *Acta Odontol. Scand.* **20,** 225–232.

Strasia, C. A. 1971. Vanadium: Essentiality and toxicity in the laboratory rat. Ph.D. thesis. University Microfilms, Ann Arbor, Michigan.

Sunderman, F. W., Jr. 1965. Measurements of nickel in biological materials by atomic absorption spectrometry. *Amer. J. Clin. Pathol.* **44,** 182–188.

Sunderman, F. W., Jr., Decsy, M. I., and McNeely, M. D. 1972a. Nickel metabolism in health and disease. *Ann. N.Y. Acad. Scie.* **199,** 300–312.

Sunderman, F. W., Jr., Nomoto, S., Morang, R., Nechay, M. W., Burke, C. N., and Nielsen, S. W. 1972b. Nickel deprivation in chicks. *J. Nutr.* **102,** 259–267.

Tal, M. 1968. On the role of Zn^{2+} and Ni^{2+} in ribosome structure. *Biochim. Biophys. Acta* **169,** 564–565.

Tal, M. 1969a. Thermal denaturation of ribosomes. *Biochemistry* **8,** 424–435.

Tal, M. 1969b. Metal ions and ribosomal conformation. *Biochim. Biophys. Acta* **195,** 76–86.

Tiffin, L. O. 1971. Translocation of nickel in xylem exudate of plants. *Plant Physiol.* **48,** 273–277.

Underwood, E. J. 1971. *Trace Elements in Human and Animal Nutrition,* 3rd ed. Academic Press, New York, pp. 369 and 416.

Vohra, P., Gray, G. A., and Kratzer, F. H. 1965. Phytic-acid–metal complex. *Proc. Soc. Exp. Biol. Med.* **120,** 447–449.

Wacker, W. E. C., and Vallee, B. L. 1959. Nucleic acids and metals. I. Chromium, manganese, nickel, iron, and other metals in ribonucleic acid from diverse biological sources. *J. Biol. Chem.* **234,** 3257–3262.

Wacker, W. E. C., Gordon, M. P., and Huff, J. W. 1963. Metal content of tobacco mosaic virus and tobacco mosaic virus RNA. *Biochemistry* **2,** 716–718.

Webster, L. T., Jr. 1965. Studies of the acetyl coenzyme A synthetase reaction. III. Evidence of a double requirement for divalent cations. *J. Biol. Chem.* **240,** 4164–4169.

CHAPTER 9

SELENIUM

INTRODUCTION

Selenium has been shown to be essential for several animal species (McCoy and Weswig, 1969; Thompson and Scott, 1970). Its essentiality for man has not been proved. However, selenium has been shown to be an essential constituent of erythrocyte glutathione peroxidase in several species (Rotruck *et al.,* 1973), and such an enzyme is known to be present in human red cells (Steinberg and Necheles, 1971).

There have been major recent advances in our basic knowledge of selenium in addition to its discovery as part of glutathione peroxidase. The protective effect against mercury toxicity in animals (Ganther *et al.,* 1972) could be extremely important if it is found to be operative in man. Two bacterial enzyme systems (Turner and Stadtman, 1973; Andreesen and Ljungdahl, 1973) and a sheep muscle cytochrome (Whanger *et al.,* 1973) have been shown to contain selenium. Future research may show that selenium is indeed important for certain enzymes required for human metabolism (Burk, 1976).

BIOCHEMISTRY

Glutathione peroxidase (GSH-Px) was discovered by Mills (1957), who demonstrated the presence in bovine erythrocytes of an enzyme that catalyzed the breakdown of hydrogen peroxide, with glutathione serving as the hydrogen donor. Mills (1959) later purified the enzyme and confirmed that the peroxidase and catalase activities of the red cell were attributable to two different enzymes. GSH-Px is not inhibited by cyanide or azide, unlike catalase and various other peroxidases. Cohen and Hochstein (1963) compared the role of erythrocyte GSH-Px and catalase in hydrogen peroxide destruction and concluded that under physiological conditions, the major pathway of hydrogen peroxide destruction involved GSH-Px. Through the investigations of Little and O'Brien (Little and O'Brien, 1968; O'Brien and Little, 1969) and Christophersen (1968, 1969), it was learned that GSH-Px also catalyzed the reduction of hydroperoxides formed from fatty acids and from other substances. Thus, the general reaction catalyzed by this enzyme can be described by

$$ROOH + 2\ GSH \rightarrow R\text{-}OH + HOH + GSSG$$

A wide role for GSH-Px in protecting tissues from oxidative damage is thus apparent (Ganther *et al.,* 1976).

Major contributions to the knowledge about the chemistry and biological function of GSH-Px have come from the work of Flohe and his co-workers in Germany. By the early 1970's, this group had succeeded for the first time in isolating weighable quantities of the pure enzyme (Flohe *et al.,* 1971; Ganther *et al.,* 1976).

In the early 1970's, Rotruck, Hoekstra, and co-workers (Ganther *et al.,* 1976) began an investigation of GSH-Px in relation to the overlapping nutritional roles of selenium, vitamin E, and sulfur amino acids (Ganther *et al.,* 1976). The same year that GSH-Px was discovered, selenium was reported to be a beneficial trace element for animals (Schwarz and Foltz, 1957; Patterson *et al.,* 1957). It was demonstrated that selenium, as the active component of factor 3, prevented liver necrosis in rats, a nutritional disorder also prevented by vitamin E and delayed by the sulfur-containing amino acids (Schwarz, 1961, 1965). By the late 1960's, the essentiality of selenium, even in the presence of vitamin E in the diet, had been firmly established (Thompson and Scott, 1969), but no specific biochemical role had been discovered. In 1973, erythrocyte GSH-Px was identified as a selenoprotein. This protein was shown to contain 4 gram atoms of selenium per mole. Although the selenium atoms have not yet been shown to function in catalysis, the unique chemical properties of selenium and its presence in stoichiometric amounts with the number of subunits make it attractive to propose a mechanism based on selenium functioning at the active site (Ganther *et al.,* 1974, 1976).

In studies of long-term selenium deficiency, some decrease in GSH-Px activity is observed in all body components studied, but the magnitude of decrease varies greatly for different tissues. Short-term studies show rapid depletion of GSH-Px in some components such as plasma and liver, but little or no depletion in tissues such as testis and lens. The body components in which GSH-Px activity appears to be most extensively depleted due to dietary selenium deficiency include plasma, liver, heart, lungs, stomach mucosa, and skeletal muscle. Components showing moderate decreases in GSH-Px include kidney, adrenal glands, and erythrocytes, and those that appear to be least affected are testis and brain.

Information on the subcellular localization of GSH-Px is available for liver. Green and O'Brien (1970) found that of the nuclei-free homogenate of rat liver, 60% of the total GSH-Px was recovered in the soluble or cytosolic fraction and 28% in the mitochondrial fraction. The soluble fraction had a specific activity for GSH-Px of 31 units/mg protein, while the mitochondrial fraction had 17 units/mg protein, and the microsomal and lysosomal fractions had much lower amounts, which could be accounted for by contamination. No values were given for the nuclear fraction. It was also concluded that within the mitochondria, GSH-Px was located within the mitochondrial matrix and may be responsible for protecting the inner membrane, while cytosolic GSH-Px may protect the outer membrane (Ganther *et al.,* 1976). Reports in which rather large amounts of GSH-Px activity are associated with other particulate fractions, such as the nuclear fraction (Demus-Oole and Swierczewski, 1969; Noguchi *et al.,* 1973), must be viewed with caution until more highly purified and carefully characterized preparations are studied. In erythrocytes, some GSH-Px activity is found in the isolated membrane (or ghost) fraction, but it appears to be loosely bound, as it is in the case of hemoglobin (Duchon and Collier, 1971; Ganther *et al.,* 1976).

Iron-deficiency anemia is accompanied by decreased erythrocyte GSH-Px activity, and supplementation with iron causes a rapid increase in GSH-Px (MacDougall, 1972; Hopkins, J., and Tudhope, 1973; Rodvien *et al.,* 1974). While the studies in humans suggest that the decrease in GSH-Px parallels the decrease in hemoglobin (MacDougall, 1972; Hopkins and Tudhope, 1973), a study in rabbits demonstrated that the decrease in GSH-Px was manifest even when expressed in terms of per unit of hemoglobin (Rodvien *et al.,* 1974). It has been suggested that the depressed erythrocyte GSH-Px may be the possible cause of the shortened life span of erythrocytes in iron deficiency. The effect of iron deficiency on GSH-Px was not caused by anemia *per se,* since anemia induced by bleeding or phenylhydrazine did not depress the GSH-Px level (Rodvien *et al.,* 1974), and pernicious anemia was accompanied by an increased level of erythrocyte GSH-Px (Hopkins, J. and Tudhope, 1973). The relationship of iron to GSH-Px remains to be clarified. Iron is apparently not a component of GSH-Px, so that its effect must be by some other mechanism. Studies on the effect of iron deficiency on GSH-Px in tissues other than erythrocytes are lacking (Ganther *et al.,* 1976).

ERYTHROCYTES

The glutathione-dependent pathway concerned with the protection of the red blood cell from oxidative damage due to hydrogen peroxide and other peroxides is shown schematically in Fig. 7. The preferential oxidation of glutathione by peroxides is catalyzed by GSH-Px. The oxidized glutathi-

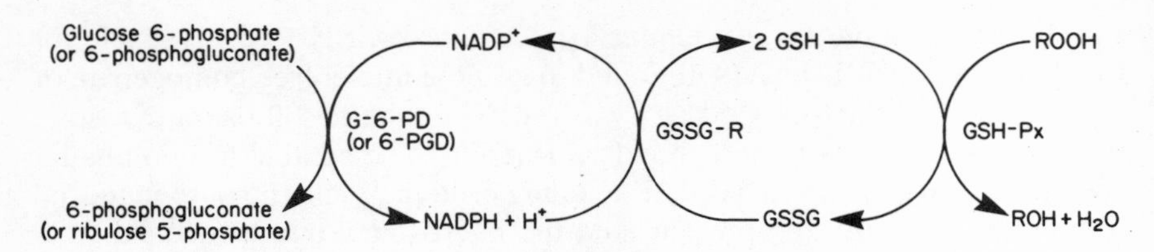

Fig. 7. Glutathione-peroxidase-dependent peroxide decomposition in relation to hexose monophosphate shunt. (G-6-PD) glucose-6-phosphate dehydrogenase; (6-PGD) 6-phosphogluconate dehydrogenase; (GSSG-R) glutathione reductase; (GSH-Px) glutathione peroxidase. From Ganther *et al.* (1976).

one is then reduced by NADPH in a reaction catalyzed by glutathione reductase. The only known mechanism for the reduction of NADP in the mature erythrocyte is by oxidation of glucose via the hexose monophospate shunt pathway. Decreased activity of any of the four enzymes in the pathway or the enzymes of glutathione synthesis due to genetic deficiency, the presence of inhibitors, deficiency of dietary factors necessary for their synthesis or activity (certain amino acids, riboflavin, selenium), or deficiency of any of the building blocks of the substrates involved (niacin, sulfur amino acids) might be expected to result in impaired functioning of this protective pathway, leading to oxidative damage to hemoglobin, precipitation of Heinz bodies, and hemolytic anemia subsequent to oxidative challenge (Ganther *et al.,* 1976).

Genetic deficiencies of each of the enzymes in the pathway as well as the enzymes of glutathione synthesis have been implicated as causes for increased sensitivity to oxidant drugs. Glucose-6-phosphate dehydrogenase (G-6-PD) deficiency is by far the most common of these deficiencies (Beutler, 1965, 1969a; Carson and Frischer, 1966) and results in lack of sufficient NADPH to reduce the oxidized glutathione produced in oxidative stress. Reports of oxidant sensitivity with 6-phosphogluconate dehydrogenase deficiency have also appeared (Brewer, 1969; Scialom *et al.,* 1966; Lausecker *et al.,* 1965). Deficiency of this activity would not only block another NADP-reducing step, but also could cause accumulation of 6-phosphogluconate, leading to product inhibition of G-6-PD. Glutathione reductase deficiency was originally thought to be a genetic disorder (Carson *et al.,* 1961; Waller, 1968), but subsequent reports (Glatzle *et al.,* 1968; Beutler, 1969a,b) have indicated that in a majority of cases, glutathione reductase deficiency is due to mild riboflavin deficiency, and that animals and human subjects made deficient in glutathione reductase by a partial riboflavin deficiency do not show increased sensitivity to oxidant drugs (Beutler and Srivastava, 1970; Jaffe *et al.,* 1968; Paniker *et al.,* 1970). Likewise, GSH-Px deficiency, although previously attributed to genetic causes, could be due to selenium deficiency in some cases. Several clinical cases of GSH-Px deficiency associated with hemolysis have been described (Gharib *et al.,* 1969; Necheles *et al.,* 1967, 1969, 1970; Boivin *et al.,* 1969; Steinberg *et al.,* 1970; Steinberg and Necheles, 1971; Nishimura *et al.,* 1972), and when the deficiency is sufficiently severe, extensive hemolysis has resulted even in the absence of external oxidative challenge. A lack of reduced glutathione caused by deficiency of glutathione synthesis has also been reported to result in severe drug-induced anemia (Waller and Gerok, 1964) or congenital hemolytic anemia (Prins *et al.,* 1966; Boivin *et al.,* 1966; Ganther *et al.,* 1976).

In view of the presence of relatively large amounts of catalase in the red blood cells, Nicholls, in his earlier publication (Nicholls, 1965), discounted the role of GSH-Px in protecting hemoglobin from peroxidation, but later modified this position (Nicholls, 1972), and now believes that both are important. Paniker and Iyer (1965, 1969, 1972), Aebi *et al.* (1964a,b), Aebi and Suter (1966), and Jacob *et al.* (1965) all favor nearly equal roles for the two, with GSH-Px being more important at low concentrations and catalase at high concentrations of hydrogen peroxide, but with either being capable of protecting adequately in the absence of the other. Cohen and Hochstein (1963) and Tudhope and Leece (1971), on the other hand, maintain that GSH-Px is the primary agent for eliminating hydrogen peroxide at the low concentrations found *in vivo.* In support of the latter view, erythocytes having normal levels of catalase but deficient in G-6-PD are more susceptible to oxidant drugs than are normal erythocytes. Many of these drugs, however, have been shown to inhibit catalase to varying degrees (Tudhope and Leece, 1971), and glutathione may function in other ways to enhance the stability of the erythrocyte and its hemoglobin. The GSH-Px activity of erythrocytes has been shown to vary with species, and the relative amounts of GSH-Px and catalase and hence their relative importance in removing hydrogen peroxide may vary widely in different species (Ganther *et al.,* 1976).

In addition to catalyzing the destruction of hydrogen peroxide, GSH-Px catalyzes the reduction of a wide variety of hydroperoxides other than hydrogen peroxide against which catalase is inactive. The role of these other hydroperoxides in promoting the destruction of red cells and hemoglobin is unclear. In a reevaluation of the kinetics of GSH-Px, Flohe *et al.* (1972) concluded that catalase and GSH-Px are equally effective in competing for hydrogen peroxide. The increased sensitivity of GSH-Px-deficient erythrocytes to oxidation in the presence of catalase in the red blood cell may be due to the ability of GSH-Px to reduce hydroperoxides of nearly any structure, such as might be produced by free-radical reactions (Pryor, 1973) involving the oxidant drugs known to produce hemolysis (Ganther *et al.,* 1976).

PHAGOCYTES

Because GSH-Px functions to protect cells from hydrogen peroxide and lipid hydroperoxides, the enzyme is of particular interest in regard to phagocytic cells, which greatly increase their peroxide production and lipid turnover during particle ingestion (phagocytosis). These cells include granulocytes (neutrophils, basophils, eosinophils) and monocytes in the blood, as well as specialized tissue macrophages such as alveolar and peritoneal macrophages. Following the ingestion of foreign objects, oxygen consumption increases markedly (respiratory burst), hydrogen peroxide is formed, and hexose monophosphate shunt activity increases (Klebanoff, 1971). Highly reactive forms of oxygen such as singlet oxygen and the superoxide radical also appear to be generated and may be directly or indirectly involved in the killing process (Allen *et al.,* 1972; Babior *et al.,* 1973; Curnutte and Babior, 1974). Although the ingested object is completely enclosed in a membranous structure (the phagolysosome), peroxides and other substances may diffuse from the phagolysosomes into the surrounding cytoplasm. Thus, the phagocytic cell may bring about its own destruction in the process of attacking the foreign particle. The protective enzymes in the phagocytic cells include catalase (Baehner, 1972), superoxide dismutase (Fridovich, 1974) and GSH-Px (Flohe, 1971). Inasmuch as GSH-Px has not been reported to occur in bacteria, the presence of GSH-Px in phagocytic cells of the host organism may offer an advantage for the host (Ganther *et al.,* 1976).

There is a comparatively high activity of GSH-Px in most phagocytic cells. Where studies permit a reasonably direct comparison of erythrocyte and phagocyte activities, human leukocytes possess the higher specific activity (units/mg protein) by a factor of about 2 (Holmes *et al.,* 1970), and rat macrophages twofold the specific activity of erythrocytes (Ganther *et al.,* 1976; Serfass *et al.,* 1974).

Because of its requirement for reducing equivalents in the form of glutathione, GSH-Px is coupled to the hexose monophosphate shunt via glutathione reductase (Fig. 8), which oxidizes NADPH to $NADP^+$. The rate of glucose oxidation by the hexose monophosphate shunt is controlled by the amount of $NADP^+$ present (Beck, 1958). Thus, the oxidation of glutathione by GSH-Px will cause a certain amount of NADPH to be oxidized to $NADP^+$, and glucose oxidation will take place to restore the NADPH/$NADP^+$ ratio to its initial level. The results of several investigations (Reed, 1969; Strauss *et al.,* 1969; Baehner *et al.,* 1970; Mandell, 1972) confirm the importance of the GSH-Px-dependent coupled system for hexose monophosphate shunt stimulation in normal PMNs from various species. Also, in several cases of hereditary GSH-Px deficiency in human leukocytes, hexose monophosphate shunt stimulation was greatly diminished during

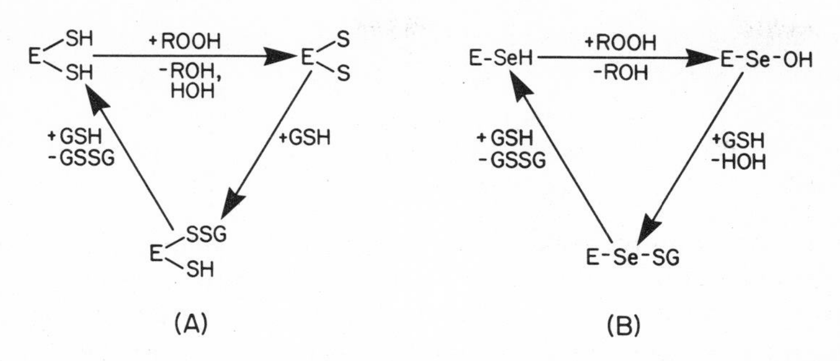

Fig. 8. Proposed mechanisms for glutathione peroxidase. (A) Flohe (1971); (B) Ganther *et al.* (1974). From Ganther *et al.* (1976).

phagocytosis (Ganther *et al.*, 1976; Holmes *et al.*, 1970; Nishimura *et al.*, 1972).

Although resting levels of NADPH and hexose monophosphate shunt activity may suffice for the initial phase of killing, additional shunt activity may be needed to maintain an adequate level of glutathione for the destruction of lipoperoxides and hydrogen peroxide produced as a consequence of the killing process. Thus, for the cell to kill maximal numbers of bacteria before its own demise, hexose monophosphate shunt stimulation may be vital to maintain glutathione levels so that GSH-Px can provide sustained protection of the cell (Ganther *et al.*, 1976).

PLATELETS

A single study describing relatively high levels of glutathione and GSH-Px in platelets has been published (Karpatkin and Weiss, 1972). These authors noted that a deficiency of platelet GSH-Px was associated with a defect in platelet function in three patients with Glanzmann's thrombasthenia, a bleeding disorder (Ganther *et al.*, 1976).

In the absence of direct experimental studies, one cannot evaluate the possible importance of platelet GSH-Px in a glutathione-dependent system protecting platelets from oxidative damage analogous to the case of erythrocytes. Platelets have neither the presence of hemoglobin nor the copious production of peroxides to contend with, in contrast to erythrocytes and phagocytic cells. Nevertheless, as Beutler (1972) commented, the observations of Karpatkin and Weiss (1972) have focused attention on platelet glutathione and GSH-Px, an aspect of platelet metabolism that has not been explored in depth. Beutler suggests that if glutathione levels do affect platelet function, riboflavin deprivation should cause abnormalities inasmuch as platelet glutathione reductase is dependent on riboflavin intake. Certainly, an even more direct approach for experimentally investigating the cellular role of the glutathione GSH-Px system in platelets would be to deplete platelet GSH-Px levels by feeding animals a selenium-deficient diet (Ganther *et al.,* 1976).

PLASMA

The first reported study of plasma GSH-Px appears to be that of Noguchi *et al.* (1973), who were investigating the possible role of GSH-Px in the development of exudative diathesis in chicks. This condition, which is prevented by selenium (or vitamin E under some conditions), is characterized by severe edema due to an increase in capillary permeability (Dam and Glavind, 1940; Ganther *et al.,* 1976). In day-old chicks fed a diet containing 0.1 ppm selenium as sodium selenite for 6–12 days, the specific activity (units per milligram nitrogen) of plasma GSH-Px was as high as that of erythrocytes and liver (Noguchi *et al.,* 1973). In chicks fed the same diet lacking selenium, plasma GSH-Px had decreased to nearly zero after only 5 days of depletion, while GSH-Px in liver had decreased about 50% in this period, and erythrocytes showed little change. Plasma GSH-Px levels were roughly proportional to dietary selenium levels between 0 and 0.06 ppm (Ganther *et al.,* 1976).

A primary role of plasma GSH-Px in preventing peroxidation of the plasma membrane of capillary endothelial cells was proposed by Noguchi *et al.* (1973), who observed that a drop in plasma GSH-Px to almost zero levels occurred just before the onset of exudative diathesis in chicks. They hypothesized a role of GSH-Px in plasma together with vitamin E in the plasma membrane and GSH-Px in the cytosol of capillary endothelial cells in the prevention of exudative diathesis (Ganther *et al.,* 1976).

LIVER

GSH-Px is present in the liver of some species in rather large amounts (Mills, 1960). Liver is also rich in catalase. Hochstein and Utley (1968) demonstrated that GSH-Px and catalase competed equally for the hydrogen peroxide produced at a low steady-state level by glucose oxidase and glucose. However, when hydrogen peroxide was present in high concentration, catalase was mainly responsible for its decomposition. Since hepatic catalase is predominantly localized in peroxisomes (deDuve and Baudhuin, 1966), GSH-Px is likely to have an appreciable role in utilizing extraperoxisomally generated hydrogen peroxide (Ganther *et al.,* 1976).

The major role of GSH-Px may not be its role in hydrogen peroxide metabolism, but rather its ability to catalyze the decomposition of lipid hydroperoxides. Catalase has no activity toward these substrates, although it can act on low-molecular-weight organic peroxides such as methyl and ethyl hydroperoxides (O'Brien, 1969; Nicholls and Schonbaum, 1963). GSH-Px, in comparison, reacts with many organic peroxides with very little specificity.

The nutritional benefit of selenium was first realized because of its ability to prevent liver necrosis in rats fed a diet suboptimal in the sulfur-containing amino acids and deficient in vitamin E (Schwarz and Foltz, 1957). The disease becomes fatal after the diet is fed for 3–4 weeks to weanling rats. It is characterized by massive hepatic necrosis; degeneration of the endoplasmic reticulum and mitochrondrial swelling can be observed by electron microscopy (Piccardo and Schwarz, 1958). Liver tissue from rats deficient in vitamin E and selenium fails to maintain normal respiration *in vitro,* a phenomenon that has been termed "respiratory decline" (Chernick *et al.,* 1955; Schwarz, 1965). Lack of liver GSH-Px and vitamin E may be responsible for this liver disease. Rat liver GSH-Px declined to 20% of that found in selenium-supplemented controls after the deficient diet was fed for only 10 days to weanling rats (Ganther *et al.,* 1976). The enzyme is undetectable ($< 1\%$ of the control level) by the twenty-fourth day of the deficiency (Hafeman *et al.,* 1974).

Either dietary selenium or vitamin E prevents liver necrosis as well as respiratory decline in liver slices *in vitro*. In homogenates of the same tissue, only vitamin E affords protection against respiratory failure (Schwarz, 1962). It is possible that the lack of protection by selenium in homogenates results from dilution of cytosolic GSH-Px and glutathione in the homegenate medium. Glutathione, when present in adequate concentration, can protect in the absence of vitamin E or dietary selenium (Schwarz, 1962). The effect of glutathione may be attributed to nonenzymatic reduction of hydrogen peroxide by glutathione. This reaction is appreciable at neutral or elevated pH, and is also promoted by high levels of glutathione (Flohe, 1971; Ganther *et al.,* 1976).

Certain environmental factors can apparently increase the need for cellular agents preventing peroxidation. Carbon tetrachloride and ethanol are examples of such compounds that induce peroxidation (DiLuzio. 1968; Ganther *et al.,* 1976).

The mechanism of carbon tetrachloride toxicity has received considerable study. It causes fatty liver due to inhibition of triglyceride transport out of this organ (Recknagel, 1967). Centrolobular necrosis is also observed, and if the dosage is sufficiently high, death is the final result. Free radicals generated during the oxidation of carbon tetrachloride to carbon dioxide and inorganic chloride are believed to initiate lipid peroxidation, ultimately leading to disruption of cellular membranes and decreased protein synthesis (Ganther *et al.,* 1976; Recknagel, 1967; Slater, 1972; Ugazio *et al.,* 1973).

Vitamin E, synthetic antioxidants, selenium, and the sulfur-containing amino acids all provide some degree of protection against carbon tetrachloride poison (Hove, 1948; Muth, 1960; Gallagher, 1962; Fodor and Kemény, 1965; Seward *et al.,* 1966). Vitamin E reduces the amount of lipid diene conjugation in liver microsomes, and also decreases carbon-tetrachloride-induced steatosis (Comporti and Benedetti, 1972). Whether selenium and the sulfur-containing amino acids protect by reducing lipid peroxidation is not known. It is plausible that GSH-Px mediates selenium's protective effect by inhibiting the lipid peroxidation reaction. The sulfur-containing amino acids may protect by increasing the level of liver glutathione (Linden and Work, 1953) to serve as substrate for the reduction of lipid peroxides (Ganther *et al.,* 1976).

LENS

The lens fibers are similar to red blood cells in many respects (Kinoshita, 1964; Jacob, 1971), including the lack of mitochondria and therefore the citrate-cycle enzymes. The glutathione-dependent pathway for destruction of peroxides that is operative in erythrocytes is also responsible for their removal in the lens (Kinoshita, 1955, 1964; van Heyningen and Pirie, 1953; Pirie, 1965). The conditions that result in precipitation of the hemoglobin into Heinz bodies and hemolysis of red cells might therefore be expected to result in cataract formation. The existence of this pathway in lens may explain the importance of the extremely high glutathione content of lens tissue (Ganther *et al.,* 1976).

In support of this hypothesis, cataracts have been observed in patients with severe G-6-PD deficiency (Westring and Pisciotta, 1966; Harley *et al.,* 1966; Helge and Barness, 1966). GSH-Px activity has been demonstrated in the lenses of various animal species (Pirie, 1965b; Holmberg, 1968; Lawrence *et al.,* 1974), and has been partially purified from cattle lens (Holmberg, 1968). This activity decreased to very low levels with selenium deficiency (Lawrence *et al.,* 1974), and cataracts have been observed in the second- and third-litter offspring of selenium-deficient female rats (Sprinker *et al.,* 1971). In addition, Swanson and Truesdale (1971) presented data showing that selenium concentration increased about fourfold in normal human lenses between birth and age 85, while in cataractous lenses, the selenium concentration was less than one sixth that of normal lenses from the same age groups (Ganther *et al.,* 1976).

Cataractogenic drugs and chemicals may exert their effects by producing peroxides in amounts too great to be handled by the GSH-Px protective mechanism, or by impairing the ability of this mechanism to protect against endogenously produced peroxides, or both. Naphthalene (Pirie, 1965) and many of the antimalarials (Bernstein, 1967; Cohen and Hochstein, 1964) have been shown to produce peroxides in the course of their metabolism in the body. A rather large group of cataractogenic chemicals is known as radiomimetics (Paterson, 1971; van Heyningen, 1969; Kuck, 1970); these chemicals, like ionizing radiation, probably produce free radicals or are themselves metabolized to free radicals (Pirie *et al.,* 1970). Free radicals can cause peroxidation of unsaturated lipids, nucleic acids, and other cell components (Pryor, 1973; Meyers, 1973), and these may be produced in amounts sufficient to overwhelm the protective mechanisms, especially if these mechanisms are in some way defective (Ganther *et al.,* 1976).

GLUTATHIONE PEROXIDASE IN HUMAN DISEASES

RED-CELL DISORDERS

Several clinical cases of hemolytic anemia attributed to GSH-Px deficiency have been reported in the literature. Necheles *et al.* (1967, 1969) described an 18-year-old Puerto Rican male who suffered a hemolytic episode following autotransfusion after surgery. During the hemolytic crisis, his blood contained numerous red cells with Heinz bodies, but these disappeared within a few weeks. Incubation with acetylphenylhydrazine continued to produce five or more Heinz bodies in 53% of his red cells, however. Following recovery from the hemolytic episode, about 3 months later, the reticulocyte count remained at 2.8–5%, suggesting a compensated hemolysis. The erythrocyte GSH-Px activity was approximately one third of normal, and hemolysates of his red cells did not show the characteristic stimulation of the hexose monophosphate shunt pathway on incubation with hydrogen peroxide in the presence of glucose. Both of his parents and one of three siblings had GSH-Px activities slightly lower than normal, which the authors interpreted as indicative of heterozygous genetic deficiency (Ganther *et al.,* 1976).

Necheles *et al.* (1970) summarized data on infants with neonatal jaundice as well as sick adults with drug-induced hemolytic anemia in whom GSH-Px activities ranged from 47–78% of normal (mean, 66%) and nine others without hemolysis whose GSH-Px activities averaged 69% of normal, all of whom were classified as heterozygous genetic deficiency on the basis of family studies. In addition, one adult (described in the previous paragraph) with low GSH-Px activities (34% of normal) was classified as homozygous genetically deficient. No other cause for hemolysis could be found in those who suffered from it. Drug-induced hemolytic episodes were precipitated by high doses of acetylsalicylic acid, sulfisoxazole, or nitrofurantoin (Ganther *et al.,* 1976).

Although several investigators (Gharib *et al.,* 1969; Boivin *et al.,* 1969; Nishimura *et al.,* 1972) attributed the GSH-Px deficiency to genetic causes, dietary selenium deficiency may have played a significant role in GSH-Px deficiency. It is also known that the activity of GSH-Px is greatly decreased in cases of iron-deficiency anemia. It is evident from several studies that GSH-Px activity is important in preventing damage to human red cells, even in the presence of normal catalase activity (Ganther *et al.,* 1976).

The increased susceptibility of the erythrocytes of newborn infants and especially premature infants to oxidative stress is well known and has been attributed to various causes, including greater susceptibility of fetal hemoglobin to oxidation and vitamin E deficiency (Cornblath and Hartman, 1948; Gasser, 1953; Allison, 1955; Betke *et al.,* 1956; Kravitz *et al.,* 1956; Gross and Schroeder, 1963; Hassan *et al.,* 1966; Oski and Barness, 1967; Ritchie *et al.,* 1968; Bracci *et al.,* 1970; Melhorn and Gross, 1971a,b; Flohe, 1971; Abrams *et al.,* 1973; Lo, 1973). Recent work however, has focused on a reduced activity of GSH-Px in erythrocytes from newborns as a possible explanation (Ganther *et al.,* 1976).

Most investigators have found reduced GSH-Px activity in the erythrocytes of premature and full-term newborn infants (Gross *et al.,* 1967; Necheles *et al.,* 1968; Swierczewski *et al.,* 1969; Whaun and Oski, 1970; Emerson *et al.,* 1972; Glader and Conrad, 1972; Konrad *et al.,* 1972; Lie-Injo *et al.,* 1973), but two groups from Germany did not (Vetrella *et al.,* 1970; Butenandt, 1971; Vetrella and Barthelmai, 1971). The original report by Gross *et al.* (1967) showed that erythrocyte GSH-Px activity (units per gram of hemoglobin) in premature and full-term infants averaged approximately two thirds that of adults, and they suggested an important role of GSH-Px in the resistance to oxidative stress. Necheles *et al.* (1968) confirmed this finding. Necheles *et al.* (1970) studied 11 infants in whom neonatal jaundice was associated with a "moderately severe" decrease in erythrocyte GSH-Px, and in whom no other cause for hyperbilirubinemia was evident. Eight showed signs of mild hemolysis with reticulocytosis (some also had increased Heinz body formation after incubation with acetylphenylhydrazine); in these infants, they postulated an inherited partial deficiency of GSH-Px. In addition, one infant with very low erythrocyte GSH-Px (15% of normal) was described and was classified as homozygous-deficient. In a survey of 100 consecutive full-term newborns, two cases of apparent hereditary deficiency of GSH-Px were uncovered. Emerson *et al.* (1972), commenting on the studies of Necheles *et al.* (1970), thought that "this incidence of a genetically transmitted defect would appear to be exceedingly high when compared with most other congenital enzyme deficiency states. . . ." Whaun and Oski (1970) also found that the average GSH-Px activity was decreased in infants.

It is clear that GSH-Px activity is frequently lower in the newborn when expressed in terms of number per cell (Emerson *et al.,* 1972). The work of Konrad *et al.* (1972) confirmed this observation.

There is a good possibility that some of the variations in the degree of

GSH-Px deficiency in newborns as a group, as well as the apparent existence of genetically related deficiencies of GSH-Px in individual cases, are related to the dietary selenium intake. It is interesting that most of the reports of low GSH-Px activity in the United States were from areas in which the selenium content of the forages is known to be low (Kubota *et al.,* 1967). Although the dietary histories of the mothers of these infants were not investigated, the selenium content in human blood tends to vary with the selenium content of plants (Allaway *et al.,* 1968).

PLATELET DISORDERS

A study by Karpatkin and Weiss (1972) of a number of enzymes in platelet extracts of three unrelated patients with Glanzmann's thrombasthenia revealed a markedly decreased level of GSH-Px in all three patients and a twofold increase in acid-soluble thiol concentration in two of the three cases. These results indicate that enzymatic pathways for maintaining glutathione were normal, but utilization of glutathione for destruction was impaired, making the platelet more susceptible to oxidative damage.

HERMANSKI–PUDLAK SYNDROME

A triad of symptoms consisting of oculocutaneous albinism, mild hemorrhagic symptoms, and accumulation of ceroid pigment in reticuloendothelial cells was first described by Hermansky and Pudlak (1959). Witkop *et al.* (1973) stated that many patients with this disorder have had spontaneous gingival hemorrhage and prolonged bleeding following tooth extraction, childbirth, or surgery, and that aspirin may enhance these tendencies. The authors postulate that a hereditary deficiency of GSH-Px may be the cause of Hermansky–Pudlak syndrome, but unfortunately no measurements of GSH-Px activity in such patients have yet been made (Ganther *et al.,* 1976).

CHRONIC INFECTION

Patients with chronic granulomatous disease (CGD) respond normally to infection in terms of an appropriate leukocytosis. The particle ingestion is normal in CGD, and these patients are immunologically competent (Holmes *et al.,* 1966). The cellular defect consists of a diminished microbicidal capacity of the PMNs (polymorphonuclear leukocytes), associated with one or more enzyme defects in the pathways known to be involved in the bactericidal process.

Deficiencies of G-6-PD, NADH-or NADPH-dependent primary oxidases, or myeloperoxidase in human leukocytes have been extensively studied (Johnson and Baehner, 1971). GSH-Px is another important enzyme in the leukocytes, but very few studies have been done in relation to diminished microbicidal capacity in disease states (Ganther *et al.*, 1976).

Leukocyte GSH-Px deficiency was reported to be associated with CGD of childhood in two female patients (Holmes *et al.*, 1970). This deficiency distinguishes their disease from that of male patients with the more common X-linked disorder. Leukocytes from the male patients were found to possess normal levels of GSH-Px. Erythrocyte GSH-Px activity was normal in patients of both sexes. Leukocytes of both male and female patients were not deficient in glutathione reductase or G-6-PD activity in comparison with controls (Ganther *et al.*, 1976).

Metabolic studies on leukocytes from these patients (Quie *et al.*, 1968) demonstrated that the increases in oxygen consumption and hexose monophosphate shunt activity characteristic of normal leukocytes undergoing phagocytosis were lacking in both the male and female patients. However, hydrogen peroxide production, myeloperoxidase, and primary oxidase activities in these patients were not reported. It is therefore not possible to ascertain whether the GSH-Px deficiency was the primary determinant of CGD in the female patients or a secondary result of some other enzyme deficiency (Ganther *et al.*, 1976).

If GSH-Px is present only to protect the phagocyte rather than being involved in the killing process *per se*, one might expect that patients with no defect other than leukocyte GSH-Px deficiency would experience milder abnormalities than the CGD cases referred to above. Syndromes have been described in which the metabolic abnormalities are similar to CGD, but the clinical signs are not as marked and the infections are milder (Rodey *et al.*, 1970; Shmerling *et al.*, 1969; Bannatyne *et al.*, 1969). It is interesting that lipopigments, which may represent end products of lipid peroxidation, are observed in patients susceptible to chronic infections (Rodey *et al.*, 1970) and in Batten's disease, a form of cerebral degeneration with an associated deficiency of leukocyte peroxidase (Armstrong *et al.*, 1974). It will be of great interest to correlate GSH-Px activities in the neutrophils of such cases with their clinical status with respect to the infections.

OTHER DISEASES

J. Hopkins and Tudhope (1973) assayed erythrocyte GSH-Px in 163 patients with various diseases. In 55 patients with carcinoma, there was a wide variation in red cell GSH-Px, but the mean value was significantly lower compared the values in 62 normal subjects. GSH-Px was also decreased in hepatomatous livers of rats treated with diethylnitrosamine (Pinto and Bartley, 1973). Abnormally high values for erythrocyte GSH-Px were found in acute myeloblastic leukemia and in myelofibrosis, whereas the enzyme activity tended to be low in chronic lymphocytic and myeloid leukemia (Hopkins, J., and Tudhope, 1973).

Certain carcinogenic substances are metabolized to electrophilic derivatives such as epoxides that may be the actual carcinogenic agents. Since many of these agents are detoxified by glutathione-linked conjugation reactions, it is possible that selenium derivatives of glutathione such as the selenopersulfides (GSSeH), with their greater nucleophilic character compared to glutathione, might help detoxify carcinogenic metabolites (Ganther *et al.*, 1976).

METABOLISM

DIETARY INTAKE

Chemical Form and Availability

Selenium occurs in a number of forms in food, but its biological availability is not known. Ion-exchange chromatography of pronase hydrolysates of gluten and seeds from wheat grown in soil containing [^{75}Se]selenate indicated that over 40% of the ^{75}Se was present as protein-bound selenomethionine (Olson *et al.*, 1970). No other major ^{75}Se-containing peak was identified. Thus, if wheat can be regarded as representative of plants eaten by human beings, about half the element in plant food sources is present as selenomethionine. The nature of the other half is unknown.

Very little is known about the form of selenium in animal tissues. The original recognition of the nutritional significance of selenium was its identification as the essential component of factor 3 against dietary liver necrosis (Schwarz and Foltz, 1957). This factor can be extracted from animal tissues and is a biologically highly active form of selenium, but its chemical structure has not been elucidated.

Selenoamino acids can be incorporated into animal protein (Ochoa-Solano and Gitler, 1968), but their origin is probably in plants, since currently available evidence suggests that mammals and birds are unable to synthesize these compounds (Cummins and Martin, 1967; Jenkins, 1968). Another form of selenium, the selenotrisulfide, has been found in animal tissues (Jenkins, 1968), but more recent work suggests that this form may be present only in situations of selenium excess (Burk, 1973); it may not be found in significant amounts in food. An association of selenium with mercury in certain fish and marine mammals has been noted (Ganther *et al.*, 1972; Koeman *et al.*, 1973), and evidence that a chemical bond exists between selenium and mercury in animal tissues has been presented (Burk *et al.,* 1974). Thus, many foods containing mercury will also contain appreciable quantities of selenium (Burk, 1976).

It appears that in the presence of adequate selenium, a relatively fixed amount of this element is present in selenoenzymes in animals. The amount present as selenoamino acids most likely depends on the ingestion of this form, and selenotrisulfide formation may be the result of excess intake of selenium. The presence of selenium in association with mercury may depend on mercury intake. Thus, a number of factors can influence the form of selenium found in animal tissues used for food by human subjects (Burk, 1976).

Several factors modify the biological availability of dietary selenium. Extensive studies have been reported by Schwarz and co-workers (Schwarz and Foltz, 1958; Schwarz *et al.,* 1972) on the biological effectiveness of dozens of selenium compounds in the prevention of dietary liver necrosis. It is obvious that some forms of selenium are more available than others. Selenium as selenite, DL-selenomethionine, and DL-selenocystine was equally effective in preventing liver necrosis, but factor 3 selenium was three times more effective than these forms (Burk, 1976; Schwarz and Foltz, 1958).

Selenium associated with mercury may be relatively unavailable. This view is based on the report of low availability of selenium in fish meal (Miller *et al.,* 1972) and the knowledge that selenium is sometimes associated with mercury in fish (Ganther *et al.,* 1972). There is some evidence that high dietary sulfate levels decrease selenium availability, at least in selenium toxicity (Halverson and Monty, 1960). Tri-*o*-cresyl phosphate (Shull and Cheeke, 1973) and silver (Swanson *et al.,* 1974) in the diet are known antagonists of selenium (Burk, 1976).

Quantity in Foods

Food selenium content is related to protein content and geographical origin. In most biological material, selenium is found largely in the protein fraction (Olson *et al.,* 1970; Burk, 1973); indeed, foods low in protein, such as fruits, have been shown to contain very little of this element (Morris and Levander, 1970). Geographical areas have been delineated in which the soil content of selenium is high, intermediate, or low; the selenium content of plant and animal products from those areas corresponds generally to the soil selenium levels (Allaway, 1973; Millar *et al.,* 1973b). Cooking does not cause major losses of selenium from most foods (Higgs *et al.,* 1972). However, up to 23% loss was noted when cereals were dry heated, and a few vegetables lost even more selenium than this (Burk, 1976).

Various fish and fish products may contain more than 1 μg selenium g. Grains from seleniferous areas contained about 1 μg selenium g, but the same products from low-selenium areas were selenium-poor. Animal meats contained about 0.2 μg selenium g (Burk, 1976).

Selenium in municipal water supplies is usually very low and does not differ from one area to another (Jaffé *et al.,* 1972). Thus, it appears that food is the only significant source of selenium for man (Burk, 1976).

Several authors have provided values for daily selenium intake. No selenium could be detected in five total diet samples collected in Baltimore in 1963 and 1964 (Hopkins, L. L., and Majaj, 1967). Analysis of a hospital diet in Vermont indicated a daily selenium intake of 31 μg (Schroeder *et al.,* 1970). Measurement of dietary selenium intake of 13 New Zealand women revealed a range of 6–70 μg/day (Griffiths, 1973). All these measurements were made in low-selenium areas. At present, it is not possible to judge the adequacy of selenium intake, inasmuch as the availability of selenium from food is not known.

Animal experiments have demonstrated that retention of a dose of ^{75}Se is inversely related to the dietary selenium level (Ewan *et al.,* 1967; Burk *et al.,* 1972). Although this variable has not yet been studied in human subjects, some whole-body retention data are available. A study of three cancer patients using [^{75}Se]selenite gave a biological half-life of 65 days (Cavalieri *et al.,* 1966). The corresponding figure for [^{75}Se]selenomethionine was 70 days as calculated from data collected from 24 subjects (Burk, 1976; Lathrop *et al.,* 1972).

Comparatively little is known regarding the intestinal absorption of selenium. Human absorption of [^{75}Se]selenite has been reported to be 70, 64, and 44% in three healthy subjects, which compares with over 90% absorption in rats (Thomson and Stewart, 1972). On the basis of the limited data available, it appears likely that selenium absorption is less efficient in man than in the rat (Burk, 1976).

In rats under physiological conditions, selenium homeostasis is achieved by the regulation of urinary selenium excretion (Burk *et al.,* 1972). When large quantities of selenium are ingested, some of the element is lost in the breath as dimethyl selenide, but in other circumstances, this route of excretion is negligible. Fecal losses are not governed by selenium intake as is urinary selenium (Burk, 1976).

Available human data show that 11.2% of the ^{75}Se in an intravenous dose of [^{75}Se]L-selenomethionine appeared in the urine in the 120 hr after administration, while 2.5% appeared in the feces (Lathrop *et al.,* 1972); when [^{75}Se]selenite was given intravenously, urinary excretion was 11% in 24 hr and 16.5% in 72 hr in one study (Cavalieri *et al.,* 1966) and 5.5–9.4% in 24 hr in another (Burk, 1974, 1976).

Measurement of urinary selenium content has been used for identifying groups at risk of selenium toxicity (Smith and Westfall, 1937; Mondragón and Jaffé, 1971). Urinary selenium has been estimated to account for approximately half the dietary intake (Thomson, 1972). This conclusion, however, is based on data obtained from only four subjects consuming from 7.8 to 15.7 μg selenium/day, and thus may not be valid for higher intakes of selenium. The determination of selenium in urine is more difficult than in blood (Burk, 1976).

Urinary selenium in the rat consists largely of trimethylselenonium ion and an unidentified substance called U-2 (Palmer *et al.,* 1969). These substances can be separated by two-dimensional paper chromatography and quantitated (Kiker and Burk, 1974). Such a chromatogram of urine from a young man with a testicular tumor who had been given [^{75}Se]selenite suggested that trimethylselenonium ion may also be produced in man (Burk, 1976).

Selenium absorption does not appear to depend on the selenium status of the rats. Homeostasis is maintained by urinary excretion of selenium metabolites, including trimethylselenonium ion and U-2. The excretion of these two metabolites is directly proportional to dietary selenium level. When large quantities of selenium are supplied, dimethyl selenide is excreted in expired air. In man, urinary selenium appears to be controlled by dietary selenium as in the rat (Burk, 1976).

Distribution of ^{75}Se

The distribution of ^{75}Se from a single intravenous dose has been studied in rats and found to be highly dependent on dietary selenium intake, amount of selenium injected with the ^{75}Se, and time between ^{75}Se administration and study (Hopkins, L. L. *et al.,* 1966; Atkins *et al.,* 1971; Burk *et al.,* 1972; Brown and Burk, 1973). ^{75}Se distribution studies in human subjects have not been adequately controlled, and thus their results should be interpreted with care (Burk, 1976).

Human tissue distribution of ^{75}Se after [^{75}Se]L-selenomethionine administration intravenously was reviewed by Lathrop *et al.* (1972). The uptake of ^{75}Se by the liver and pancreas was prompt. Pancreas ^{75}Se decreased to blood level in 2 days, but liver ^{75}Se concentration remained about twice the blood level at 100 days. Skin and muscle ^{75}Se concentration never reached as high as the blood level (Burk, 1976).

Penner (1966) demonstrated incorporation of ^{75}Se into hemoglobin following [^{75}Se]selenomethionine administration. He was able to study red cell turnover by measuring the ^{75}Se content of red cells, and also demonstrated significant reutilization of this label. ^{75}Se may have been incorporated into the GSH-Px of the red cell (Burk, 1976).

Much less is known regarding the time distribution of ^{75}Se when it is administered as inorganic selenium. In three cancer patients, the liver ^{75}Se (monitored externally) rose for 2 hr and then fell gradually, while muscle ^{75}Se fell throughout the observation period (Cavalieri *et al.*, 1966). In a similar study of six patients, biological half-times of 100 days for muscle, 70 days for tumor, 50 days for liver, 32 days for kidney, and 28 days for serum were obtained (Wenzel *et al.*, 1971). Eight days after [^{75}Se]selenate injection in a patient with a hepatoma, the greatest ^{75}Se concentrations of the ten tissues studied were found in the kidney and liver (Burk, 1976; Hirooka and Galambos, 1966).

Only a small amount of ^{75}Se as selenite is bound to plasma proteins after incubation with plasma. If, however, the incubation is done using whole blood, a substantial amount of the ^{75}Se will bind to the plasma proteins. It appears that ^{75}Se is first taken up by the red cells and then released for binding by the plasma proteins (Lee *et al.*, 1969). Dialysis of the plasma proteins against a bath containing cysteine resulted in release of the ^{75}Se. This finding suggests that the ^{75}Se was associated with protein sulfhydryl groups (Burk, 1976).

^{75}Se incorporation into plasma proteins was studied following [^{75}Se]selenomethionine injection (Awwad *et al.*, 1966). Virtually all the plasma ^{75}Se was trichloroacetic-acid-precipitable 10 hr after injection. The decline in plasma protein specific activity was shown to follow a multiexponential pattern during the 25 days of observation (Burk, 1976).

Paper electrophoresis of serum from patients with liver disease who had received [^{75}Se]selenate showed that the α_2- and β-globulins had the greatest affinity for ^{75}Se (Hirooka and Galambos, 1966). After intravenous injection of [^{75}Se]selenite into patients with various forms of cancer, plasma ^{75}Se decreased rapidly during the first hour and then rose slightly between 1 and 6 hr due to a marked increase in protein-bound ^{75}Se (Cavalieri *et al.*, 1966; Burk, 1974). Gel filtration of the human plasma showed that large amounts of the ^{75}Se were unbound in the early samples, but by 6 hr, about 85% was protein-bound. It has been suggested that selenium is bound to specific human plasma proteins (Burk, 1976).

Significant amounts of the ^{75}Se were associated with very-low-density and low-density lipoproteins, especially shortly after injection, but very little was found in the high-density lipoproteins (Burk, 1974). The very-low-density lipoprotein ^{75}Se activity declined more rapidly than low-density lipoprotein ^{75}Se activity. These findings are intriguing, since it is known that very-low-density lipoproteins are catabolized to low-density lipoproteins (Bilheimer *et al.*, 1972). Selenium has not been found in rat lipoproteins under similar conditions (Burk, 1973). Further investigations must be carried out to establish whether selenium is a natural constituent of human very-low-density and low-density lipoproteins (Burk, 1976).

TISSUE LEVELS

A recent report indicates that over 75% of ovine red cell selenium is in the enzyme GSH-Px (Oh *et al.,* 1974). Dickson and Tomlinson (1967), using a neutron-activation method, found 18.2 μg selenium/100 ml blood, 23.6 μg/100 ml cells, and 14.4 μg/100 ml plasma in 253 Canadian subjects. They noted a gradual decline in both plasma and cell selenium with age. Allaway *et al.* (1968) studied the selenium content of blood from blood banks across the United States using a fluorimetric method. They found slightly higher values in blood from seleniferous areas, but the range of their 210 samples was only 10–34 μg/100 ml blood, with a mean of 20.6. Kasperek *et al.* (1972) studied serum selenium levels in 184 normal persons using neutron-activation analysis and found a mean value of 9.8 μg/100 ml. They noted a gradual rise of serum selenium to age 35, and then a gradual decline in older individuals (Burk, 1976).

Blood selenium levels in a few pathological conditions have been measured. Plasma but not cell selenium was decreased in three patients with extensive burns (Dickson and Tomlinson, 1967). Guatemalan children with kwashiorkor had a mean blool selenium content of 11 μg/100 ml compared with 23 μg/100 ml in controls (Burk *et al.,* 1967). In this study also, the plasma selenium was decreased and red cell selenium content was unaltered. Similar data were obtained in Thai infants with kwashiorkor and marasmus (Levine and Olson, 1970). Jaffé *et al.* (1972) reported a level of 81.3 μg selenium/100 ml blood in Venezuelan children living in a seleniferous zone vs 35.5 μg/100 ml blood in a control group in Caracas.

Shamberger *et al.* (1973) found 22.9 μg selenium/100 ml blood in 48 normal subjects, whereas patients with colonic cancer had 15.8, gastric cancer 15.3, and pancreatic cancer 13.2 μg/100 ml. Patients with cirrhosis had a blood level of 13.6 μg/100 ml, and those with hepatitis had 14.5 μg/100 ml. Blood selenium levels were normal in patients with a number of other disorders, including rectal cancer and diabetes (Burk, 1976).

Low blood selenium levels seem to be associated with low plasma levels and normal red cell content. Measurement of plasma or serum selenium level may be a more sensitive indicator of selenium status than whole-blood measurement (Burk, 1976).

Organ Levels

Kidney and liver generally have the highest concentrations of selenium (Dickson and Tomlinson, 1967; Schroeder *et al.,* 1970). Dickson and Tomlinson (1967) measured liver, skin, and muscle selenium in tissues from ten autopsies, and the values they reported were very variable.

SELENIUM DEFICIENCY

Experimental selenium deficiency has been produced in several animal species by prolonged feeding of rations low in selenium. Selenium-deficient rats grow slowly, develop cataracts, lose their hair, and have aspermatogenesis (Sprinker *et al.,* 1971). Pancreatic degeneration is a prominent feature in selenium-deficient chicks (Burk, 1976; Gries and Scott, 1972).

Conditions under which human dietary selenium deficiency is likely to occur can be inferred from what is known about selenium in food and animal studies. Since selenium is associated with protein in food, a low-protein diet is probably also low in selenium. Crops produced in areas with low soil selenium are low in selenium, so that people in such an area subsisting on locally grown foods are likely to have a low selenium intake. Finally, inasmuch as growing animals have been shown to be more susceptible to development of selenium deficient than mature ones, it is likely that children may be more susceptible to selenium deficiency. It is also possible that human selenium deficiency might occur as a consequence of an acquired or inherited metabolic defect analogous to copper deficiency in the kinky hair syndrome (Burk, 1976; Danks *et al.,* 1972).

Schwarz (1961) reported a significant weight gain in response to feeding selenium to children with protein–calorie malnutrition. Two children with protein–calorie malnutrition who were not gaining weight in response to apparently adequate treatment, were administered 25 μg selenium daily as γ,γ'-diselenodivaleric acid. They gained 450 and 660 g over 10 and 14 days posttreatment (Burk, 1976).

L. L. Hopkins and Majaj (1967) reported similar results in three infants given 25 μg selenium as sodium selenite daily, and demonstrated a reticulocyte response following the institution of selenium treatment in three of five anemic infants. Unfortunately, since neither of these studies included nontreated control patients, no firm conclusions can be drawn regarding the effects of selenium therapy in protein–calorie malnutrition (Burk, 1976).

Decreased plasma and whole-blood selenium contents have been reported in protein–calorie malnutrition (Burk *et al.,* 1967; Levine and Olson, 1970). Blood selenium levels rose slowly to reach the normal after many months, in contrast to plasma proteins, which rapidly returned to normal levels after the institution of an adequate diet. These findings imply that selenium stores were severely depleted in these children.

ASSESSMENT OF SELENIUM STATUS

Blood levels of selenium have been widely used as an index of selenium status. Many studies have demonstrated that blood selenium levels were lower in animals fed a selenium-deficient diet than in controls. It has been shown that when rats are fed a selenium-deficient diet, blood selenium concentration falls in the same way as liver selenium does, although not quite as precipitously (Burk *et al.*, 1968). This suggests that blood selenium levels may mirror tissue stores when they are subnormal. Once adequate selenium intake is achieved, however, the blood level does not rise with further increases in dietary selenium until toxic selenium intake occurs unless organic forms of selenium such as selenomethionine are ingested (Burk, 1976; Burk *et al.*, 1968; Scott and Thompson, 1971).

Studies in human beings suggest that plasma or serum levels may be a more sensitive indicator of selenium status than whole-blood levels. No studies have been reported in which human beings were fed selenium-deficient diets to study changes in selenium levels (Burk, 1976).

The *in vitro* uptake of [^{75}Se]selenite by ovine red cells was shown to increase with the length of time the animals were fed a selenium-deficient diet (Wright and Bell, 1963). This technique was used in a study of children with protein–calorie malnutrition, and the results correlated inversely with the blood selenium concentration (Burk *et al.*, 1967). This is a simple procedure, but needs further evaluation before it can be accepted as a useful diagnostic aid (Burk, 1976).

Urinary selenium excretion in rats seems to reflect dietary intake of the element until pulmonary excretion begins at high selenium intakes. Attempts to correlate urinary excretion of the element with dietary intake in man is warranted. Twenty-four-hour urine collections should be used, as they are not subject to error from meal and dilution effects (Burk, 1976).

Erythrocyte GSH-Px activity in rats has been shown to fall in response to a selenium-deficient diet and rise in response to a diet containing mildly toxic amounts of the element (Hafeman *et al.*, 1974). If this can be shown to occur in man also, it could eventually prove to be the most sensitive and useful indicator of human selenium status (Burk, 1976).

SELENIUM TOXICITY

The toxic effects of selenium have been recognized for a long time. The discovery in the 1930's that certain geographical areas are seleniferous and produce plants with high selenium content explained observations dating back centuries that the population consuming food grown in these areas suffered from toxicity. In addition to the generalized increase of selenium in vegetation from such areas, a few species of plants were identified that thrived in them and were called "selenium indicator plants" (Rosenfeld and Beath, 1964). These plants characteristically accumulate selenium to extremely high levels in the form of nonprotein selenoamino acids such as Se-methylselenocysteine (Nigam and McConnell, 1969) and produce acute toxicity in animals following ingestion (Burk, 1976).

A number of syndromes of selenium toxicity in animals have been described (Rosenfeld and Beath, 1964). The pathology in acute toxicity consists of widespread necrosis and hemorrhage, and death is probably due to hypoxia secondary to these lesions in the lungs. Manifestations of chronic toxicity are often species-dependent and related to the form and amount of selenium ingested. In almost all species, the liver is affected and cirrhosis develops. Frequently, a cardiomyopathy is found. Loss of hair and sloughing of hoofs occurs (Burk, 1976).

The biochemical mechanism of selenium toxicity has not been established. Recent *in vitro* studies demonstrated glutathione-dependent inhibition of amino acid incorporation into polyribosomes by nanomole quantities of selenite (Vernie *et al.,* 1974).

Several moderating influences on selenium toxicity are known. Increasing dietary protein generally decreases toxicity (Lewis *et al.,* 1940). The combination of methionine and vitamin E apparently facilitates excretion of this element (Levander and Morris, 1970); while a nonprotein factor in linseed oil meal increases tissue levels of selenium, the toxicity is decreased (Levander *et al.,* 1970). Arsenic protects by increasing biliary excretion of selenium (Burk, 1976; Levander and Baumann, 1966).

Although selenium toxicity has had a tremendous impact on animals in seleniferous areas, very little effect on human populations has been demonstrated. Smith and his colleagues (Smith *et al.,* 1936; Smith and Westfall, 1937) surveyed rural populations of seleniferous areas in South Dakota and Nebraska. They found high concentrations of selenium in urine from many subjects, but were unable to demonstrate signs or symptoms that could be attributed to selenium toxicity. However, their study lacked a control population (Burk, 1976).

Jaffé *et al.* (1972) studied Venezuelan children clinically and biochemically, and compared a group living in a seleniferous area with a control population. Blood and urinary selenium were much higher in the seleniferous area. The liver function tests, serum glutamic oxaloacetic transaminase (SGOT) and alkaline phosphatase, were normal in both groups. Pathological symptoms, such as history of nausea and vomiting, skin depigmentation, and hair loss, were more frequent and hemoglobin values were lower in the group exposed to selenium, but the authors believed that this may not have been due solely to difference in selenium intake. They concluded that this level of selenium intake was not likely to pose severe health hazards to children (Burk, 1976).

An isolated instance of selenium poisoning by well water containing 9 ppm selenium was reported (Rosenfeld and Beath, 1964). The Indian family affected had alopecia, abnormal nails, and lassitude, and recovered when use of the contaminated water was stopped (Burk, 1976).

Selenium is widely used in the electronics, glass, and paint industries, and safeguards against worker exposure must be employed. Glover (1970) had the opportunity to observe for 15 years men exposed to selenium in their work, and concluded on the basis of a statistical study that selenium exposure did not alter the death rate. It was further pointed out that an early sign of excessive selenium exposure was garlicky breath due to dimethyl selenide excretion (Burk, 1976).

Dental caries has been attributed to high selenium intake, and several epidemiological studies have indicated a slightly higher overall caries incidence in seleniferous areas than in control populations (Hadjimarkos, 1965; Ludwig and Bibby, 1969). Animal studies have not yielded consistent production of caries except when selenium was administered during tooth development (Bowen, 1972). The conclusion that selenium is cariogenic for human beings cannot yet be made (Burk, 1976).

Selenium has known teratogenic effects in chickens (Moxon and Rhian, 1943), and it was reported by Robertson (1970) that a higher number of abortions than expected were noted in a group of laboratory technicians handling selenite. No differences in urinary selenium levels between the technicians and nonexposed subjects were found. This report indicates a need for a controlled study of women of childbearing age exposed to selenium (Burk, 1976).

Recently, the Food and Drug Administration approved the use of selenite as an animal feed additive in an amount of up to 0.2 ppm selenium. This was done to combat widespread selenium deficiency in farm animals. Although this level of selenium in organic forms has been shown to cause accumulation of more selenium in muscle tissue, such is not the case with selenite (Carey *et al.,* 1973). This being the case, consumption of meat from these animals is unlikely to cause selenium toxicity in man (Burk, 1976).

No specific treatment for selenium toxicity exists except the removal from selenium exposure. BAL (British anti-lewisite), penicillamine, and bromobenzene have all been evaluated for use in selenium toxicity but found ineffective or impractical for one reason or another (Burk, 1976; Rosenfeld and Beath, 1964; Levander, 1972).

Selenium toxicity in animals has been a major problem in the past, and a few cases of selenium toxicity in human beings have been reported. Although large land areas contain excessive quantities of the element and selenium is extensively used in industry, there is no firm evidence of a significant selenium toxicity problem in human subjects (Burk, 1976).

MEDICAL APPLICATIONS

THERAPEUTIC USES

Selenium sulfide is incorporated into shampoos and ointments and sold for the treatment of seborrheic dermatitis. Selenium sulfide and zinc pyrithione shampoos were found to be equally effective and better than an unmedicated shampoo in the treatment of dandruff (Orentreich *et al.*, 1969). Selenium sulfide is water-insoluble and possesses a very low toxicity in comparison with selenite (Cummins and Kumura, 1971). However, toxicity due to prolonged use of the agent on open skin lesions has been reported, and elevated urinary selenium levels were documented (Ransone *et al.*, 1961). Symptoms included tremor and loss of appetite. It seems reasonable to avoid the use of this compound when the integument is not intact (Burk, 1976).

DIAGNOSTIC USES

Selenium in the form of [^{75}Se]selenomethionine has been used to scan the pancreas and the parathyroid glands (Bachrach *et al.*, 1972). The use of these scans at present should be restricted to major research centers for further evaluation (Bachrach *et al.*, 1972; Burk, 1976; Giulio and Morales, 1969).

Several reports of the use of [^{75}Se]selenomethionine in the diagnosis and staging of lymphoma have appeared (Herrera *et al.*, 1965; Ferrucci *et al.*, 1970). A negative study by this technique was not a reliable indicator of the absence of disease, but an abnormal study indicated a 70–80% probability that disease was present. A reduced brain uptake of [^{75}Se]-selenomethionine was reported in phenylketonuria (Oldendorf *et al.*, 1971).

The use of [^{75}Se]selenite as a scanning agent for a variety of tumors has been recommended. Cavalieri and Steinberg (1971) advocate using it in conjunction with another isotope to take advantage of selenium's greater uptake in rapidly metabolizing cells. Thus, it can be used with strontium in bone. A positive strontium scan with a negative [^{75}Se]selenite scan would suggest a noncancerous lesion, while ^{75}Se uptake in the area would suggest cancer. Detection of lung cancer (Jereb *et al.*, 1972) and many other tumors (Thiemann *et al.*, 1971) has been accomplished with the use of [^{75}Se]selenite and other isotopes, but not enough control data are available to make recommendations on their use (Burk, 1976).

[^{75}Se]Selenomethionine has been used to measure erythrocyte life span (Penner, 1966), but its use has not been widespread due to the greater radiation exposure than with ^{51}Cr. Attempts have been made to use it to study protein turnover in human beings (Waterlow *et al.*, 1969), but these attempts have failed, probably because of the reutilization of the ^{75}Se after the amino acid is catabolized (Burk, 1976).

REFERENCES

Abrams, B. A., Gutteridge, J. M. C., Stocks, J., Friedman, M., and Dormandy, T. L. 1973. Vitamin E in neonatal hyperbilirubinaemia. *Arch. Dis. Child.* **48,** 721–724.

Aebi, H., and Suter, H. 1966. Peroxide sensitivity of acatalatic erythrocytes. *Humangenetik* **2,** 328–343.

Aebi, H., Baggiolini, M., Dewald, B., Lauber, E., Suter, H., Micheli, A., and Frei, J. 1964a. Observations on two Swiss families with acatalasia II. *Enzymol. Biol. Clin.* **4,** 121–151.

Aebi, H., Heiniger, J. T., and Lauber, E. 1964b. Methemoglobin formation in erythrocytes due to peroxide action: Experiments on the evaluation of the protective function of catalase and glutathione peroxidase. *Helv. Chim. Acta* **47,** 1428–1440.

Allaway, W. H. 1973. Selenium in the food chain. *Cornell Vet.* **63,** 151–170.

Allaway, W. H., Kubota, J., Losee, F., and Roth, M. 1968. Selenium, molybdenum, and vanadium in human blood. *Arch. Environ. Health* **16,** 343–348.

Allen, R. C., Stjerholm, R. L., and Steele, R. H. 1972. Evidence for the generation of an electron excitation state(s) in human polymorphonuclear leukocytes and its participation in bactericidal activity. *Biochem. Biophys. Res. Commun.* **47,** 679–684.

Allison, A. C. 1955. Danger of vitamin K to the newborn. *Lancet* **268,** 669.

Andreesen, J. R., and Ljungdahl, L. G. 1973. Formate dehydrogenase of *Clostridium thermoaceticum:* Incorporation of selenium-75, and the effects of selenite, molybdate, and tungstate on the enzyme. *J. Bacteriol.* **116,** 867–873.

Armstrong, D., Dimmitt, S., and VanWormer, D. E. 1974. Studies in Batten disease. I. Peroxidase deficiency in granulocytes. *Arch. Neurol. (Chicago)* **30,** 144–152.

Atkins, H. L., Hauser, W., and Klopper, J. F. 1971. Effects of carrier on organ distribution of ^{75}Se-selenomethionine. *Metab. Clin. Exp.* **20,** 1052–1056.

Awwad, H. K., Potchen, E. J., Adelstein, S. J., and Dealy, J. B. 1966. Se^{75}-selenomethionine incorporation into human plasma proteins and erythrocytes. *Metab. Clin Exp.* **15,** 626–640.

Babior, B. M., Kipnes, R. S., and Curnutte, J. T. 1973. Biological defense mechanisms: The production by leukocytes of superoxide, a potential bactericidal agent. *J. Clin. Invest.* **52,** 741–744.

Bachrach, W. H., Birsner, J. W., Izenstark, J. L., and Smith, V. L. 1972. Pancreatic scanning: A review. *Gastroenterology* **63,** 890–910.

Baehner, R. L. 1972. Disorders of leukocytes leading to recurrent infection. *Pediatr. Clin. North. Amer.* **19,** 935–956.

Baehner, R. L., Gilman, N., and Karnovsky, M. L. 1970. Respiration and glucose oxidation in human and guinea pig leukocytes: Comparative studies. *J. Clin. Invest.* **49,** 692–700.

Bannatyne, R. M., Skowron, P. N., and Weber, J. L. 1969. Job's syndrome—a variant of chronic granulomatous disease. *J. Pediatr.* **75,** 236–242.

Beck, W. S. 1958. Occurrence and control of the phosphogluconate oxidation pathway in normal and leukemic leukocytes. *J. Biol. Chem.* **232,** 271–287.

Bernstein, H. N. 1967. Chloroquine ocular toxicity. *Surv. Opthalmol.* **12,** 415–447.

Betke, K., Kleinhauer, E., and Lipps, M. 1956. Vergleichende Untersuchungen über die spontan Oxydation von Nableschnar and Erwachsenenhämoglobin. *Z. Kinderheilkd.* **77,** 549–553.

Beutler, E. 1965. Glucose-6-phosphate dehydrogenase deficiency and non-spherocytic congenital hemolytic anemia. *Semin. Hematol.* **2,** 91–138.

Beutler, E. 1969a. Drug-induced hemolytic anemia. *Pharmacol. Rev.* **21,** 73–103.

Beutler, E. 1969b. Effect of flavin compounds on GSSG-R activity: *In vivo* and *in vitro* studies. *J. Clin. Invest.* **48,** 1957–1966.

Beutler, E. 1972. Glanzmann's thrombasthenia and reduced glutathione. *N. Engl. J. Med.* **287,** 1094–1095.

Beutler, E., and Srivastava, S. K. 1970. Relationship between glutathione reductase activity and drug-induced haemolytic anemia. *Nature (London)* **226,** 759–760.

Bilheimer, D. W., Eisenberg, S., and Levy, R. I. 1972. The metabolism of very low density lipoprotein proteins. I. Preliminary *in vitro* and *in vivo* observations. *Biochim. Biophys. Acta* **260,** 212–221.

Boivin, P., Galand, C., André, R., and Debray, J. 1966. Anémies hémolytiques congénitales avec déficit isolé en glutathion réduit par déficit en glutathion synthétase. *Nouv. Rev. Franc. Hematol.* **6,** 859–866.

Boivin, P., Galand, C., Hakim, J., Rogé, J., and Guéroult, N. 1969. Anémie hémolytique avec déficit en glutathion peroxydase chez un adulte. *Enzymol. Biol. Clin.* **10,** 68–80.

Bowen, W. H. 1972. The effect of selenium and vanadium on caries activity in monkeys *(M. Irus). J. Ir. Dent. Assoc.* **18,** 83.

Bracci, R., Calabri, G., Bettini, F., and Princi, P. 1970. Glutathione peroxidase in human leukocytes. *Clin. Chim. Acta* **29,** 345–348.

Brewer, G. J. 1969. 6-Phosphogluconate-dehydrogenase and glutathione reductase. In: *Biochemical Methods in Red Cell Genetics* (G. J. Yunis, ed.). Academic Press, New York, pp. 139–165.

Brown, D. G., and Burk, R. F. 1973. Selenium retention in tissues and sperm of rats fed a Torula yeast diet. *J. Nutr.* **103,** 102–108.

Burk, R. F. 1973. ^{75}Se-binding by rat plasma proteins after injection of $^{75}SeO_3^{2-}$. *U.S. Army Med. Res. Nutr. Lab. Rep. 334.*

Burk, R. F. 1974. *In vivo* ^{75}Se binding to human plasma proteins after administration of $^{75}SeO_3^{2-}$. *Biochim. Biophys. Acta* **372,** 255–265.

Burk, R. F. 1976. Selenium in man. In: *Trace Elements in Human Health and Disease,* Vol II (A. S. Prasad, ed.). Academic Press, New York, pp. 105–133.

Burk, R. F., Pearson, W. N., Wood, R. P., and Viteri, F. 1967. Blood-selenium levels and *in vitro* red blood cell uptake of ^{75}Se in kwashiorkor. *Amer. J. Clin. Nutr.* **20,** 723–733.

Burk, R. F., Whitney, R., Frank, H., and Pearson, W. N. 1968. Tissue selenium levels during the development of dietary liver necrosis in rats fed torula yeast diets. *J. Nutr.* **95,** 420–428.

Burk, R. F., Brown, D. G., Seely, R. J., and Scaief, C. C. 1972. Influence of dietary and injected selenium on whole-body retention, route of excretion, and tissue retention of $^{75}SeO_3^{2-}$ in the rat. *J. Nutr.* **102,** 1049–1056.

Burk, R. F., Foster, K. A., Greenfield, P. M., and Kiker, K. W. 1974. Binding of simultaneously administered inorganic selenium and mercury to a rat plasma protein. *Proc. Soc. Exp. Biol. Med.* **145,** 782–785.

Butenandt, O. 1971. Glutathione, glutathione peroxidase, glutathione reductase, glucose-6-phosphate dehydrogenase, lactic dehydrogenase, and catalase in erythrocytes of newborns, infants, and children and their relation to the formation of Heinz bodies. *Z. Kinderheilkd.* **111,** 149–161.

Carson, P. E., and Frischer, H. 1966. Glucose-6-phosphate dehydrogenase deficiency and related disorders of the pentose phosphate pathway. *Amer. J. Med.* **41,** 744–761.

Carson, P. E., Brewer, G. J., and Ickes, C. 1961. Decreased glutachione reductase with susceptibility to hemolysis. *J. Lab. Clin. Med.* **58,** 804 (abstract).

Cary, E. E., Allaway, W. H., and Miller, M. 1973. Utilization of different forms of dietary selenium. *J. Anim. Sci.* **36,** 285–292.

Cavalieri, R. R., and Steinberg, M. 1971. Selenite (Se^{75}) as a tumor-scanning agent. *J. Surg. Oncol.* **3,** 617–724.

Cavalieri, R. R., Scott, K. G., and Sairenji, E. 1966. Selenite (^{75}SE) as a tumor-localizing agent in man. *J. Nucl. Med.* **7,** 197–208.

Chernick, S. S., Moe, J. G., Rodman, G. P., and Schwarz, K. 1955. A metabolic lesion in dietary necrotic liver degeneration. *J. Biol. Chem.* **217,** 829–843.

Christophersen, B. O. 1968. Formation of monohydroxypolyenic fatty acids from lipid peroxides by a glutathione peroxidase. *Biochim. Biophys. Acta* **164,** 35–46.

Christophersen, B. O. 1969. Reduction of X-ray induced DNA and thymine hydroperoxides by rat liver glutathione peroxidase. *Biochim. Biophys. Act* **186,** 387–389.

Cohen, G., and Hochstein, P. 1963. Glutathione peroxidase: The primary agent for the elimination of hydrogen peroxide in erythrocytes. *Biochemistry* **2,** 1420–1428.

Cohen, G., and Hochstein, P. 1964. Generation of hydrogen peroxide in erythrocytes by hemolytic agents. *Biochemistry* **3,** 895–900.

Comporti, M., and Benedetti, A. 1972. Carbon tetrachloride-induced peroxidation of liver lipids in vitamin E pretreated rats. *Biochem. Pharmacol.* **21,** 418–420.

Cornblath, M., and Hartman, A. F. 1948. Methemoglobinemia in young infants. *J. Pediatr.* **33,** 421–425.

Cummins, L. M., and Kimura, E. T. 1971. Safety evaluation of selenium sulfide antidandruff shampoo. *Toxicol. Appl. Pharmacol.* **20,** 89–96.

Cummins, L. M., and Martin, J. L. 1967. Are selenocystine and selenomethionine synthesized *in vivo* from sodium selenite in mammals? *Biochemistry* **6,** 3162–3168.

Curnutte, J., and Babior, B. M. 1974. The effect of bacteria and serum on superoxide production by granulocytes. *J. Clin. Invest.* **53,** 1662–1672.

Dam, H., and Glavind, J. 1940. Vitamin E and capillary permeability. *Naturwissenschaften* **28,** 207.

Danks, D. M., Campbell, P. E., Walker-Smith, J., Stevens, B. J., Gillespie, J. M., Blomfield, J., and Turner, B. 1972. Menkes' kinky hair syndrome. *Lancet* **1,** 1100–1104.

deDuve, C., and Baudhuin, P. 1966. Peroxisomes (microbodies and related particles). *Physiol. Ref.* **46,** 323–357.

Demus-Oole, A., and Swierczewski, E. 1969. Glutathione peroxidase in rat liver during development. I. Localization and characterization of the enzyme in the subcellular liver fractions of newborn and adult rat. *Biol. Neonate* **14,** 211–218.

Dickson, R. C., and Tomlinson, R. H. 1967. Selenium in blood and human tissues. *Clin. Chim. Acta* **16,** 311–321.

DiLuzio, N. R. 1968. The role of lipid peroxidation and antioxidants in ethanol-induced lipid alterations. (letter to the editor). *Exp. Mol. Pathol.* **8,** 394–402.

Duchon, G., and Collier, H. B. 1971. Enzyme activities of human erythrocyte ghosts: Effects of various treatments. *J. Membrane Biol.* **6,** 138–157.

Emerson, P. M., Mason, D. Y., and Cuthbert, J. E. 1972. Erythrocyte glutathione peroxidase content and serum tocopherol levels in newborn infants. *Brit. J. Haematol.* **22,** 667–680.

Ewan, R. C., Pope, A. L., and Baumann, C. A. 1967. Elimination of fixed selenium by the rat. *J. Nutr.* **91,** 547–554.

Ferrucci, J. T., Berke, R. A., and Postsaid, M. S. 1970. Se^{75}-selenomethionine isotope lymphography to lymphoma: Correlation with lymphangiography. *Amer. J. Roetgenol.* **109,** 793–802.

Flohe, L. 1971. Die Glutathionperoxidase: Enzymologie und biologische Aspekte. *Klin. Wochenschr.* **49,** 669–683.

Flohe, L., Eisele, B., and Wendel, A. 1971. Glutathioneperoxidase. I. Reindarstellung and Molekulargewichtsbestimmungen. *Hoppe-Zeyler's Z. Physiol. Chem.* **352,** 151–158.

Flohe, L., Loschen, G., Gunzler, W. A., and Eichele, E. 1972. Glutathione peroxidase. V. The kinetic mechanism. *Hoppe-Zeyler's Z. Physiol. Chem.* **353,** 987–999.

Fodor, G., and Kemény, G. L. 1965. On the hepatoprotective effect of selenium in carbon tetrachloride poisoning in albino rats. *Experientia* **21,** 666–667.

Fridovich, I. 1974. Superoxide radical and the bactericidal action of phagocytes. *N. Engl. J. Med.* **290,** 624–625.

Gallagher, C. H. 1962. The effect of antioxidants on poisoning by carbon tetrachloride. *Aust. J. Exp. Biol. Med. Sci.* **40,** 241–253.

Ganther, H. E., Goudie, C., Sunde, M. L., Kopecky, M. J., Wagner, P., Oh, S. H., and Hoekstra, W. G. 1972. Selenium: Relation to decreased toxicity of methylmercury added to diets containing tuna. *Science* **175,** 1122–1124.

Ganther, H. E., Oh, S. H., Chittaranjan, D., and Hoekstra, W. G. 1974. Studies on selenium in glutathione peroxidase. *Fed. Proc. Fed. Amer. Soc. Exp. Biol.* **33,** 694 (abstract).

Ganther, H. E., Hafeman, D. G., Lawrence, R. A., Serfass, R. E., and Hoekstra, W. G. 1976. Selenium and glutathione peroxidase in health and disease—A review. In: *Trace Elements in Human Health and Disease,* Vol. II (A. S. Prasad, ed.). Academic Press, New York, pp. 165–234.

Gasser, C. 1953. The hemolytic anemia of premature infants with spontaneous Heinz-body formation, a new syndrome observed in 14 cases. *Helv. Pediatr. Acta* **8,** 491–529.

Gharib, H., Fairbanks, V. F., and Bartholomew, L. G. 1969. Hepatic failure with acanthocytosis associated with hemolytic anemia and deficiency of glutathione peroxidase. *Proc. Staff Meet. Mayo Clin.* **44,** 96–101.

Giulio, W. D., and Morales, J. O. 1969. The value of the selenomethionine Se^{75} scan in preoperative localization of parathyroid adenomas. *J. Amer. Med. Ass.* **209,** 1873–1880.

Glader, B. E., and Conrad, M. E. 1972. Decreased glutathione peroxidase in neonatal erythrocytes: Lack of relation to hydrogen peroxide metabolism. *Pediatr. Res.* **6,** 900–904.

Glatzle, D., Weber, F., and Wiss, O. 1968. Enzymatic test for detection of a riboflavin deficiency: NADPH-dependent glutathione reductase of red blood cells and its activation by FAD *in vitro*. *Experientia* **24,** 1122.

Glover, J. R. 1970. Selenium and its industrial toxicology. *Ind. Med. Surg.* **39,** 50–54.

Green, R. C., and O'Brien, P. J. 1970. The cellular localization of glutathione peroxidase and its release from mitochondria during swelling. *Biochim. Biophys. Acta* **197,** 31–39.

Gries, C. L., and Scott, M. L. 1972. Pathology of selenium deficiency in the chick. *J. Nutr.* **102,** 1287–1296.

Griffiths, N. M. 1973. Dietary intake and urinary excretion of selenium in some New Zealand women. *Proc. Univ. Otago Med. Sch.* **51,** 8–9.

Gross, R. T., and Schroeder, E. A. R. 1963. The relationship of TPNH content to abnormalities in the erythrocytes of premature infants. *J. Pediatr.* **63,** 823–825.

Gross, R. T., Bracci, R., Rudolph, N., Schroeder, E., and Kochen, J. A. 1967. Hydrogen peroxide toxicity and detoxification in erythrocytes of newborn infants. *Blood* **29,** 481–493.

Hadjimarkos, D. M. 1965. Effect of selenium on dental caries. *Arch. Environ. Health* **10,** 893–899.

Hafeman, D. G., Sunde, R. A., and Hoekstra, W. G. 1974. Effect of dietary selenium on erythrocyte and liver glutathione peroxidase in the rat. *J. Nutr.* **104,** 580–586.

Halverson, A. W., and Monty, K. J. 1960. An effect of dietary sulfate on selenium poisoning in the rat. *J. Nutr.* **70,** 100–102.

Harley, J. D., Robin, H., Meuser, M. A., and Hertzberg, R. 1966. Cataracts in glucose-6-phosphate dehydrogenase deficiency. *Brit. Med. J.* **1,** 421.

Hassan, H. A., Hashim, S. A., Van Itallie, T., and Sebrell, W. H. 1966. Syndrome in premature infants associated with low plasma vitamin E levels and high polyunsaturated fatty acids in the diet. *Amer. J. Clin. Nutr.* **19,** 147–157.

Helge, H., and Barness, K. 1966. Congenital hemolytic anemia, cataract, and glucose-6-phosphate dehydrogenase deficiency. *Dsch. Med. Wochenschr.* **91,** 1584–1590.

Hermansky, F., and Pudlak, P. 1959. Albinism associated with hemorrhagic diathesis and unusual pigmented reticular cells in the bone marrow: Report of two cases with histochemical studies. *Blood* **14,** *162–169.*

Herrera, N. E., Gonzalez, R., Schwartz, R. D., Diggs, A. M. and Belsky, J. 1965. ^{75}Se methionine as a diagnostic agent in malignant lymphoma. *J. Nucl. Med.* **6,** 792–804.

Higgs, D. J., Morris, V. C., and Levander, O. A. 1972. Effect of cooking on selenium content of foods. *J. Agric. Food Chem.* **20,** 678–680.

Hirooka, T., and Galambos, J. T. 1966. Selenium metabolism. III. Serum proteins, lipoproteins, and liver injury. *Biochim. Biophys. Acta* **130,** 321–328.

Hochstein, P., and Utley, H. 1968. Hydrogen peroxide detoxification by glutathione peroxidase and catalase in rat liver homogenates. *Mol. Pharmacol.* **4,** 574–579.

Holmberg, N. J. 1968. Purification and properties of glutathione peroxidase from bovine lens. *Exp. Eye Res.* **7,** 570–580.

Holmes, B., Quie, P. G., Windhorst, D. B., and Good, R. A. 1966. Fatal granulomatous disease of childhood: An inborn abnormality of phagocytic function. *Lancet* **1,** 1225.

Holmes, B., Park, B. H., Malawista, S. E., Quie, P. G., Nelson, D. L., and Good, R. A. 1970. Chronic granulomatous disease in females. *N. Engl. J. Med.* **283,** 217–221.

Hopkins, L. L., and Majaj, A. S. 1967. Selenium in human nutrition. In: *Selenium in Biomedicine* (O. H. Muth, ed.). Avi Publications, Westport, Connecticut, pp. 203–211.

Hopkins, J., and Tudhope, G. R. 1973. Glutathione peroxidase in human red cells in health and disease. *Brit. J. Haematol.* **25,** 563–575.

Hopkins, L. L., Pope, A. L., and Baumann, C. A. 1966. Distribution of microgram quantities of selenium in the tissues of the rat, and effects of previous selenium intake. *J. Nutr.* **88,** 61–65.

Hove, E. L. 1948. Interrelation between α-tocopherol and protein metabolism. III. The protective effect of vitamin E and certain nitrogenous compounds against CCl_4 poisoning in rats. *Arch. Biochem.* **17,** 467–474.

Jacob, H. S. 1971. Mechanism of hemoglobin precipitation into Heinz bodies: Possible relevance to cataract formation. *Exp. Eye Res.* **11,** 356–364.

Jacob, H. S., Ingbar, S. H., and Jandl, J. H. 1965. Oxidative hemolysis and erythrocyte metabolism in hereditary actalasia. *J. Clin. Invest.* **44,** 1187–1199.

Jaffe, E. R., Rieber, E. E., Anderson, H. M., Kosower, N. S., and Penny, J. L. 1968. Glutathione reductase activity and hemolysis in hemoglobin C disease. *J. Clin. Invest.* **47,** 51a.

Jaffé, W. G., Ruphael' D. M., Mondragon, M. C., and Cuevas, M. A. 1972. Estudio clínico y bioquímico en niños escolares de una zona selenífera. *Arch. Latinoamer. Nutr.* **22,** 595–611.

Jenkins, K. J. 1968. Evidence for the absence of selenocystine and selenomethionine in the serum proteins of chicks administered selenite. *Canad. J. Biochem.* **46,** 1417–1425.

Jereb, M., Jereb, B., and Unge, G. 1972. Radionuclear selenite (^{75}Se) for scintigraphic demonstration of lung cancer and metastases in the mediastinum. *Scand. J. Respir. Dis.* **53,** 331–337.

Johnson, R. B., Jr., and Baehner, R. L. 1971. Chronic granulomatous disease: Correlation between pathogenesis and clinical findings. *Pediatrics* **48,** 730–748.

Karpatkin, S., and Weiss, H. J. 1972. Deficiency of glutathione peroxidase associated with high levels of reduced glutathione in Glanzmann's thrombasthenia. *N. Engl. J. Med.* **287,** 1062–1066.

Kasperek, K., Shicha, H., Siller, V., and Feinendegen, L. E. 1972. Normalverte von Spurenelementen im menschlichen Serum und Korrelation zum Lebensalter und zur Serum-Eiweiss-Konzentration. *Strahlentherapie* **143,** 468–472.

Khandwala, A., and Gee, J. B. L. 1973. Linoleic acid hydroperoxide: Impaired bacterial uptake by alveolar macrophages, a mechanism of oxidant lung injury. *Science* **182,** 1364–1365.

Kiker, K. W., and Burk, R. F. 1974. Production of urinary selenium metabolites in the rat following $^{75}SeO_3^{2-}$ administration. *Amer. J. Physiol.* **227,** 643–646.

Kinoshita, J. H. 1955. Carbohydrate metabolism of the lens. *AMA Arch. Opthalmol.* **54,** 360–368.

Kinoshita, J. H. 1964. Selected topics in ophthalmic biochemistry. *AMA Arch. Opthalmol.* **72,** 554–572.

Klebanoff, S. 1971. Intraleukocytic microbicidal defects. *Annu. Rev. Med.* **22,** 39–62.

Koeman, J. H., Peeters, W. H. M., Koudstaal-Hol, C. H. M., Tjioe, P. S., and deGoeij, J. J. M. 1973. Mercury–selenium correlations in marine mammals. *Nature (London)* **245,** 385–386.

Konrad, P. N., Valentine, W. N., and Paglia, D. E. 1972. Enzymatic activities and glutathione content of erythrocytes in the newborn: Comparison with red cells of older normal subjects and those with comparable reticulocytosis. *Acta Haematol.* **48,** 193–201.

Kravitz, H., Elegant, L. D., Kaiser, E., and Kagan, B. M. 1956. Methemoglobin values in premature and mature infants and children. *Amer. J. Dis. Child.* **91,** 1–5.

Kubota, J., Allaway, W. H., Carter, D. L., Carey, E. E., and Lazar, V. A. 1967. Selenium in crops in the United States in relation to the selenium-responsive diseases of livestock. *J. Agric. Food Chem.* **15,** 448–453.

Kuck, J. F. R., Jr., 1970. The lens. In: *Biochemistry of the Eye* (C. N. Graymore, ed.). Pergamon Press, Oxford, pp. 319–371.

Lathrop, K. A., Johnston, R. E., Blau, M., and Rothschild, E. O. 1972. Radiation dose to humans from ^{75}Se-L-selenomethionine. *J. Nucl. Med.* **13,** (Suppl. 6), 7–30.

Lausecker, C., Heidt, P., Fischer, D., Hartleyb, H., and Lohr, G. W. 1965. Anémie hémolytique constitutionnelle avec déficit in 6-phospho-gluconate-déshydrogénase. *Arch. Franc. Pediatr.* **22,** 789–797.

Lawrence, R. A., Sunde, R. A., Schwartz, G. L., and Hoekstra, W. G. 1974. Glutathione peroxidase activity in rat lens and other tissues in relation to dietary selenium intake. *Exp. Eye Res.* **18,** 563–569.

Lee, M., Dong, A., and Yano, J. 1969. Metabolism of ^{75}Se-selenite by human whole blood *in vitro. Canad. J. Biochem.* **47,** 791–797.

Levander, O. A. 1972. Metabolic interrelationships and adaptations in selenium toxicity. *Ann. N. Y. Acad. Sci.* **192,** 181–192.

Levander, O. A., and Baumann, C. A. 1966. Selenium metabolism. VI. Effect of arsenic on the excretion of selenium in the bile. *Toxicol. Appl. Pharmacol.* **9,** 106–115.

Levander, O. A., and Morris, V. C. 1970. Interactions of methionine, vitamin E, and antioxidants in selenium toxicity in the rat. *J. Nutr.* **100,** 1111–1117.

Levander, O. A., Young, M. L., and Meeks, S. A. 1970. Studies on the binding of selenium by liver homegenates from rats fed diets containing either casein or casein plus linseed oil meal. *Toxicol. Appl. Pharmacol.* **16,** 79–87.

Levine, R. J., and Olson, R. E. 1970. Blood selenium in Thai children with protein–calorie malnutrition. *Proc. Soc. Exp. Biol. Med.* **134,** 1030–1034.

Lewis, H. B., Schultz, J., and Gortner, R. A. 1940. Dietary protein and the toxicity of sodium selenite in the white rat. *J. Pharmacol. Exp. Ther.* **68,** 292–299.

Lie-Injo, L. E., Wong, W. P., and Ng, T. 1973. Reduced glutathione, glutathione reductase, glutathione peroxidase, and pyruvate kinase in the erythrocytes of human newborns and adults in Malaysia. *Brit. J. Haematol.* **25,** 577–584.

Linden, O., and Work, E. 1953. Experimental liver necrosis in rats. I. Changes in liver, blood, and spleen glutathione and ascorbic acid levels in dietetic liver necrosis. *Biochem. J.* **55,** 554–562.

Little, C., and O'Brien, P. J. 1968. An intracellular GSH-peroxidase with a lipid peroxide substrate. *Biochem. Biophys. Res. Commun.* **31,** 145–150.

Lo, S. S. 1973. Vitamin E and hemolytic anemia in premature infants. *Arch. Dis. Child.* **48,** 360–365.

Ludwig, T. G., and Bibby, B. G. 1969. Geographic variations in the prevalence of dental caries in the United States of America. *Caries Res.* **3,** 32–43.

MacDougall, L. G. 1972. Red cell metabolism in iron deficiency anemia. III. The relationship between glutathione peroxidase, catalase, serum vitamin E and susceptibility of iron-deficient red cells to oxidative hemolysis. *J. Pediatr.* **80,** 775–782.

Mandell, G. L. 1972. Functional and metabolic derangements in human neutrophils induced by a glutathione antagonist. *J. Reticuloendothel. Soc.* **11,** 129–137.

McCoy, K. E. M., and Weswig, P. H. 1969. Some selenium responses in the rat not related to vitamin E. *J. Nutr.* **98,** 383–389.

Melhorn, D. K. and Gross, R. T. 1971a. Vitamin E-dependent anemia in the premature infant. I. Effect of large doses of medicinal iron. *J. Pediatr.* **79,** 569–580.

Melhorn, D. K., and Gross, R. T. 1971b. Vitamin E-dependent anemia in the premature infant. II. Relationships between gestational age and absorption of vitamin E. *J. Pediatr.* **79,** 581–588.

Meyers, L. S., Jr. 1973. Free radical damage of nucleic acids and their components by ionizing radiation. *Fed. Proc. Fed. Amer. Soc. Exp. Biol.* **32,** 1882–1894.

Millar, K. R., Gardiner, M. A., and Sheppard, A. D. 1973b. A comparison of the metabolism of intravenously injected sodium selenite, sodium selenate, and selenomethionine in rats. *N. Z. J. Agric. Res.* **16,** 115–127.

Miller, D., Soares, J. H., Bauersfeld, P., and Cuppett, S. L. 1972. Comparative selenium retention by chicks fed sodium selenite, selenomethionine, fish meal, and fish solubles. *Poultry Sci.* **51,** 1669– 1673.

Mills, G. C. 1957. Hemoglobin catabolism. I. Glutathione peroxidase, an erythrocyte enzyme which protects hemoglobin from oxidative breakdown. *J. Biol. Chem.* **229,** 189–197.

Mills, G. C. 1959. The purification and properties of glutathione peroxidase of erythrocytes. *J. Biol. Chem.* **234,** 502–506.

Mills, G. C. 1960. Glutathione peroxidase and the destruction of hydrogen peroxide in animal tissues. *Arch. Biochem. Biophys.* **86,** 1–5.

Mondragón, M. C., and Jaffé, W. G. 1971. Selenio en alimentos y en orína de escolares de diferentes zonas de Venezuela. *Arch. Latinoamer. Nutr.* **21,** 185–195.

Morris, V. C., and Levander, O. A. 1970. Selenium content of foods. *J. Nutr.* **100,** 1383–1388.

Moxon, A. L., and Rhian, M. 1943. Selenium poisoning. *Physiol. Rev.* **23,** 305–337.

Muth, O. H. 1960. Carbon tetrachloride poisoning of ewes on a low selenium ration. *Amer. J. Vet. Res.* **21,** 86–87.

Necheles, T. F., Maldonado, N., Barquet-Chediak, A., and Allen, D. M. 1967. Homozygous erythrocyte glutathione peroxidase deficiency. *Blood* **30,** 880–881 (abstract).

Necheles, T. F., Boles, T. A., and Allen, D. M. 1968. Erythrocyte glutathione peroxidase deficiency and hemolytic disease of the newborn infant. *J. Pediatr.* **72,** 319–324.

Necheles, T. F., Maldonado, N., Barquet-Chediak, A., and Allen, D. M. 1969. Homozygous erythrocyte glutathione peroxidase deficiency: Clinical and biochemical studies. *Blood* **33,** 164–169.

Necheles, T. F., Stimberg, M. H., and Cameron, D. 1970. Erythrocyte glutathione peroxidase deficiency. Brit. *J. Haematol.* **19,** 605–612.

Nicholls, P. 1965. Activity of catalase in the red cell. *Biochim. Biophys. Acta* **99,** 286–297.

Nicholls, P. 1972. Contributions of catalase and glutathione peroxidase to red blood cell peroxide removal. *Biochim. Biophys. Acta* **279,** 306–309.

Nicholls, P., and Schonbaum, G. R. 1963. Catalases. In: *The Enzymes,* 2nd ed., Vol. 8 (P. D. Boyer, H. Lardy, and K. Myrbäck, eds.). Academic Press, New York, pp. 147–225.

Nigam, S. N., and McConnell, W. B. 1969. Seleno amino compounds from *Astragalus bisulcatus.* Isolation and identification of γ-L-glutamyl-Se-methyl-seleno-L-cysteine and Se-methylseleno-L-cysteine. *Biochim. Biophys. Act* **192,** 185–190.

Nishimura, Y., Chida, N., Hayashi, T., and Arakawa, T. 1972. Homozygous glutathione-peroxidase deficiency of erythrocytes and leukocytes. *Tohoku J. Exp. Med.* **108,** 207–217.

Noguchi, T., Cantor, A. H., and Scott, M. L. 1973. Mode of action of selenium and vitamin E in prevention of exudative diathesis in chicks. *J. Nutr.* **103,** 1502–1511.

O'Brien, P. J. 1969. Intracellular mechanisms for the decomposition of a lipid peroxide. I. Decomposition of a lipid peroxide by metal ions, heme compounds, and nucleophiles. *Canad. J. Biochem.* **47,** 485–492.

O'Brien, P. J., and Little, C. 1969. Intracellular mechanisms for the decomposition of a lipid peroxide. II. Decomposition of a lipid peroxide by subcellular fractions. *Canad. J. Biochem.* **47,** 493–499.

Ochoa-Solano, A., and Gitler, C. 1968. Incorporation of ^{75}Se-selenomethionine and ^{35}S-methionine into chicken egg white proteins. *J. Nutr.* **94,** 243–248.

Oh, S. H., Ganther, H. E., and Hoekstra, W. G. 1974. Selenium as a component of glutathione peroxidase isolated from ovine erythrocytes. *Biochemistry* **13,** 1825–1829.

Oldendorf, W. H., Sisson, W. B., and Silverstein, A. 1971. Brain uptake of selenomethionine Se^{75}. II. Reduced brain uptake in phenylketonuria. *Arch. Neurol. (Chicago)* **24,** 524–528.

Olson, O. E., Novacek, E. J., Whitehead, E. I., and Palmer, I. S. 1970. Investigations on selenium in wheat. *Phytochemistry* **9,** 1181–1188.

Orentreich, N., Taylor, E. H., Berger, R. A., and Auerbach, R. 1969. Comparative study of two antidandruff preparations. *J. Pharm. Sci.* **58,** 1279–1280.

Oski, F. A., and Barness, L. A. 1967. Vitamin E deficiency: A previously unrecognized cause of hemolytic anemia in the premature infant. *J. Pediatr.* **70,** 211–220.

Palmer, I. S., Fischer, D. D., Halverson, A. W., and Olson, O. E. 1969. Identification of a major selenium excretory product in rat urine. *Biochim. Biophys. Acta* **177,** 336–342.

Paniker, N. V., and Iyer, G. Y. N. 165. Erythrocyte catalase and detoxification of hydrogen peroxide. *Canad. J. Biochem.* **43,** 1029–1039.

Paniker, N. V., and Iyer, G. Y. N. 1969. Protective factors in the detoxication of hydrogen peroxide in the red blood cell. *Canad. J. Biochem.* **47,** 405–410.

Paniker, N. V., and Iyer, G. Y. N. 1972. Role of red blood cell catalase in the protection of hemoglobin against hydrogen peroxide. *Indian J. Biochem. Biophys.* **9,** 176–178.

Paniker, N. V. Srivastava, S. K., and Beutler, E. 1970. Glutathione metabolism of the red cells. Effect of glutathione reductase deficiency on the stimulation of hexose monophosphate shunt under oxidative stress. *Biochim. Biophys. Acta* **215,** 456–460.

Paterson, C. A. 1971. Effects of drugs on the lens. *Int. Ophthalmol. Clin.* **11(2),** 63–97.

Patterson, E. L., Milstrey, R., and Stokstad, E. L. R. 1957. Effect of selenium in preventing exudative diathesis in chicks. *Proc. Soc. Exp. Biol. Med.* **95,** 617–620.

Penner, J. A. 1966. Investigation of erythrocyte turnover with selenium-75-labeled methionine. *J. Lab. Clin. Med.* **67,** 427–438.

Piccardo, M. G., and Schwarz, K. 1958. The electron microscopy of dietary necrotic liver degeneration. In: *Liver Function* (R. W. Brauer, ed.). American Institute of Biological Science, Washington, D.C., pp. 528–540.

Pinto, R. E., and Bartley, W. 1973. Glutathione reductase and glutathione peroxidase activities in hepatomatous livers of rats treated with diethylnitrosamine. *FEBS Lett.* **32,** 307–309.

Pirie, A. 1965. Glutathione peroxidase in lens and a source of H_2O_2 in aqueous humor. *Biochem. J.* **96,** 244–253.

Pirie, A., Rees, J. R., and Holmberg, N. J. 1970. Diquat cataract: Formation of the free radical and its reaction with constituents of the eye. *Exp. Eye Res.* **9,** 204–218.

Prins, H. K., Oort, M., Loos, J. A., Zurcher, C., and Beckers, T. 1966. Congenital nonspherocytic hemolytic anemia associated with glutathione deficiency of the erythrocytes: Hematological and biochemical studies. *Blood* **27,** 145–166.

Pryor, W. A. 1973. Free radical reactions and their importance in biochemical systems. *Fed. Proc. Fed. Amer. Soc. Exp. Biol.* **32,** 1862–1869.

Quie, P. G., Kaplan, E. L., Page, A. R., Gruskay, F. L., and Malawista, S. E. 1968. Defective polymorphonuclear leukocyte function and chronic granulomatous disease in two female children. *N. Engl. J. Med.* **278,** 976–979.

Ransone, J. W., Scott, N. M., and Knoblock, E. C. 1961. Selenium sulfide intoxication. *N. Engl. J. Med.* **264,** 384–385.

Recknagel, R. O. 1967. Carbon tetrachloride hepatotoxicity. *Pharmacol. Rev.* **19,** 145–208.

Reed, P. W. 1969. Glutathione and the hexose monophosphate shunt in phagocytizing and hydrogen peroxide-treated rat leukocytes. *J. Biol. Chem.* **244,** 2459–2464.

Ritchie, J. H., Mathews, B. F., McMasters, V., and Grossman, M. 1968. Edema and hemolytic anemia in premature infants: A vitamin E deficiency syndrome. *N. Engl. J. Med.* **270,** 1185–1190.

Robertson, D. S. F. 1970. Selenium—a possible teratogen? *Lancet* **1,** 518–519.

Rodey, G. E., Park, B. H., Ford, D. K., Gray, B. H., and Good, R. A. 1970. Defective bactericidal activity of peripheral blood leukocytes in lipochrome histiocytosis. *Amer. J. Med.* **49,** 322–327.

Rodvien, R., Gillum, A., and Weintraub, L. R. 1974. Decreased glutathione peroxidase activity secondary to severe iron deficiency: A possible mechanism responsible for the shortened life span of the iron-deficient cell. *Blood* **43,** 281–289.

Rosenfeld, S., and Beath, O. A. 1964. *Selenium: Geobotany, Biochemistry, Toxicity, and Nutrition.* Academic Press, New York.

Rotruck, J. T., Pope, A. L., Ganther, H. E., Swanson, A. B., Hafeman, D. G., and Hoekstra, W. G. 1973. Selenium: Biochemical role as a component of glutathione peroxidase. *Science* **179,** 588–590.

Said, A. K., and Hegsted, D. M. 1970. ^{75}Se-selenomethionine in the study of protein and amino acid metabolism of adult rats. *Proc. Soc. Exp. Biol. Med.* **133,** 1388–1391.

Schroeder, H. A., Frost, D. V., and Balassa, J. J. 1970. Essential trace metals in man: Selenium. *J. Chronic Dis.* **23,** 227–243.

Schwarz, K. 1961. Development and status of experimental work on factor 3-selenium. *Fed. Proc. Fed. Amer. Soc. Exp. Biol.* **20,** 666–673.

Schwarz, K. 1962. Vitamin E, trace elements, and sulfhydryl groups in respiratory decline. *Vitam. Horm. (N.Y.)* **20,** 463–484.

Schwarz, K. 1965. Role of vitamin E, selenium, and related factors in experimental nutritional liver disease. *Fed. Proc. Fed. Amer. Soc. Exp. Biol.* **24,** 58–67.

Schwarz, K., and Foltz, C. M. 1957. Selenium as an integral part of factor 3 against deitary necrotic liver degeneration. *J. Amer. Chem. Soc.* **79,** 3292–3293.

Schwarz, K., and Foltz, C. M. 1958. Factor 3 activity of selenium compounds. *J. Biol. Chem.* **233,** 245–251.

Schwarz, K., Porter, L. A., and Fredga, A. 1972. Some regularities in the structure–function relationship of organoselenium compounds effective against dietary liver necrosis. *Ann. N.Y. Acad. Sci.* **192,** 200–214.

Scialom, C., Najeau, Y., and Bernard, J. 1966. Anémie hémolytique congénitale non-sphérocytoire avec déficit incomplet en 6-phosphogluconate déshydrogenase. *Nouv. Rev. Franc. Hematol.* **6,** 452–457.

Scott, M. L., and Thompson, J. N. 1971. Selenium content of feedstuffs and effects of dietary selenium levels upon tissue selenium in chicks and poults. *Poultry Sci.* **50,** 1742–1748.

Serfass, R. E., Hinsdill, R. D., and Ganther, H. E. 1974. Protective effect of dietary selenium on *Salmonella* infection: Relation to glutathione peroxidase and superoxide dismutase activities of phagocytes. *Fed. Proc. Fed. Amer. Soc. Exp. Biol.* **33,** 694 (abstract).

Seward, C. R., Vaughan, G., and Hove, E. L. 1966. Effect of selenium on incisor depigmentation and carbon tetrachloride poisoning in vitamin E-deficient rats. *Proc. Soc. Exp. Biol. Med.* **121,** 850–852.

Shamberger, R. J., Rukovena, E., Longfield, A. K., Tytko, S. A., Deodhar, S., and Willis, C. E. 1973. Antioxidants and cancer. I. Selenium in the blood of normals and cancer patients. *J. Natl. Cancer Inst.* **50,** 863–870.

Shmerling, D. H., Prader, A., Hitzig, W. H., Giedion, A., Hadorn, B., and Kuhni, M. 1969. The syndrome of exocrine pancreatic insufficiency, neutropenia, metaphyseal dysostosis and dwarfism. *Helv. Faediatr. Acta* **24,** 547–553.

Shull, L. R., and Cheeke, P. R. 1973. Antiselenium activity of tri-*o*-cresyl phosphate in rats and Japanese quail. *J. Nutr.* **103,** 560–568.

Slater, T. F. 1972. *Free Radical Mechanisms in Tissue Injury.* Pion, London.

Smith, M. I., and Westfall, B. B. 1937. Further field studies on the selenium problem in relation to public health. *Public Health Rep.* **52,** 1375–1384.

Smith, M. I., Franke, K. W., and Westfall, B. B. 1936. The selenium problem in relation to public health: A preliminary survey to determine the possibility of selenium intoxication in the rural population living on seleniferous soil. *Public Health Rep.* **51,** 1496–1505.

Sprinker, L. H., Harr, J. R., Newberne, P. M., Whanger, P. D., and Weswig, P. H. 1971. Selenium deficiency lesions in rats fed vitamin E supplemented rations. *Nutr. Rep. Int.* **4,** 335–340.

Steinberg, M. H., and Necheles, T. F. 1971. Erythrocyte glutathione peroxidase deficiency: Biochemical studies on the mechanisms of drug-induced hemolysis. *Amer. J. Med.* **50,** 542–546.

Steinberg, M. H., Brauer, M. J., and Necheles, T. F. 1970. Acute hemolytic anemia associated with glutathione-peroxidase deficiency. *Arch. Intern. Med.* **125,** 302–303.

Strauss, R. R., Paul, B. B., Jacobs, A. A., and Sbarra, A. J. 1969. The role of the phagocyte in host–parasite interactions. XIX. Leukocytic glutathione reductase and its involvement in phagocytosis. *Arch. Biochem. Biophys.* **135,** 265–271.

Swanson, A. A., and Truesdale, A. W. 1971. Elemental analysis in normal and cataractous human lens tissue. *Biochem. Biophys. Res. Commun.* **45,** 1488–1496.

Swanson, A. B., Wagner, P. A., Ganther, H. E., and Hoekstra, W. G. 1974. Antagonistic effects of silver and tri-*o*-cresyl phosphate on selenium and glutathione peroxidase in rat liver and erythrocytes. *Fed. Proc. Fed. Amer. Soc. Exp. Biol.* **33,** 693 (abstract).

Swierczewski, E., Demus-Oole, A. M., and Minkowski, A. 1969. Glutathione peroxidase and catalase in the erythrocytes of premature, full term, and hypotrophic infants. *Z. Klin. Chem.* **7,** 208–209.

Thiemann, G., Holldorf, M., and Schwartz, K. D. 1971. Ergebnisse der Se^{75}-Selenite-Tumorszintigraphie. *Radiobiol. Radiother.* **12**, 109–116.

Thompson, J. N., and Scott, M. L. 1969. Role of selenium in the nutrition of the chick. *J. Nutr.* **97**, 335–342.

Thompson, J. N., and Scott, M. L. 1970. Impaired lipid and vitamin E absorption related to atrophy of the pancreas in selenium-deficient chicks. *J. Nutr.* **100**, 797–809.

Thomson, C. D. 1972. Urinary excretion of selenium in some New Zealand women. *Proc. Univ. Otago Med. Sch.* **50**, 31–33.

Thomson, C. D., and Stewart, R. D. H. 1972. Measurement of intestinal absorption of selenium. *Proc. Univ. Otago Med. Sch.* **50**, 63–64.

Tudhope, G. R., and Leece, S. P. 1971. Red cell catalase and the production of methemoglobin, Heinz bodies, and changes in osmotic fragility due to drugs. *Acta Haematol.* **45**, 290–302.

Turner, D. C., and Stadtman, T. C. 1973. Purification of protein components of the clostridial glycine reductase system and characterization of protein A as a selenoprotein. *Arch. Biochem. Biophys.* **154**, 366–381.

Ugazio, G., Koch, R. R., and Recknagel, R. O. 1973. Reversibility of liver damage in rats rendered resistant to carbon tetrachloride by prior carbon tetrachloride administration: Bearing on the lipoperoxidation hypothesis. *Exp. Mol. Pathol.* **18**, 281–289.

van Heyningen, R. 1969. The lens: Metabolism and cataract. In: *The Eye,* 2nd ed., Vol. 1 (H. Davson, ed.). Academic Press, London, pp. 381–388.

van Heyningen, R., and Pirie, A. 1953. Reduction of glutathione coupled with oxidative decarboxylation of malate in cattle lenses. *Biochem. J.* **53**, 436–444.

Vernie, L. N., Bont, W. S., and Emmelot, P. 1974. Inhibition of *in vitro* amino acid incorporation by sodium selenite. *Biochemistry* **13**, 337–341.

Vetrella, M., and Barthelmai, W. 1971. Erythrocyten Enzyme bei menschlichen Feten. *Monatsschr. Kinderheilkd.* **119**, 265–267.

Vetrella, M., Barthelmai, W., and Reitkolter, J. 1970. Erythrocyte glutathione peroxidase activity from fetal to adult ages. *Klin. Wochenschr.* **48**, 85–88.

Waller, H. D. 1968. Glutathione reductase deficiency. In: *Hereditary Disorders of Erythrocyte Metabolism* (E. Beutler, ed.). Grune and Stratton, New York, pp. 185–208.

Waller, H. D., and Gerok, W. 1964. Schwere strahleninduzierte Hämolyse bei hereditärem Mangel an reduziertem Glutathion in Blutzellen. *Klin. Wochenschr.* **47**, 948–954.

Waterlow, J. C., Garrow, J. S., and Millward, D. J. 1969. The turnover of (^{75}Se) selenomethionine in infants and rats measured in a whole body counter. *Clin. Sci.* **36**, 489–504.

Wenzel, M., Otto, R., and Riehle, I. 1971. Der Einbau von ^{75}Se nach Applikation von radioaktivem Natriumselenit in Normalgewebe und in Tumoren *in vitro* und *in vivo*. *Int. J. Appl. Radiat. Isotopes* **22**, 361–369.

Westring, D. W., and Pisciotta, A. V. 1966. Anemia, cataract, and seizures in a patient with glucose-6-phosphate dehydrogenase deficiency. *Arch. Intern. Med.* **118**, 385–390.

Whanger, P. D., Pedersen, N. D., and Weswig, P. H. 1973. Selenium proteins in ovine tissue. II. Spectral properties of a 10,000 molecular weight selenium protein. *Biochem. Biophys. Red. Commun.* **53**, 1031–1035.

Whaun, J. M., and Oski, F. A. 1970. Relation of red cell glutathione peroxidase to neonatal jaundice. *J. Pediatr.* **76**, 555–560.

Witkop, C. J., Jr., White, J. G., Gerritsen, S. M., Townsend, D., and King, R. A. 1973. Hermansky–Pudlak syndrome (HPS): A proposed block in glutathione peroxidase. *Oral Surg.* **35**, 790–806.

Wright, P. L., and Bell, M. C. 1963. Selenium and vitamin E invluence upon the *in vitro* uptake of Se^{75} by ovine blood cells. *Proc. Soc. Exp. Biol. Med.* **114**, 379–382.

Zeller, E. A. 1953. Contribution to the enzymology of the normal and cataractorus lens. III. On the catalase of the crystalline lens. *Amer. J. Opthalmol.* **38**, 51–53.

CHAPTER 10

ZINC

INTRODUCTION

Raulin (1869) first showed in 1869 that zinc was essential for the growth of *Aspergillus niger*. This essentiality was confirmed almost 40 years later by Bertrand and Javillier (1911). In 1926, the essentiality of zinc for higher forms of plant life was established (Sommer, 1928; Sommer and Lipman, 1926).

Todd *et al.* (1934) published evidence indicating that zinc was necessary for the growth and well-being of the rat. Tucker and Salmon (1955) reported that zinc cures and prevents parakeratosis in swine. In 1958, O'Dell and co-workers (O'Dell and Savage, 1957; O'Dell *et al.*, 1958) showed that zinc was required for growth and various other functions in birds. Zinc deficiency occured in suckling mice that were deprived of colostrum (Nishimura, 1953). The manifestation consisted of retarded growth and ossification, alopecia, thickening and hyperkeratinization of the epidermis, clubbed digits, deformed nails, and moderate congestion in certain viscera. Experimental zinc deficiency in calves was produced by J. K. Miller and Miller (1960, 1962). The main features were retarded growth, testicular atrophy, and hyperkeratosis. Deficiency of zinc in the diet of breeding hens results in (1) lowered hatchability, (2) gross embryonic anomalies characterized by impaired skeletal development, and (3) varying degrees of weakness in chicks that hatch (Blamberg *et al.*, 1960). Zinc deficiency in dogs was produced by feeding a diet low in zinc and high in calcium (Robertson and Burns, 1963). Signs of zinc deficiency in dogs included retardation of growth, emaciation, emesis, conjuctivitis, keratitis, general debility, and skin lesions on the abdomen and extremities. Zinc deficiency was produced in young Japanese quail by feeding a zinc-low purified diet containing soybean protein (Fox and Harrison, 1964). Slow growth, abnormal feathering, labored respiration, incoordinate gait, and low content of zinc in the liver and tibias were noted.

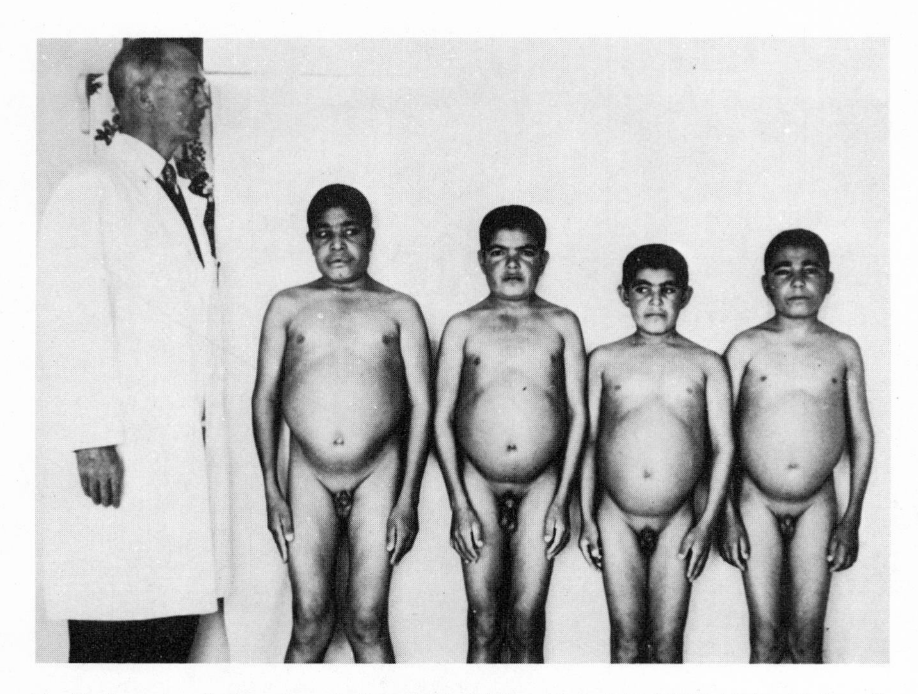

Fig. 9. Four dwarfs from Iran. Left to right: (1) Age 21, height 4 ft 11 1/2 in; (2) Age 18, height 4 ft 9 in; (3) Age 18, height 4 ft 7 in; (4) Age 21, height 4 ft 7 in. Staff physician at left is 6 ft in height. From Prasad *et al.* (1961).

Deficiency of zinc was first suspected in 1961 to occur in man (Prasad *et al.*, 1961) in Iranian males, and was established following detailed studies in Egypt in 1963 (Prasad *et al.*, 1963a–d; Sandstead *et al.*, 1967). In the fall of 1958, a 21-year-old patient at Saadi Hospital, Shiraz, Iran, who looked like a 10-year-old boy and had severe anemia was brought to my attention (Fig. 9). In addition to dwarfism and anemia, he had hypogonadism, hepatosplenomegaly, rough and dry skin, mental lethargy, and geophagia. This patient ate only bread made of wheat flour, and the intake of animal protein was negligible. He consumed nearly one pound of clay daily. The habit of geophagia is not uncommon in the villages around Shiraz. The patient had severe iron deficiency, although there was no evidence of blood loss. Hookworm and schistosomiasis infestations are not seen in that part of Iran. Shortly thereafter, ten additional similar cases were investigated in detail.

The probable factors responsible for anemia in these patients were: (1) the amount of available iron in the diet was insufficient; (2) excessive sunburn and sweating probably caused greater iron loss from the skin than would occur in a temperate climate; and (3) geophagia may have further decreased iron absorption, as was observed by Minnich *et al.* (1968). In every case, the anemia was completely corrected by administration of oral iron (Prasad *et al.,* 1961).

This clinical syndrome was previously observed in 1910 by Lemann (1910) in the United States. However, it was not related to a nutritional deficiency. Similar patients from Turkey were reported (Reimann, 1955), but detailed descriptions were not given, and a genetic defect as a possible explanation for certain aspects of the clinical picture was considered. Our detailed clinical report from Iran was published in 1961 (Prasad *et al.,* 1961). Although we had no data to document zinc deficiency in our patients, this possibility was considered at that time. Subsequently, our studies in Egypt established that such patients were zinc-deficient (Prasad *et al.,* 1963a,b; Sandstead *et al.,* 1967), thus demonstrating for the first time that deficiency of zinc may occur in man.

BIOCHEMISTRY AND PHYSIOLOGY

Various studies by Vallee (1959) showed that zinc is a constituent of a number of metalloenzymes. Although iron and copper enzymes, owing to their characteristic colors, have been recognized for some time, zinc metalloenzymes have emerged on the scene only recently.

The first demonstration of a specific biological function critically dependent on the presence of zinc came with the discovery of Keilin and Mann (1940) showing that carbonic anhydrase contained zinc essential to its mechanism of action. Over the next 20 years, only five additional zinc metalloenzymes were identified, but in the last 15 years, the total number has risen to about two dozen (Table VI). If related enzymes from different species are included, then more than 70 zinc metalloenzymes are now on record (Riordan and Vallee, 1976).

Zinc metalloenzymes exhibit great diversity both of catalytic function and of the role played by the metal atom (Keilin and Mann, 1940; Parisi and Vallee, 1969; Vallee and Wacker, 1970). They are now known to be present throughout all phyla and to participate in a wide variety of metabolic processes including carbohydrate, lipid, protein, and nucleic acid synthesis or degradation. Each of the six categories of enzymes designated by the IUB (International Union of Biochemistry) Commission on Enzyme Nomenclature contains at least one example of a zinc metalloenzyme. The metal is present in several dehydrogenases, aldolases, peptidases, and phosphatases. Since the zinc cation has a d_{10} electronic configuration, it exists in the +2 oxidation state and does not undergo oxidation or reduction. The development of highly precise, rapid, and convenient means for

Table VI. Zinc Metalloenzymes[a]

Enzyme	IUB No.	Source
Alcohol dehydrogenase	1.1.1.1	Yeast; horse, human liver
D-Lactate cytochrome reductase	1.1.2.4	Yeast
Glyceraldehyde-phosphate dehydrogenase	1.2.1.13	Beef, pig muscle
Phosphoglucomutase	2.7.5.1	Yeast
RNA polymerase	2.7.7.6	*E. coli*
DNA polymerase	2.7.7.7	*E. coli;* sea urchin
Reverse transcriptase	2.7.7.	Avian myeloblastosis virus
Mercaptopyruvate sulfurtransferase	2.8.1.2	*E. coli*
Alkaline phosphatase	3.1.3.1	*E. coli*
Phospholipase C	3.1.4.3	*B. cereus*
Leucine aminopeptidase	3.4.1.1	Pig kidney; lens
Carboxypeptidase A	3.4.2.1	Beef, human pancreas
Carboxypeptidase B	3.4.2.2	Beef, pig pancreas
Carboxypeptidase C	3.4.2.	*Pseudomonas Stutzeri*
Dipeptidase	3.4.3.	Pig kidney
Neutral protease	3.4.4.	*Bacillus sp.*
Alkaline protease	3.4.4.	*E. freundii*
AMP aminohydrolase	3.5.4.6	Rabbit muscle
Aldolase	4.1.2.13	Yeast; *A. niger*
Carbonic anhydrase	4.2.1.1	Erythrocytes
δ-Aminolevulinic acid dehydratase	4.2.1.24	Beef liver
Phosphomannose isomerase	5.3.1.8	Yeast
Pyruvate carboxylase	6.4.1.1	Yeast

[a] From Riordan and Vallee (1976).

zinc analysis no doubt accounts for much of the increase in the recognition of zinc metalloenzymes.

Chemical stability may be an essential aspect of the utilization of zinc in diverse biological processes such as hydrolysis, transfer, and addition to double bonds and even oxidoreduction. However, the role of zinc in redox enzymes, such as alcohol dehydrogenase, is not to donate or accept electrons; rather, it serves as a Lewis acid. It is this capacity to serve as a super acid that likely underlies the function of zinc in many zinc metalloenzymes (Riordan and Vallee, 1976). A zinc metalloenzyme is defined as a catalytically active metalloprotein containing stoichiometric amounts of zinc firmly bound at its active site (Vallee, 1955). The metal atoms are so tightly bound that they do not dissociate from the protein during the isolation procedure. When the metal is loosely bound, the association is chemically and functionally more tenuous, and the designation metal–enzyme complex has been employed to convey this distinction (Riordan and Vallee, 1976).

In zinc metalloenzymes, the metal is located at the active site and participates in the actual catalytic process. This is not, however, the only function that zinc may have in enzymes. It may serve to stabilize structure, as in *B. subtilis* α-amylase (Vallee, 1959), or it may have a regulatory role as in aspartate transcarbamylase (Rosenbusch and Weber, 1971). It can serve in both catalysis and structure, e.g., horse liver alcohol dehydrogenase (Drum *et al.,* 1967), or in both catalysis and regulation, e.g., bovine lens aminopeptidase (Carpenter and Vahl, 1973).

In the past few years, zinc has been found in both DNA and RNA polymerases. The recent demonstration that RNA-dependent DNA polymerase in the reverse transcriptase of avian myeloblastosis and other viruses is also a zinc metalloenzyme indicates a direct relationship between zinc metabolism and cancer and opens up new approaches to the investigation of this disease (Riordan and Vallee, 1976). Recent studies in biological experiments indicate that thymidine kinase is also a zinc-dependent enzyme, and that this enzyme is very sensitive to a lack of zinc (Prasad and Oberleas, 1974). The activity of RNase is regulated by exogenous zinc; thus, zinc appears to play a very important role in RNA and DNA metabolism.

ZINC ENZYMES IN ZINC DEFICIENCY

Since zinc is needed for many enzymes, one may speculate that the level of zinc in cells controls the physiological processes through the formation or regulation of activity, or both of zinc-dependent enzymes. Until 1965, however, there was no evidence in the literature to support this concept (Prasad, 1966). Since that time, studies have been reported showing that in zinc-deficient rats, the activity of various zinc-dependent enzymes (as judged by histochemical techniques) was reduced in testes, bones, esophagus, and kidneys in comparison with their pair-fed controls (Prasad, 1966; Prasad *et al.,* 1967; Prasad and Oberleas, 1971). These results correlated with the decreased zinc content in the aforenamed tissues of the zinc-deficient rats and with the clinical manifestations of testicular atrophy, reduced growth rate, and esophageal parakeratosis. This suggests that the likelihood of detecting any biochemical changes is greatest in tissues that are sensitive to zinc depletion.

The activity of alkaline phosphatase was reported to decrease in the serum of zinc-deficient rats, pigs, dairy cows, calves, and chicks (Kirchgessner *et al.,* 1976). Only in the study of Kfoury *et al.* (1968) was there no reduction in the activity of the serum alkaline phosphatase in the plasma of zinc-deficient rats. In some studies, the serum or plasma activities were not different from those of zinc-supplemented pair-fed control rats, but were significantly lower than those of ad-libitum-fed controls (Macapinlac *et al.,* 1966; Luecke and Baltzer, 1968; Luecke *et al.,* 1968).

The alkaline phosphatase activity in serum declines rapidly as a result of zinc depletion. In the studies by Roth and Kirchgessner (1974a), the activity of this enzyme decreased significantly within 2–4 days after the feeding of the zinc-deficient diet was initiated. Since the activity of this enzyme decreased before any signs of a lowered food intake or reduced growth rate were evident, it can be concluded that the activity loss was directly attributable to zinc deficiency.

In zinc-deficient subjects, as reported from the Middle East by Prasad (Prasad *et al.*, 1961; Sandstead *et al.*, 1967), serum alkaline phosphatase activity consistently increased following supplementation with zinc. Thus, it appears that an induction of serum alkaline phosphatase activity following zinc supplementation may indicate a zinc-deficient state in man retrospectively.

In almost all studies, the activity of the alkaline phosphatase was found to be reduced in bones from zinc-deficient rats, pigs, cows, chicks, turkey poults, and quails. In disagreement with this finding are only the early report by Day and McCollum (1940) and the studies by Shrader and Hurley (1972), who did not detect a reduced activity in the bone marrow of depleted rats.

Besides the bone and the intestine, the kidneys and stomach may also have reduced activity of alkaline phosphatase in zinc deficiency. Not only may there be a loss of activity due to a lack of sufficient zinc for maintaining the enzyme activity, but also the amount of apoenzyme present may be diminished because of either decreased synthesis or increased degradation. This possibility was suggested by Kfoury *et al.* (1968), Luecke *et al.* (1968), and M. J. Davies and Motzok (1971), who added zinc to homogenates of intestinal mucosa and were unable to raise the alkaline phosphatase activity in the tibiae of chicks by preincubation with zinc to the level of the zinc-supplemented controls. The study by Igbal (1971), using pair-fed animals, indicates that the lowered activity of the intestinal alkaline phosphatase is probably not caused by reduced food intake. Furthermore, Williams (1972) noted decreased activity of this enzyme in intestinal tissue as early as 3 days after rats were given a zinc-deficient diet, indicating that the activity of alkaline phosphatase depended on zinc and not on the intake of protein or calories.

PANCREATIC CARBOXYPEPTIDASES

Two enzymes of importance in protein digestion are pancreatic carboxypeptidases A and B. A loss of activity of pancreatic carboxypeptidase A in zinc deficiency is a consistent finding (Hsu, J. M., *et al.*, 1966; Prasad and Oberleas, 1971). According to studies by Roth and Kirchgessner (1974b), this enzyme lost 24% of its activity in the rat pancreas within 2 days of a dietary zinc depletion. Zinc repletion rapidly restored the activity of carboxypeptidase A within 3 days to the normal levels of pair-fed animals. The level of food intake had no influence.

With regard to carboxypeptidase B, J. M. Hsu *et al.* (1966) did not find reduced activities in the zinc-deficient pancreas. Roth and Kirchgessner (1974b), however, reported a loss of activity for this pancreatic enzyme of about 50% in zinc-depleted rats compared with pair-fed and ad-libitum-fed control animals.

CARBONIC ANHYDRASE

In tissues such as blood, stomach, and intestine in which carbonic anhydrase has a major functional role, reduced activities have been observed. However, the decreased activities that were found in the blood of rats (Roth and Kirchgessner, 1974c), of calves (Miller, J. K., and Miller, 1962), and of lambs (Ott *et al.,* 1965) are in contrast to other studies that did not report such changes (Huber and Gershoff, 1973a). In the studies by Roth and Kirchgessner (1974c), the activity of carbonic anhydrase was reduced by 41% after 4 days of zinc depletion. After 30 days, however, there was no longer any difference noted between the deficient and the zinc-supplemented animals. At the same time, the erythrocyte count expressed per cubic millimeter of blood had increased by 41% in the deficient group. Therefore, when the enzyme activity was expressed per unit of erythrocytes, a reduction in the activity of the carbonic anhydrase of blood could be demonstrated both at the beginning of the dietary zinc depletion and in later stages of zinc deficiency. Igbal (1971) found that zinc deficiency reduced the carbonic anhydrase activity of gastric and intestinal tissue of rats by 47 and 33%.

Recently, in sickle cell disease patients, an example of a conditioned zinc-deficient state, the content of carbonic anhydrase in the red cells was found to be decreased and correlated with the zinc content of the red cells (Prasad *et al.,* 1975a). Inasmuch as this technique measured the apoenzyme content, it appears that zinc may have a specific effect on the synthesis of this protein. The precise mechanism by which zinc may affect the synthesis of the apoenzyme is not understood at present.

ALCOHOL DEHYDROGENASE

Primarily, the studies by Prasad *et al.* (1967, 1969a,b, 1971) and Prasad and Oberleas (1971) showed that zinc deficiency lowers the activity of this enzyme in the liver, bone, testes, kidneys, and esophagus of rats and pigs. Roth and Kirchgessner (1974d) found a 28% lower activity of the alcohol dehydrogenase in the liver of rats in an extreme stage of zinc deficiency.

Similarly, Kfoury *et al.* (1968) observed reduced activity of the liver enzyme only in severely zinc-depleted rats. Other workers, however, did not detect reduced activities in the liver (Macapinlac *et al.*, 1966; Hsu, J. M., *et al.*, 1966; Swenerton, 1971) or in the femur muscle of zinc-deficient rats (Roth and Kirchgessner, 1974e).

EXPRESSION OF ENZYME ACTIVITY IN ZINC DEFICIENCY

It is customary to express enzyme activities in terms of units per milligram of protein. Prasad and Oberleas (1971), however, pointed out that impaired growth is one of the major effects of zinc deficiency, and therefore the protein content of the cells of certain body tissues may be altered. Thus, it is unsatisfactory to express enzyme activities per milligram of protein. These authors therefore suggested expressing enzyme activities in terms of DNA, which is a most stable cellular constituent. Evidence has been provided, however, that zinc deficiency also affects the DNA and RNA content of tissues. As was previously stated, the activities of alkaline phosphatase and pancreatic carboxypeptidase A were reduced before growth retardation and inappetence became evident. Thus, it seems justified to assume that the protein content of the tissues was not yet affected. Furthermore, evidence for the conclusion that the response of these enzymes is specific for zinc is provided by the observation that the activities of only zinc-dependent enzymes are altered by zinc deficiency compared with control levels of pair-fed animals. There was no difference between zinc-deficient and pair-fed animals in activities of other enzymes for which zinc is not required (Table VII). This has been shown to be true for sorbitol dehydrogenase and manganese-dependent isocitric dehydrogenase, glutamic-pyruvic transaminase, glutamic-oxalacetic transaminase of rats (Roth and Kirchgessner, 1974d), and isocitric dehydrogenase and iron-dependent succinic dehydrogenase of rats and pigs (Prasad *et al.*, 1971; Prasad and Oberleas, 1971).

DIFFERENCES IN THE RESPONSE OF INDIVIDUAL ZINC METALLOENZYMES TO ZINC DEPLETION

The research results presented in this review clearly reveal that among the zinc metalloenzymes, only specific ones change their activity and then only in certain tissues. The probability of detecting biochemical changes, therefore, is highest in those tissues that respond rather sensitively to a lack of available zinc, as, for example, serum, bones, pancreas, and intestinal mucosa (Prasad *et al.*, 1971).

It is not to be expected that zinc-dependent enzymes are affected to the same extent in all tissues of a zinc-deficient animal. Differences in the sensitivity of enzymes are evidently the result of differences both in the zinc-ligand affinity of the various zinc metalloenzymes and in their turnover rates in the cells of the affected tissues (Prasad *et al.,* 1971). Thus, it is to be expected that those zinc metalloenzymes that bind zinc with a very high affinity are still fully active even in extreme stages of zinc deficiency.

Swenerton and co-workers (Swenerton, 1971; Swenerton *et al.* 1972; Swenerton and Hurley, 1968) could not find reduced activities of the lactic or glutamic dehydrogenases in the liver of zinc-depleted rats, nor were there reduced activities of the malic and lactic dehydrogenases in the testes showing histological lesions. They therefore did not favor the hypothesis that reduced enzyme activities are responsible for the severe physiological and morphological changes observed in zinc-deficient animals. The complete lack of responsiveness of the activity of these enzymes, even when symptoms of severe zinc deficiency are apparent, again may be explained on the basis that the affinity of zinc for these enzymes is high, and consequently the turnover rate in these tissues remains unaltered.

REDUCED ENZYME ACTIVITIES AND ZINC SYMPTOMS

Severe zinc deficiency is associated with reduced activities of a number of zinc-containing enzymes. Since tissues bind zinc with different affinities, dietary zinc depletion may rapidly lead to a deficiency in labile zinc, especially in certain organs, and is therefore associated with a corresponding loss in the activity of specific zinc metalloenzymes. Adequate supplementation with zinc rapidly overcomes this deficiency and raises the activity of these zinc metalloenzymes to normal levels. The extent to which the metalloenzymes lose their activity also depends on the functional role that zinc plays in maintaining the enzyme structure. In some zinc-dependent enzymes, e.g., alkaline phosphatase, zinc deficiency may induce structural changes that increase the chance for degradation. The consequence is an increased turnover rate and a lower activity of the enzymes in the tissues (Reinhold and Kfoury, 1969).

Mills *et al.* (1969) and Prasad and co-workers (Prasad *et al.,* 1971; Prasad and Oberleas, 1970b) suggested that the rapidity with which biochemical changes arise in response to zinc depletion and the response on repletion help to identify the primary site of metabolic functions of zinc. In studies applying dietary zinc depletion, the early changes in enzyme activities that are detectable before a general depletion becomes evident from tissue zinc levels indicate that the primary role of zinc must be associated with a tissue component with an extremely high turnover, or that zinc is essential at a site where it is freely exchangeable (Prasad *et al.,* 1969a).

According to Prasad *et al.* (1969a,b), many metabolic processes are regulated by zinc metalloenzymes the synthesis and activity of which are in

Table VII. Zinc and Specific Activities of Various Enzymes in Tissues of Controls and Zinc-Deficient Rats[a]

Tissue[b]	Zinc (μg/g dry wt)	Activity of enzymes (ΔOD/min per mg protein)[c]					Alkaline phosphatase (sigma U/mg protein)	CPD (μmol β-naphthol liberated/mg protein)[c]
		ADH	Aldolase	LDH	ICDH	SDH		
Liver								
A	91.7 ± 4.7	0.021 ± 0.0022	0.107 ± 0.0064		0.43 ± 0.02			
B	107.3 ± 3.1	0.022 ± 0.0013	0.134 ± 0.0098		0.38 ± 0.03	0.151 ± 0.012		
C	87.6 ± 3.5	0.013 ± 0.0008	0.124 ± 0.0100		0.38 ± 0.02	0.152 ± 0.017		
A vs. B[d]	$P < 0.025$	NS	$P < 0.05$		NS			
A vs. C	NS	$P < 0.001$	NS		NS			
B vs. C	$P < 0.001$	$P < 0.001$	NS		NS	NS		
Kidney								
A	93 ± 2.2	0.0031 ± 0.00025	0.20 ± 0.01	2.9 ± 0.27	0.57 ± 0.03		3.3 ± 0.22	
B	87 ± 0.8	0.0031 ± 0.00012	0.22 ± 0.01	2.67 ± 0.07	0.48 ± 0.03	0.188 ± 0.0075	4.5 ± 0.25	
C	80 ± 0.9	0.0014 ± 0.00013	0.21 ± 0.01	2.53 ± 0.04	0.49 ± 0.04	0.187 ± 0.0056	2.3 ± 0.17	
A vs. B	NS	NS	NS	NS	NS		$P < 0.005$	
A vs. C	$P < 0.001$	$P < 0.001$	NS	NS	NS		$P < 0.005$	
B vs. C	$P < 0.001$	$P < 0.001$	NS	NS	NS	NS	$P < 0.001$	
Testis								
A	191.0 ± 3.1	0.022 ± 0.0018	0.161 ± 0.0034		0.063 ± 0.0067		2.75 ± 0.11	
B	197.1 ± 2.9	0.028 ± 0.0030	0.161 ± 0.0047	1.20 ± 0.08	0.046 ± 0.0052	0.128 ± 0.0046	2.80 ± 0.10	
C	114.7 ± 4.9	0.012 ± 0.0014	0.164 ± 0.0112	1.22 ± 0.09	0.090 ± 0.0076	0.127 ± 0.0054	1.70 ± 0.10	
A vs. B	NS	NS	NS		$P < 0.025$		NS	
A vs. C	$P < 0.001$	$P < 0.001$	NS		$P < 0.025$		$P < 0.001$	
B vs. C	$P < 0.001$	$P < 0.001$	NS	NS	$P < 0.001$	NS	$P < 0.001$	

Pancreas							
A	79.5 ± 3.2				0.18 ± 0.02	1.8 ± 0.18	64.8 ± 11.2
B	88.9 ± 3.7				0.16 ± 0.02	1.7 ± 0.11	61.19 ± 10.29
C	74.4 ± 3.2				0.14 ± 0.01	1.4 ± 0.05	10.69 ± 6.41
A vs. B	NS				NS	NS	NS
A vs. C	NS				NS	$P < 0.5$	$P < 0.001$
B vs. C	$P < 0.01$				NS	$P < 0.025$	$P < 0.001$
Bone							
A	180 ± 7.7	0.0020 ± 0.0001	0.128 ± 0.000			3.46 ± 0.23	
B	211 ± 5.4	0.0026 ± 0.0001	0.068 ± 0.006	0.82 ± 0.04		4.69 ± 0.16	
C	139 ± 9.6	0.0009 ± 0.0001	0.078 ± 0.009	0.76 ± 0.04		2.69 ± 0.14	
A vs. B	$P < 0.01$	$P < 0.001$	$P < 0.001$			$P < 0.001$	
A vs. C	$P < 0.01$	$P < 0.001$	$P < 0.001$			$P < 0.025$	
B vs. C	$P < 0.001$	$P < 0.001$	NS	NS		$P < 0.001$	
Thymus							
A	83.7 ± 1.9		0.079 ± 0.008			6.2 ± 0.54	
B	98.8 ± 3.5		0.080 ± 0.006	4.41 ± 0.34		5.7 ± 0.62	
C	81.1 ± 2.2		0.077 ± 0.005	6.78 ± 0.52		3.5 ± 0.25	
A vs. B	$P < 0.005$		NS			NS	
A vs. C	NS		NS			$P < 0.001$	
B vs. C	$P < 0.005$		NS	NS		$P < 0.001$	

[a]From Prasad and Oberleas (1971). Values are means ± S.E. (NS) Not significant ($P > 0.05$).
[b](A) Ad-libitum-fed controls; (b) pair-fed controls; (c) zinc-deficient rats.
[c](ADH) Alcohol dehydrogenase; (LDH) lactic dehydrogenase; (ICDH) isocitric dehydrogenase; (SDH) succinic dehydrogenase; (CPD) carboxypeptidase.
[d]Comparison of means.

turn controlled by the tissue levels of available zinc. Pancreatic carboxypeptidase A, alkaline phosphatase, and thymidine kinase are enzymes that reduce their activity before food intake and growth are affected or even before lesions appear. Though no causal connection between the reduced activities and the deficiency symptoms has yet been demonstrated one can at least draw inferences regarding the state of supply and the zinc requirement of man and animal from the changes in the enzyme activities (Kirchgessner and Roth, 1975a,b).

TOTAL PROTEIN IN ZINC DEFICIENCY

Several investigators (Prasad *et al.,* 1971; Macapinlac *et al.,* 1968; Sandstead *et al.,* 1971a) reported that the total protein content of various tissues of zinc-deficient rats was lowered in comparison with that in the tissues of zinc-supplemented pair-fed animals. Somers and Underwood (1969a) demonstrated that zinc-deficient rat testes contain a higher level of nonprotein nitrogen. In lambs, the retention of dietary amino acids was reduced as indicated by an increased urinary excretion of nitrogen and sulfur in comparison with that of pair-fed control animals. Biochemical changes in protein metabolism are also indicated by abnormalities in the protein pattern of plasma and serum (Fox and Harrison, 1965; Miller, E. R., *et al.,* 1968; Tao and Hurley, 1971). On the basis of their data, Macapinlac *et al.* (1968) and Somers and Underwood (1969a) suggested that zinc deficiency stimulates protein catabolism. Other reports, however, indicated that protein synthesis is impaired (Theuer and Hoekstra, 1966; Mills *et al.,* 1967). More recent investigations show that zinc deficiency induces changes in nucleic acid metabolism that may limit protein biosynthesis, growth, and tissue regeneration.

CHANGES IN NUCLEIC ACID METABOLISM

It was shown some time ago that zinc deficiency may affect the RNA and DNA metabolism of microorganisms and plants and thus be responsible for impaired protein synthesis (Schneider and Price, 1962; Wacker, 1962; Wegener and Romano, 1963, 1964; Kessler and Monselise, 1959). This was recently demonstrated to be true for animals also.

The biochemical changes brought about by zinc deficiency in animals may be so extensive that they are indicated by gross alterations in the cellular composition of certain tissues. Thus, the testes and connective tissue of zinc-deficient rats were found to contain significantly less RNA and DNA than those of pair-fed and ad-libitum-fed control animals (Somers and Underwood, 1969a; Fernandez-Madrid *et al.,* 1973; Macapinlac *et al.,* 1968). In rapidly regenerating connective tissue, RNA was affected more than DNA, as indicated by a significantly lower RNA/DNA ratio (Fernandez-Madrid *et al.,* 1973). Similarly, lower RNA/DNA ratios were observed in the liver, kidneys, and pancreas of zinc-deficient young pigs in comparison with pair-fed control animals, while the DNA content per unit weight of tissue remained largely unaltered (Prasad *et al.,* 1971) (see Table VIII). In the thymus of the young pig, however, the DNA content seems to be consistently depressed (Ku *et al.,* 1970).

Recent studies provide evidence that such changes in tissue levels of RNA and DNA of zinc-deficient animals may be the result of both increased catabolism and impaired biosynthesis of these polynucleotides. As shown in Table IX, increased activities of ribonuclease were found in several tissues of the zinc-deficient rat (Somers and Underwood, 1969a; Prasad and Oberleas, 1973). Zinc at a concentration of 10^{-4} M was previously shown to inhibit the activity of yeast ribonuclease completely (Ohtaka *et al.,* 1963). Thus, an enhanced ribonuclease activity may explain the lower RNA levels and RNA/DNA ratios observed in certain zinc-deficient animals tissues (Table IV). Although this response may also account, at least in part, for the impaired protein synthesis and growth retardation, which are common manifestations of zinc deficiency, it is not an early and sensitive effect (Prasad and Oberleas, 1973). Deoxyribonuclease activity assayed in the testes, kidney, bone, and thymus of zinc-deficient rats was comparable to that of the pair-fed control animals (Prasad and Oberleas, 1973) (Table IX).

In sickle cell disease patients (an example of a conditioned deficiency of zinc), plasma RNase activity was increased (Prasad *et al.,* 1975a). This observation suggests that measurement of plasma RNase activity may be a helpful diagnostic test for zinc deficiency in man.

Several investigators have studied the effects of zinc deficiency on the biosynthesis of RNA and DNA. Although some investigators failed to find differences in the *in vivo* incorporation of precursors into the polynucleotides of the testes and brain of zinc-deficient and restricted-fed zinc-supplemented rats (Macapinlac *et al.,* 1968; O'Neal *et al.,* 1970), there is sufficient evidence to implicate essential functions for zinc in both RNA and DNA synthesis.

Livers from zinc-deficient rats incorporated less phosphorus-32 into the nucleotides of RNA and DNA than did livers from pair-fed control animals (Williams *et al.,* 1965). Zinc injected intraperitoneally into partially hepatectomized rats stimulated the incorporation of labeled orotic acid into rapidly synthesized nuclear RNA (Weser *et al.,* 1969a,b). Zinc was found to be necessary for RNA and DNA synthesis in monolayer animal cell cultures (Rubin, 1972; Rubin and Koide, 1973).

There are numerous studies showing that zinc deficiency in animals impairs the incorporation of labeled thymidine into DNA (Dreosti *et al.,*

Table VIII. Zinc, DNA, RNA, and Protein Content and Activities of Various Enzymes in Tissues of Pair-Fed Controls and Zinc-Deficient Animals[a]

Tissue[c]	Zinc (μg/g dry wt)	DNA (μg/mg wet wt)	RNA (μg/μg DNA)	Protein (mg/mg DNA)	ADH[b]			Activity of enzymes (ΔOD/min/mg DNA)[b]				AP (U/mg DNA)[b]	CPD (μg/μg DNA)[b]		
						Change from initial (%)								Change from initial (%)	
					Initial	After addition of Zn[d]	After addition of EDTA[e]	LDH	ALD	SDH	ICDH		Initial	After addition of Zn[d]	After addition of EDTA[e]
Liver															
A	150.8 ± 12	4.2 ± 0.42	3.5 ± 0.34	40 ± 2.9	6.4 ± 0.69	89 ± 2	79 ± 4	46 ± 4	5.7 + 0.7	—	—	—	—	—	—
B	96.1 ± 8	5.1 + 0.3	2.5 ± 0.18	35 ± 1.9	3.6 ± 0.39	95 ± 3	77 ± 1	50 ± 4	3.0 ± 0.3	—	—	—	—	—	—
p^f	< 0.005	NS	< 0.05	NS	<0.005	—	—	NS	< 0.005	--	—	—	—	—	—
Kidney															
A	97.8 ± 2.6	3.7 ± 0.16	1.4 ± 0.06	23.4 ± 0.8	0.162 ± 0.009	91 ± 4	NA	—	2.54 ± 0.11	1.6 ± 0.17	6.9 ± 0.72	154.8 ± 16.4	—	—	
B	87.0 ± 2.8	3.9 ± 0.20	1.1 ± 0.05	21.2 ± 1.0	0.123 ± 0.008	96 ± 8	NA	—	1.86 ± 0.09	1.7 ± 0.19	7.2 ± 0.19	80.2 ± 9.5	—	—	—
p^f	< 0.025	NS	< 0.005	< 0.05	< 0.025	—	—	—	< 0.001	NS	NS	< 0.005	—	—	—
Bone															
A	98.5 ± 2.08	0.53 ± 0.07	3.04 ± 0.26	57.5 ± 5	2.30 ± 0.35	60 ± 10	NA	81 ± 10	21 ± 3.4	—	—	2640 ± 420	—	—	—
B	48.1 ± 2.74	0.83 ± 0.13	1.81 ± 0.22	36.8 ± 5	0.64 ± 0.07	50 ± 24	NA	44 ± 7	12 ± 2.5	—	—	480 ± 120	—	—	—
p^f	< 0.001	< 0.1 > 0.05	< 0.005	< 0.025	< 0.001	—	—	< 0.025	< 0.1 > 0.05	—	—	< 0.001	—	—	—
Pancreas															
A	133.3 ± 6	4.7 ± 0.28	5.0 ± 0.15	25 ± 1.8	—	—	—	14 ± 1.6	—	—	—	—	2.8 ± 0.1	82 ± 7	40 ± 16
B	96.8 ± 4	4.0 ± 0.30	4.1 ± 0.1	22 ± 2.2	—	—	—	14 ± 1.0	—	—	—	—	1.3 ± 0.2	70 ± 12	35 ± 15
p^f	< 0.001	< 0.2 > 0.1	< 0.05	NS	—	—	—	NS	—	—	—	—	< 0.001	—	—

[a]From Prasad *et al.* (1971). Values are means ± S.E. (NS) Not significant; (NA) no activity.
[b](ADH) Alcohol dehydrogenase; (ALD) adolase; (SDH) succinic dehydrogenase; (CPD) carboxypeptidase; (LDH) lactic dehydrogenase; (ICDH) isocitric dehydrogenase; (AP) alkaline phosphatase.
[c](A) Pair-fed controls; (B) zinc-deficient animals.
[d]Final concentration of Zn: liver, 8×10^{-5} M; kidney, 3.3×10^{-5} M; bone, 1.7×10^{-5} M; pancreas, 1.8×10^{-5} M.
[e]Final concentration of EDTA: liver, 6.7×10^{-3} M; kidney, 3.3×10^{-3} M; bone, 6.7×10^{-3} M; pancreas, 7.3×10^{-3} M.
[f]Comparison of means.

Table IX. Effect of Zinc Deficiency on Activity of Enzmes Involved in Nucleic Acid Metabolism of Animals

Enzyme	Species	Tissue	Enzyme activity[a]	Reference
Ribonuclease (acid)	Rat	Testis	+	Somers and Underwood (1969a)
Ribonuclease (acid)	Rat	Testis, kidney, bone	+	Prasad and Oberleas (1973)
Ribonuclease (alkaline)	Rat	Testis, kidney, thymus	+	Prasad and Oberleas (1973)
Deoxyribonuclease (acid and alkaline)	Rat	Testis, kidney, thymus, bone	0	Prasad and Oberleas (1973)
RNA polymerase	Rat	Liver nuclei	−	Sandstead *et al.* (1971a), Terhune and Sandstead (1972)
DNA polymerase	Rabbit	Kidney cortex (cell cultures)	−	Lieberman *et al.* (1963)
Thymidine kinase	Rabbit	Kidney cortex (cell cultures)	−	Lieberman *et al.* (1963)
	Rat	Connective tissue	−	Prasad and Oberleas (1974)

[a](+) Increased; (0) unchanged; (−) decreased.

1972; Fernandez-Madrid *et al.*, 1973; Grey and Dreosti, 1972; Hsu, T. H. S., and Hsu, 1972; Prasad and Oberleas, 1974; Sandstead and Rinaldi, 1969; Sandstead *et al.*, 1972; Stephan and Hsu, 1973; Swenerton *et al.*, 1969; Weser *et al.*, 1969a; Williams and Chesters, 1970a,b). This effect was detected within a few days after the feeding of the zinc-deficient diet was begun (Dreosti *et al.*, 1972; Grey and Dreosti, 1972; Prasad and Oberleas, 1974). Williams and Chesters (1970a,b) observed a progressive fall in thymidine incorporation into DNA of liver, kidney, and spleen within 5 days after a zinc-deficient diet was fed to rats. Thus, dietary zinc deficiency may result in an immediate impairment of DNA biosynthesis. Prasad and Oberleas (1974) provided evidence that decreased activity of thymidine kinase may be responsible for this early reduction in DNA synthesis, and may ultimately relate to growth retardation (Tables X–XII). The activity of thymidine kinase, an enzyme essential for DNA synthesis, was reduced in rapidly regenerating connective tissue of zinc-deficient rats compared to pair-fed controls as early as 6 days after the animals were placed on the dietary treatment. These results were recently confirmed by Dreosti and Hurley (1975). The activity of thymidine kinase in 12-day fetuses taken from females exposed to dietary zinc deficiency during pregnancy was significantly lower than in ad-libitum- and restricted-fed controls. The

Table X. Thymidine Kinase Activity in Regenerating Tissue (nmol TMP formed/hr per mg protein)[a]

Expt.	Deficient	Pair-fed	Ad-libitum
6-Day[b]	1.04 ± 0.14 (12)	3.57 ± 0.36 (13)	3.37 ± 0.36 (12)
13-Day[b]	0.58 ± 0.02 (6)	2.40 ± 0.59 (5)	1.65 ± 0.12 (5)
17-Day	None (5)	2.70 ± 0.6 (5)	2.68 ± 0.7 (5)

[a]From Prasad and Oberleas (1974). Values are means ± S.E.
[b]6-Day: Deficient vs. either control, $p < +0.001$; 13-Day: Deficient vs. either control, $p < +0.025$.

activity of the enzyme was not restored by *in vitro* addition of zinc, whereas addition of copper severely affected the enzyme activity adversely (Dreosti and Hurley, 1975).

As summarized in Table IX, the activities of other enzymes involved in polynucleotide synthesis are also affected by zinc deficiency. In liver nuclei from suckling rats nursed by dams on a zinc-deficient diet, the DNA-dependent RNA polymerase activity increased very little from birth to day 10 of life and then started to fall, while in pups nursed by pair-fed dams, the activity of this enzyme was not suppressed (Terhune and Sandstead, 1972).

In liver nuclei of rats that had been maintained on normal diets, zinc was found to increase the RNA polymerase activity *in vivo* (Weser *et al.*, 1969b). The DNA-dependent RNA polymerase from *E. coli* was shown to be a zinc metalloenzyme (Scrutton *et al.*, 1971). According to the studies by Slater *et al.* (1971) and Springgate *et al.* (1973), zinc is also an essential constituent for the DNA polymerase of *E. coli*, sea urchins, and T^4-bacteriophages. Whether these observations are also true for mammalian and avian species needs to be determined. Lieberman *et al.* (1963) demonstrated that the activity of DNA polymerase of kidney cortex cells cultured from the rabbit did not increase when zinc was depleted by adding ethylene diaminetetraacetic acid (EDTA) to the medium. The inhibition of DNA synthesis in animal cells effected by EDTA can be reversed by the addition of zinc (Rubin, 1972; Lieberman *et al.*, 1963).

Table XI. [^{14}C]Thymidine Incorporation into DNA (DPM/mg DNA): 6-Day Experiment[a]

Expt.	Deficient	Pair-fed	t^b
I	18.0 ± 5.7 × 10^3 (4)	136.2 ± 15.2 × 10^3 (4)	7.24+
II	14.4 ± 2.9 × 10^3 (6)	54.7 ± 7.5 × 10^3 (5)	4.99+

[a]From Prasad and Oberleas (1974). Values are means ± S.E.
[b]$p < 0.001$.

Table XII. Gain in Body Weight of Rats, Sponge Connective Tissue Weight, and Concentration of DNA, RNA, Protein, and Zinc in Sponge Connective Tissue in 6-Day Experiments[a]

Rats	Total gain in body wt (g)	SCT dry wt (mg)	DNA (μg/mg T)	RNA (μg/mg T)	Protein (mg/mg T)	Zn (μg/mg T)
Zn-deficient	18 ± 1.6 (24)	117.8 ± 10.6 (16)	6.2 ± 0.39 (12)	11.3 ± 0.39 (12)	0.54 ± 0.03 (12)	0.10 ± 0.008 (12)
Pair-fed (PF) controls	14 ± 1.2 (24)	153.3 ± 16.2 (15)	7.54 ± 0.37 (12)	13.4 ± 1.0 (12)	0.56 ± 0.02 (12)	0.14 ± 0.007 (12)
Ad-libitum-fed (ALF) Controls	53 ± 2.0 (24)	176.5 ± 17.7 (15)	6.6 ± 0.26 (12)	14.6 ± 1.5 (12)	0.52 ± 0.03 (12)	0.12 ± 0.19 (12)
p Values						
Zn-Def. vs. PF	0.05	NS	0.025	NS	NS	0.005
Zn-Def. vs. ALF	0.001	0.01	NS	NS	NS	NS
PF vs. ALF	0.001	NS	NS	NS	NS	NS

[a]From Prasad and Oberleas (1974). (SCT) Sponge connective tissue; (T) tissue. Values are means ± S.E.; the numbers in parentheses are the numbers of rats. (NS) Not significant.

POLYNUCLEOTIDE CONFORMATION

Although zinc appears to have primarily an enzymatic effect on the regulation of the biosynthesis and catabolic rate of RNA and DNA, one cannot rule out the possibility that zinc is also associated more directly with the nucleic acids. Zinc may play a role in the maintenance of polynucleotide conformation (Wacker and Vallee, 1959; Tal, 1969). Sandstead *et al.* (1971a,b) observed abnormal polysome profiles in the livers of zinc-deficient rats and mice. Acute administration of zinc appeared to stimulate polysome formation both *in vivo* and *in vitro* (Sandstead et al., 1971a,b). This finding is supported by the data of Fernandez-Madrid *et al.* (1973), who noted a decrease in the polyribosome content of zinc-deficient connective tissue from rats and a concomitant increase in inactive monosomes. Weser *et al.* (1970), using normal rats, demonstrated an enhanced formation of high-molecular-weight or ribosomal RNA, or both, that was isolated 10 hr after the intraperitoneal injection of labeled zinc.

METALLOTHIONEIN

Metallothionein (MT) is a unique protein first identified in equine renal cortex (Margoshes and Vallee, 1957) and later in humans (Pulido *et al.,* 1966). It is a low-molecular-weight protein, has a high sulfhydryl and metal content, and lacks aromatic amino acids. Liver MT contains predominantly zinc, whereas renal MT has more cadmium. Although cadmium, copper, mercury, silver, and zinc have been shown to be associated with this low-molecular-weight cytoplasmic protein, the basic function of this protein is probably linked to the metabolism of dietary zinc.

MT is believed to play a role as a storage protein of zinc. Parenteral administration of zinc increases the synthesis of MT, and this effect is inhibited by prior injection of actinomycin D, an inhibitor of protein synthesis (Richards and Cousins, 1975a,b). This is in contrast to ferritin synthesis, which is not blocked by actinomycin D if administered prior to iron injection. It is believed that part of the control of zinc-thionein synthesis by zinc takes place at the transcriptional level. It is possible that zinc induces zinc-thionein synthesis by interacting, either directly or indirectly, with the cell nucleus to stimulate thionein mRNA synthesis. Recent studies indicate that the mechanism of control of zinc-thionein synthesis by zinc appears to involve changes in the amounts of a short-lived, poly-(A)-containing RNA the translation of which can be derepressed by additional exposure to zinc (Squibb *et al.,* 1977). Thus, these studies and others support the concept that MT synthesis is regulated by changes in the pool of translatable thionein mRNA (Squibb and Cousins, 1977).

It is believed that one of the biological roles of MT is involved in accumulation of excessive zinc rather than in storage of this metal for later utilization (Chen *et al.*, 1977). Zinc-thionein also functions to sequester zinc in intestinal mucosal cells, thereby decreasing dietary zinc absorption (Richards and Cousins, 1976).

ZINC AND HORMONES

Since the discovery by Scott (1934) that crystalline insulin contains considerable amounts of zinc ($\approx 0.5\%$), many studies have investigated the extent to which zinc nutrition of an animal influences the zinc content of the pancreas and its production, storage, and secretion of insulin. Inactive proinsulin is synthesized by the β-cells of the islets of Langerhans of the pancreas. By proteolytic cleavage of the connecting peptide, insulin is released.

One of the best known functions of insulin is to lower the blood glucose level. As early as 1937, Hove *et al.* (1937) published their results on the glucose tolerance of zinc-deficient rats. Only minor differences were noted between zinc-deficient and ad-libitum-fed control rats in the glucose tolerance curves after oral glucose doses. Hendricks and Mahoney (1972) found no difference between zinc-deficient and zinc-supplemented rats in the ability to metabolize orally administered glucose. However, when glucose was injected intraperitoneally into rats fasted overnight after a long period of dietary treatment, the glucose tolerance of zinc-deficient animals was depressed in comparison with that of the pair-fed controls (Quarterman *et al.*, 1966). This finding was confirmed in studies by Boquist and Lernmark (1969) using Chinese hamsters, by Hendricks and Mahoney (1972), and by Huber and Gershoff (1973a,b), using rats.

Figure 10 shows glucose tolerance curves obtained by Roth and Kirchgessner (1975) in zinc-deficient, pair-fed, and ad-libitum-fed control rats. In these studies, rats that had been depleted by being fed a semisynthetic zinc-deficient casein diet (2 ppm zinc) for 34 days received an intramuscular injection of 80 mg glucose/100 mg body weight after they had been fasted for 12 hr. The zinc-depleted rats, which had the same initial plasma glucose concentration as the pair-fed and ad-libitum-fed control animals, had a significantly lower glucose tolerance. Since the pair-fed animals exhibited a glucose tolerance that was even better than that of the ad-libitum-fed controls, the lowered glucose tolerance of the zinc-deficient animals cannot be attributed to inanition (Fig. 10).

In contrast to these findings are the reports by Macapinlac *et al.* (1966) and Quarterman and Florence (1972), who were unable to demonstrate that zinc deficiency affects the tolerance to intraperitoneally injected glucose. Quarterman and Florence (1972) suggested that the reduced glucose tolerance of zinc-deficient rats was due to the different pattern of food intake.

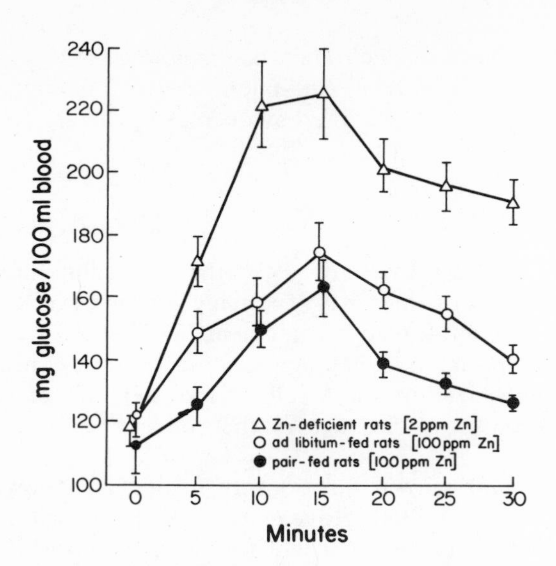

Fig. 10. Glucose tolerance curves of zinc-deficient rats in comparison to ad-libitum-fed and pair-fed control animals. The vertical bars represent the standard errors of the mean of 6 animals. From Roth and Kirchgessner (1975).

Zinc-deficient animals eat slowly and continuously throughout the day, while their meal-fed pair-mates consume their dietary allowance for the day in a rather short time. Thus, these authors consider the amount of food consumed on the day before the glucose tolerance test is made to be an important factor. The conflicting results obtained for the glucose tolerance after oral dosing on the one hand and after intraperitoneal or intravenous injection on the other may be explained by a greater stimulation of insulin secretion by glucose given orally (McIntyre *et al.*, 1965; Fasel *et al.*, 1970).

The reasons for the poorer glucose tolerance of zinc-deficient animals observed in several studies are not clear. Quarterman *et al.* (1966) demonstrated that zinc-deficient rats exhibit a reduced concentration of plasma insulin in comparison with pair-fed controls. They believe that the rate of insulin secretion in response to glucose stimulation is reduced in zinc deficiency. Furthermore, the zinc-depleted animals were less sensitive to soluble zinc-free insulin injected intraperitoneally, though there were no differences in the blood glucose levels. Huber and Gershoff (1973a,b) observed that although the serum of zinc-deficient rats contained less immunoreactive insulin than that of ad-libitum-fed control animals, there was no difference in comparison with the pair-fed controls. Total serum insulinlike activity measured by *in vitro* adipose tissue assay was significantly lower in the zinc-deficient groups than in the pair-fed and ad-libitum-fed control rats. These workers demonstrated *in vitro* that the pancreas from zinc-deficient rats incubated with glucose as stimulant released less immunoreactive insulin as well as insulinlike activity.

In another experiment, Quarterman and Florence (1972) found no difference in plasma insulin levels between zinc-deficient rats and their zinc-supplemented continuously fed or meal-fed pair-mates. Similarly, in four studies conducted by Roth and Kirchgessner (1975), the serum or plasma insulin levels were only once significantly different between the zinc-deficient and the pair-fed rats, though they were consistently lower than in the ad-libitum-fed controls. Even though there may be no difference in the insulin level, as determined by radioimmunoassay, it is possible that the physiological potency of the hormone is reduced by zinc deficiency. One must also distinguish between free active and bound inactive insulin in circulation. Zinc deficiency might affect these forms differently.

Boquist and Lernmark (1969) did not find reduced serum insulin concentration before or after the intravenous administration of glucose to zinc-deficient hamsters, although they observed lowered glucose tolerance. Since a similar reduction in glucose tolerance was found after pancreatectomy (Boquist, 1967), and after the administration of alloxan (Boquist, 1968), these workers believe that zinc deficiency causes a "prediabetic" condition. Furthermore, light- and electron-microscopic studies showed that the β-cells of the pancreas exhibit reduced granulation and thus possibly reduced insulin content. Engelbart and Kief (1970) found that acute stimulation of insulin secretion in rats also reduces the zinc content in the β-cells of the pancreas. Since it can be assumed that zinc participates in the synthesis and storage of insulin in the β-cells, it is plausible that the amount of insulin stored during zinc deficiency is lower. Hendricks and Mahoney (1972) postulated that the reduced glucose tolerance of zinc-deficient animals is caused by an increased rate of insulin degradation. This could also explain the increased insulin resistance of zinc-depleted rats observed by Quarterman *et al.* (1966). It is obvious that further research is needed to clarify the relationship between zinc deficiency and insulin.

GROWTH AND SEX HORMONES

Homan *et al.* (1954) demonstrated that the addition of zinc salts increases and prolongs the physiological potency of corticotropin preparations. In in *vitro* studies with human cell cultures, adrenal steroid hormones with glucocorticoid activity increased the uptake of Zn^{2+} (Cox and Ruckenstein, 1971). On the other hand, injections of gonadotropin and testosterone stimulated the growth of the male accessor sex organs of zinc-deficient rats, but did not prevent the tubular atrophy of the testes, which is considered to be typical for the zinc-deficient state (Millar *et al.*, 1960).

Treating zinc-deficient rats with bovine growth hormone did not result in any improvement in weight gains (Macapinlac *et al.*, 1966; Prasad *et al.*, 1969b). Similarly, Ku (1971) reported that growth hormone given to zinc-deficient pigs did not improve growth and food intake, and had no influence on the serum zinc level, the serum alkaline phosphatase activity, or the parakeratotic lesions. The administration of bovine growth hormone to zinc-deficient nonhypophysectomized rats in the studies by Prasad *et al.* (1969b) also failed to enhance growth, while the growth rates increased greatly after zinc supplementation. The growth rates of hypophysectomized rats, however, responded to both hormone and zinc supplementation irrespective of the zinc status. Here, the effects of the hormone and zinc were additive but independent of each other. Gombe *et al.* (1973) observed that the content of luteinizing hormone (LH) in pooled pituitaries of zinc-deficient female rats was not different from that of pair-fed and ad-libitum-fed control animals. The levels of LH and progesterone, however, were reduced in the plasma of not only the zinc-deficient but also the restricted-fed animals in comparison with that of the ad-libitum-fed controls. The lower plasma LH levels of zinc-deficient rats and their restricted-fed mates do not seem to be due to a lack of LH-releasing factor, since its level was comparable in all three groups.

Recently, the role of zinc in gonadal function was investigated in rats by Lei *et al.* (1976). The increase in LH, follicle-stimulating hormone (FSH), and testosterone was assayed following intravenous administration of synthetic LH-releasing hormone (LH-RH) to zinc-deficient and restricted-fed control rats. Body weight gain and the zinc content and weights of the testes were significantly lower in the zinc-deficient rats than in the controls. The serum LH and FSH responses to LH-RH administration were higher in the zinc-deficient rats, but serum testosterone response was lower than in the restricted-fed controls. These studies indicate a specific effect of zinc on testes and suggest that gonadal function in the zinc-deficient state is affected through some alteration of testicular steroidogenesis.

ZINC IN COLLAGEN METABOLISM

Since collagen is the main fibrous protein of the connective tissue and is largely responsible for the development of tensile strength in the healing wound, biochemical studies have concentrated on the question whether there is a specific effect of zinc deficiency on collagen synthesis, hydroxylation, conversion of procollagen to collagen, or some other aspect of its metabolism. Indeed, in a study of zinc deficiency in the rat, Fernandez-Madrid *et al.* (1973) found a significant reduction in total collagen in sponge connective tissue in comparison with pair-fed controls (Tables XII–XIV).

Table XIII. Final Body Weight of Rats, Connective Tissue Weight, and Content of Zinc, RNA, and DNA of Sponge Connective Tissue[a]

Expt.[b]	Final body weight (g)	SCT per rat (mg)	SCT weight/ sponge weight	Total SCT zinc per rat (μg)	SCT zinc (μg/mg T)	Total SCT DNA per rat (mg)	SCT RNA (μg/mg T)	Total SCT RNA per rat (mg)	SCT RNA (μg/mg T)	RNA/DNA
6-Day										
A	143 ± 3.0	180 ± 19	0.9 ± 0.13	8.2 ± 1.8	0.056 ± 0.009	2.533 ± 0.390	14.2 ± 1.95	3.833 ± 0.699	20.1 ± 2.7	1.4 ± 0.07
B	162 ± 2.0	263 ± 19	1.2 ± 0.16	18.5 ± 2.3	0.072 ± 0.009	2.681 ± 0.318	10.2 ± 1.08	5.569 ± 0.614	21.1 ± 1.7	2.1 ± 0.26
p Values										
A vs. B	< 0.001	< 0.025	NS	< 0.025	NS	NS	NS	NS	NS	< 0.05
10-Day										
A	110 ± 2	260.1 ± 10.7	0.5 ± 0.0489	34.5 ± 8.7	0.196 ± 0.04	2.34 ± 0.27	8.9 ± 0.89	1.93 ± 0.16	7.4 ± 0.62	0.87 ± 0.12
B	132 ± 5	479.1 ± 29.1	0.7 ± 0.051	57.3 ± 2.8	0.141 ± 0.02	4.62 ± 0.46	9.6 ± 0.79	6.33 ± 0.43	13.4 ± 0.54	1.42 ± 0.14
C	321 ± 7	601.3 ± 42.8	0.8 ± 0.032	92.8 ± 19.4	0.132 ± 0.03	6.30 ± 0.42	10.6 ± 0.80	9.24 ± 0.78	15.4 ± 0.55	1.47 ± 0.08
p Values										
A vs. B	< 0.005	< 0.001	< 0.025	< 0.05	NS	< 0.005	NS	< 0.001	< 0.001	< 0.025
A vs. C	< 0.001	< 0.001	< 0.001	< 0.05	NS	< 0.001	NS	< 0.001	< 0.001	< 0.005
B vs. C	< 0.001	< 0.05	NS	NS	NS	< 0.025	NS	< 0.01	< 0.01	NS

[a]From Fernandez-Madrid *et al.* (1973). (SCT) Sponge connective tissue; (T) tissue. Values are means ± S.E.; 8 animals per observation. (NS) Not significant.
[b](A) Zinc-deficient animals; (B) pair-fed controls; (C) ad-libitum-fed controls.

Table XIV. Protein and Collagen Content of Sponge Connective Tissue[a]

Expt.[b]	Total SCT protein per rat (mg)	SCT protein (mg/mg T)	Total SCT collagen per rat (mg)	Total SCT collagen (mg/mg T)	Collagen/protein	Percentage of total SCT collagen			
						0.15 M NaCl	1.0 M NaCl	0.5 M acetic acid	Insoluble
6-Day									
A	98.31 ± 14.62	0.54 ± 0.03	10.15 ± 1.62	0.056 ± 0.005	0.104 ± 0.007	1.44 ± 0.51	0.96 ± 0.05	41.3 ± 1.5	56.0 ± 1.27
B	195.1 ± 18.29	0.74 ± 0.04	21.53 ± 1.62	0.086 ± 0.008	0.114 ± 0.015	1.18 ± 0.11	0.63 ± 0.09	32.4 ± 1.5	74.6 ± 1.39
p Values									
A vs. B	< 0.01	< 0.01	< 0.001	< 0.01	NS	NS	< 0.025	< 0.001	< 0.001
10-Day									
A	188.6 ± 12.3	0.73 ± 0.04	27.6 ± 2.78	0.106 ± 0.008	0.148 ± 0.015	1.65 ± 0.29	1.19 ± 0.18	3.3 ± 0.59	93.9 ± 0.59
B	337.9 ± 39.4	0.70 ± 0.05	50.1 ± 5.73	0.104 ± 0.009	0.151 ± 0.017	1.89 ± 0.07	0.99 ± 0.09	2.67 ± 0.50	94.4 ± 0.54
C	425.2 ± 29.3	0.71 ± 0.03	43.9 ± 3.04	0.073 ± 0.003	0.104 ± 0.007	3.56 ± 0.23	3.14 ± 0.19	9.4 ± 0.84	83.8 ± 0.91
p Values									
A vs. B	< 0.025	NS	< 0.01	NS	NS	NS	NS	NS	NS
A vs. C	< 0.001	NS	< 0.005	< 0.01	< 0.05	< 0.001	< 0.001	<0.001	< 0.001
B vs. C	NS	NS	NS	< 0.01	< 0.05	< 0.001	< 0.001	< 0.001	< 0.001

[a]From Fernandez-Madrid *et al.* (1973). (SCT) Sponge connective tissue; (T) tissue. Values are means ± S.E.; 8 animals per observation. (NS) Not significant.
[b](A) Zinc-deficient animals; (B) pair-fed controls; (C) ad-libitum-fed controls.

In addition, there was a reduction in the total dry weight of the sponge connective tissue and of the noncollagenous protein content in the zinc-deficient tissue in comparison with the pair-fed controls. The RNA/DNA ratio was significantly lower in zinc-deficient connective tissue, and in more severe deficient states, there was also depletion of polyribosomes and a significant reduction of RNA in comparison with the connective tissue of pair-fed rats (Tables XII–XIV; Figs. 11 and 12).

These data indicate that the effect of zinc deficiency on collagen deposition was a generalized effect on protein synthesis and nucleic acid metabolism, rather than a specific effect on collagen synthesis. In fact, no differences were found with respect to level of hydroxylation, ultracentrifugation, chromatography in CM-cellulose columns, or disc-gel electrophoresis between highly purified collagen from zinc-deficient animals and pair-fed rats (Fig. 12).

Other studies have also attempted to answer the same questions. The work of J. M. Hsu *et al.* (1968) revealed that zinc deficiency drastically reduced the incorporation of labeled glycine, proline, and lysine into rat skin. This study showed that there were no marked changes in the uptake of these amino acids into liver, kidney, testes, or muscle protein. Since collagen is unusually rich in these amino acids, it was suggested that

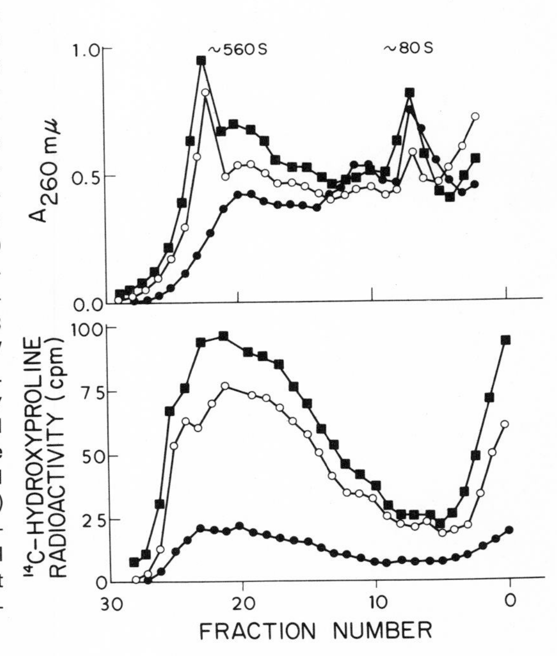

Fig. 11. Zone centrifugation through 15–60% linear sucrose gradients of polyvinyl sponge connective tissue polyribosomes. The capsules from polyvinyl sponges removed 10 days after inplantation from zinc-deficient, pair-fed, and ad-libitum-fed rats were incubated *in vitro* with [^{14}C]proline for 30 min, and the ribosomal suspensions were prepared. The suspensions were centrifuged for 3 hrs at 20,000 r.p.m. in the SW 25.1 rotor of the Spinco Model L ultracentrifuge. Absorbancy was monitored at 260 mμ, and total and [^{14}C]hydroxyproline radioactivity were determined in the individual fractions. (□—□) Ad-libitum-fed control animals; (○—○) pair-fed control animals; (●—●) Zn-deficient animals. From Fernandez-Madrid *et al.* (1973).

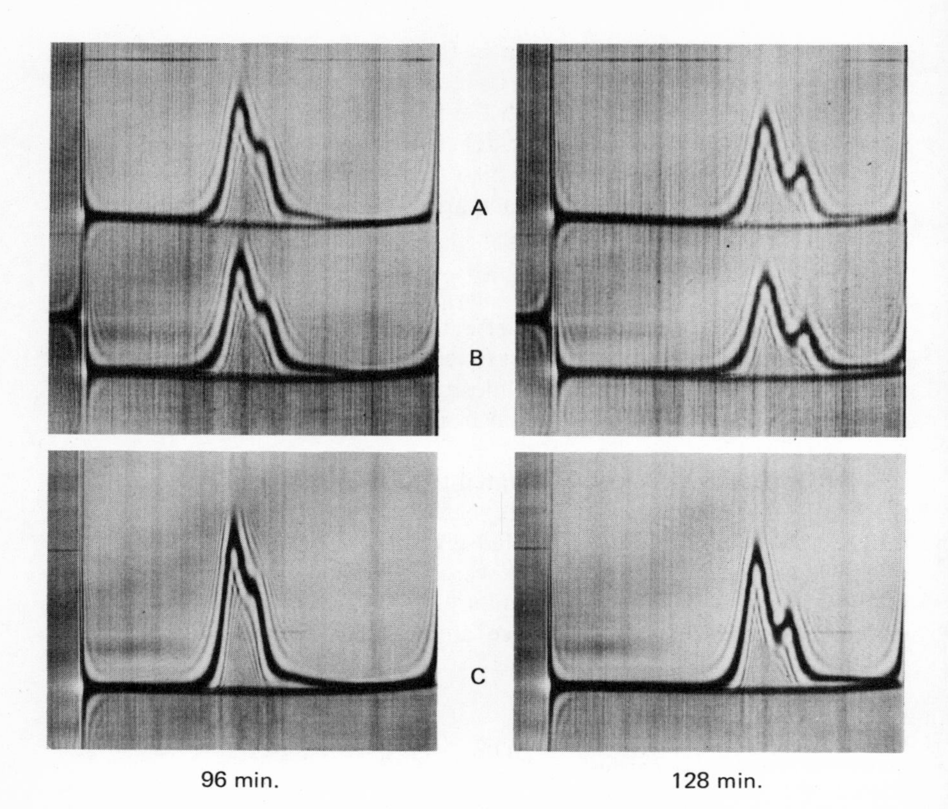

Fig. 12. Sedimentation patterns of denatured acid-extracted polyvinyl sponge connective tissue collagen, (A) Ad-libitum-fed control animals; (B) Zn-deficient animals; (C) pair-fed control animals. The samples were dissolved in 0.15 M sodium formate, pH 3.75, and incubated for 15 min at 40°C. The undissolved material was removed prior to ultracentrifugation by centrifuging at 2,000 r.p.m. for 15 min. Ultracentrifugation was done with a Spinco Model E equipped with an electronic speed control and an An-D rotor with double-sector cells, with plain and positive wedge windows. Centrifugation at 60,000 r.p.m. and 39°C was carried out for 128 min. Percentages of α- and β-chains were as follows: (A) 68.3 and 23.8; (B) 63.4 and 26.0; (C) 62.6 and 24.6. Higher aggregates in three samples were calculated to be as follows: (A) 7.9%; (B) 10.6%; (C) 12.9%. From Fernandez-Madrid *et al.* (1973).

perhaps zinc could be more important in the metabolism of skin collagen than in the metabolism of other proteins. McClain *et al.* (1973) tried to elucidate further the role of zinc in collagen metabolism. They found a decrease in the salt-soluble fraction obtained from zinc-deficient animals that was thought to be due to a reduction in protein synthesis. In support of that conclusion, they found a reduction in the incorporation of labeled glycine into α_1 and α_2 chains of salt-soluble rat-skin collagen. They did not find a significant reduction in the incorporation of labeled leucine into muscle polyribosomes, but there was an overall reduction of the polysome yield in the zinc-deficient animals. These data, in agreement with the work described above, suggested that total collagen is reduced in the zinc-deficient state as a part of a generalized impairment in protein synthesis. Elias and Chvapil (1973) explored the question whether zinc supplementation affects the rate of collagen synthesis and the extent of collagen deposition in skin wounds in normal rats. They found that the administration of zinc did not affect the mechanical properties of skin wound or total collagen content in the skin wound granulation tissue of normal rats. This lack of a stimulatory effect could be explained by assuming that normal rats were adequately supplied with the zinc required for connective tissue development, and therefore additional zinc supplementation was not necessary. Elias and Chvapil did find, however, a stimulation of collagen synthesis and an increase in the extent of collagen deposition when the same experiment was done on rats with carbon-tetrachloride-injured livers. Since experimental liver injury and various types of chronic illnesses are frequently accompanied by relative depletion of zinc (Vallee *et al.*, 1956, 1957; Serjeant *et al.*, 1970), these results are in agreement with the aforementioned reports of zinc stimulation of connective tissue development in the zinc-deficient state (Fernandez-Madrid *et al.*, 1973; McClain *et al.*, 1973).

Conflicting data were presented by Waters *et al.* (1971). These authors approached the question whether zinc might accelerate wound healing by promoting an increased production of collagen in *in vitro* studies of fibroblasts in tissue culture media. In this study, diploid human fetal fibroblasts derived from skin and muscle were incubated with the addition of 10^{-4}–10^{-8} M zinc sulfate to the experimental and control media. Newly established (low-density) rapidly growing cultures were employed to evaluate the effect of zinc on fibroblast proliferation, while confluent, stationary cultures were utilized to study the effect on collagen production. Basal levels of zinc in the experimental media were not reported. To determine the direct effect of zinc on the fibroblast, three parameters were evaluated: (1) cellular proliferation, measured by changes in total culture protein; (2) rate of collagen biosynthesis, measured by the rate of conversion of radioactively labeled proline into hydroxyproline; and (3) changes in culture collagen content, measured by total accumulation of hydroxyproline. The results showed that addition of zinc sulfate to low-density cultures in concentrations of 10^{-4}–10^{-8} M produced concentration-dependent cytotoxicity with inhibition of collagen biosynthesis, as well as of cellular proliferation. Similar addition of zinc sulfate at 10^{-4} M concentration to confluent (high-density) cultures apparently resulted in significant inhibition of collagen biosynthesis. The authors interpreted these data as indicating that zinc does not have direct acceleratory effect on either cellular proliferation or collagen biosynthesis in human fibroblasts *in vitro*. This interpretation of the data is not in agreement with several other studies suggesting the direct participation of zinc in the process of wound healing (Fernandez-Madrid *et al.*, 1973; McClain *et al.*, 1973; Elias and Chvapil, 1973). Unfortunately, the basal levels of zinc in the fibroblast cultures were not reported (Waters *et al.*, 1971), and since zinc is a notorious contaminant, it is possible that their experimental culture media already had an adequate supply of zinc. Cytotoxicity was probably seen, rather than lack of a stimulatory effect. The possibility that the reduction in the extent of collagen deposition found in the zinc-deficient state may be in part related to an increased degradation has not been studied and cannot be ruled out.

McClain *et al.* (1973) presented data interpreted as indicating a fundamental role for zinc in the process of cross-linking of collagen. Purified salt-soluble collagen from zinc-supplemented and zinc-deficient animals was subjected to disc-gel electrophoresis. It was reported that the β-components from zinc-deficient animals were increased in comparison with those from zinc-supplemented animals.

However, observation of the densitometric tracings of the disc-gel patterns showed a minimal reduction of α_1 and practically identical content of α_2 chains in the zinc-deficient collagen in comparison with that of zinc-supplemented animals. Also, the aldehyde content of the salt-soluble collagen from zinc-deficient animals was reported to be almost twice as high as that from the zinc-supplemented animals. These animals were interpreted as indicating a greater degree of intramolecular cross-linking in the salt-soluble fraction of zinc-deficient skin collagen. It was speculated that the antagonistic relationship between zinc and copper could be the basis of the postulated cross-linking abnormality. Since copper is known to be required for lysyl oxidase, the enzyme that oxidatively deaminates the precursor of the collagen intramolecular cross-link, an increased activity of this enzyme in the zinc-deficient state might possibly enhance formation of a covalent intramolecular cross-link (McClain *et al.*, 1973). Indeed, antagonism between copper and zinc has been reported (Van Campen, 1966; Magee and Matrone, 1960; Hill *et al.*, 1963). In general, zinc administration decreased the level of copper in the serum and in tissues. Also, the addition of zinc *in vitro* has been shown to interfere with the activity of lysyl oxidase (Chvapil and Walsh, 1972). It is also known that in the zinc-deficient state, the tissue concentration of copper increases (Prasad *et al.*, 1968). There is, however, no information in the literature about the activity of copper-dependent enzymes in the zinc-deficient state. In addition, accurate quantification of intramolecular cross-links cannot be reliably accomplished by the determination of the proportion of α to β chains or the aldehyde content of purified collagen. These data are of doubtful significance and cannot be interpreted as an expression of a cross-linking abnormality.

In the same study (McClain *et al.*, 1973), it was reported that the acid-soluble collagen pool from zinc-deficient animals was increased by nearly 20%, though the α/β ratios did not vary markedly between the supplemented and deficient animals. The aldehyde content of the acid-soluble collagen was not reported, but that of the insoluble skin collagen was found to be 47% lower in the zinc-deficient than in the zinc-supplemented animals. The authors interpreted these data as evidence of an inhibition of the intermolecular cross-linking mechanism induced by the deficiency of zinc. They suggested from their studies that zinc has a fundamental role in the process of cross-linking of collagen. Since solubility studies are very crude indicators of cross-linking abnormalities, and no differences were found in the acid-soluble collagen by ultracentrifugation, disc-gel electrophoresis, or CM-cellulose chromatography (Fernadez-Madrid *et al.*, 1973; McClain *et al.*, 1973), it was concluded that these data do not contribute evidence for a cross-linking defect.

Early studies of developing sponge connective tissue have shown that a spurt of DNA synthesis precedes the increase in the deposition of collagen (Kulonen, 1970). Indeed, at the time at which fibroblast proliferation as expressed by DNA synthesis is very active, there is very little accumulation of fibrous collagen in the sponge (Woessner and Boucek, 1961). It seems that this initial period of cell division preceding collagen deposition is a common denominator of developing connective tissue in most circumstances (Kulonen, 1970). It is therefore clear that any interference with the synthesis of DNA and fibroblast proliferation will profoundly influence the overall deposition of fibrous collagen in the developing connective tissue. Many studies have suggested that DNA synthesis may be impaired in zinc deficiency. Whether one enzyme is finally singled out as responsible for the inhibition of DNA synthesis or whether this effect is due to a constellation of enzymatic defects dependent on zinc remains to be established. It is obvious, however, that fibroblast proliferation is impaired, and that this defect is a major contributing factor to the abnormalities in wound healing found in the zinc-deficient state.

ZINC AND CYSTINE METABOLISM

A specific role of zinc in cystine metabolism has been observed. The increased expired $^{14}CO_2$ after injection of DL-cystine-1-^{14}C in zinc-deficient rats may be linked to a defect in the utilization of this amino acid for protein synthesis. This possibility is supported by the observation that there is a 30% reduction in the incorporation of cystine-1-^{14}C into the liver and kidney proteins of zinc-deficient rats (Hsu, J. M., *et al.*, 1970).

Zinc deficiency is also associated with enhanced urinary total ^{35}sulfur, which is comprised of inorganic sulfate-^{35}S, ethereal sulfate-^{35}S, and neutral sulfate-^{35}S after cystine-^{35}S injection. This finding is similar to the findings reported by Somers and Underwood (1969b), who observed that an increased urinary excretion of sulfur occurred in zinc-deficient ram lambs. The mechanism for these observations is not understood at present. A possible explanation is that zinc may be involved in the utilization of inorganic sulfate. The normal activity of liver ATP sulfurylase in zinc-deficient rats fails to support this view. Nevertheless, the effect of zinc deficiency on the reactions leading to incorporation of active sulfate into organic molecules requires further experimentation (Hsu, J. M., 1976).

ZINC AND THE CELL MEMBRANE

The first indication that zinc modifies the cell plasma membrane was derived from the work of cytologists who used zinc to isolate intact cell membranes (Warren *et al.*, 1966). Although no direct evidence was presented on the mechanism of the zinc effect, it was assumed that zinc interacts with thiol groups at the membrane with the formation of stable mercaptides. The same mechanism was implicated in the stabilizing effect of zinc on neurotubules from the rat brain (Nikolson and Veldstra, 1972). In this case, only the zinc and cadmium helped to isolate intact tubules, and zinc treatment produced tubules similar in structure to the ultrastructure of well-preserved neurotubules.

Peritoneal macrophages isolated from mice injected intraperitoneally with thioglycolate and treated at the same time intraperitoneally or intramuscularly with zinc (0.25 or 0.5 mg $ZnCl_2$/mouse per day) showed a significantly higher viability index than macrophages from control animals (Karl *et al.*, 1973). When zinc-treated macrophages were exposed to silica particles (1 μm) for 30 min, the cytotoxic effect of silica was significantly diminished. The reason for the decreased cytotoxicity of zinc-treated macrophages was that these cells displayed much lower phagocytosis of *Staphylococcus albus* than control macrophages. Similar results were obtained using young rats and young guinea pigs first fed, for a certain time, diets with various zinc contents amounting to 0.5, 40, and 2000 ppm zinc (Chvapil *et al.*, 1976). Mineral oil was then injected intraperitoneally for 4 consecutive days, and finally the peritoneal cavity was lavaged to harvest macropages. A striking difference in the migration capacity of macrophages isolated from animals fed the three different zinc diets was noted. Macrophages from guinea pigs fed a zinc-deficient diet (0.5 ppm zinc) displayed maximum mobility. They migrated faster than those from animals fed 40- or 2000-ppm zinc diets. Macrophages from animals fed a high-zinc diet in several experiments did not migrate at all. Still, these cells showed significantly higher viability than cells from either one of the two lower zinc groups. On the basis of these results, it was concluded that a high-zinc diet functionally immobilized macrophages.

Morphological evaluation of these cells supported this view. High-power light microscopy of macrophages from control guinea pigs fed 40 ppm zinc showed most of the cells with extrusions, long-reaching pseudopodia, or ruffling plasma membrane. In other words, these cells displayed active plasma membranes. Unlike these cells, macrophages from high-zinc-treated animals were round-shaped, only a few showed minimal ruffling, and long extrusions or pseudopodia were completely absent. Scanning microscopy provided further evidence that a high-zinc diet inactivated the mobility of plasma membranes of peritoneal macrophages (Chvapil *et al.*, 1976).

There is some evidence that zinc inhibits the activity of various forms of ATPase in alveolar macrophages (Mustafa *et al.*, 1970, 1971) or in brain microsomes (Donaldson *et al.*, 1971; Robinson, 1972). Mustafa *et al.* (1970) presented evidence that the ATPase system is membrane-bound and located predominantly in pulmonary alveolar macrophage cellular surface membranes, and others have shown that 0.5 mM zinc completely inhibits the activity of ATPase in activated macrophages (Chvapil *et al.*, 1976). The activity of macrophages has been linked to the activity of NADPH oxidase (Romeo *et al.*, 1971) as a part of the phagocytosis process. An excellent review by Sbarra *et al.* (1972) indicates that the enzymatic mechanism responsible for the stimulated metabolic activities that accompany phagocytosis appears to be directly involved with the oxidation of NADPH by its oxidase. Increased NADPH oxidase activity not only supplies pyridine nucleotides, but also forms H_2O_2 needed for the bacteriocidal activity of the phagocytes.

In a study of the effect of zinc on NADPH oxidase activity in liver microsomes and in the alveolar macrophages, it was found that zinc competitively inhibits NADPH oxidase (Chvapil *et al.*, 1976). In the liver microsomes, approximately 10 μM zinc inhibits the enzyme by 50% in whole homogenate of alveolar macrophages; the concentration of zinc required for 50% enzyme inhibition was higher, amounting to 120 μM. Inhibition of NADPH oxidation by low concentrations of zinc indicates that zinc may be in control of NADPH oxidase activity even *in vivo*. It must be pointed out, however, that these levels of zinc are much higher than normally encountered *in vivo* in man, and that, this being the case, the physiological significance of these observations remains unclear.

It is becoming evident that zinc in small quantities is present in various cell membranes. Most of the membrane-bound zinc is linked to a distinct macromolecule constituent lipoprotein fraction (Chvapil *et al.*, 1976). In this fraction, zinc is bound to the lipid moiety, whereas in the whole membrane, the distribution of zinc between the protein and lipid phase is approximately 45% to 55%. The most interesting observation, however, is that inducing lipoperoxidative damage to polyunsaturated fatty acid components of the erythrocyte membrane by ultraviolet irradiation or by introducing free radicals into the system does not cause the release of zinc from the ghost pellet into the medium, although some proteins and lipids are released into the incubation medium.

The effect of zinc and other metals on aggregation of platelets and release of [H^3]serotonin activated either by collagen or epinephrine was studied by Chvapil *et al.* (1976). The following observations were made: (1) Aggregation of platelets in dog and human platelet rich plasma (PRP) induced by either collagen or epinephrine is inhibited by zinc within a narrow range of concentrations, between 5 and 15 μM zinc. (2) Release of [H^3]serotonin from dog platelets is also significantly inhibited by zinc within the same concentration range. (3) The inhibitory effect of zinc on the release reaction depends on the presence of plasma proteins, mainly fibrinogen. Even at the lowest doses, zinc added to a suspension of washed platelets in Hank's medium enhanced the release of [H^3]serotonin, and the addition of fibrinogen restored the inhibitory effect of zinc. These observations are interesting, but their importance to human physiology must await further investigation.

In a recent publication, Sacchetti *et al.* (1974) studied the effect of manganese ion, which was shown to displace Ca^{2+}, thus modifying functions of the platelet membrane. Whether or not the role of zinc is similar to that of manganese remains to be established.

LYMPHOCYTES AND ZINC

Several authors (Ruhl *et al.,* 1971; Chesters, 1972; Alford, 1970; Berger and Skinner, 1974) have studied the role of zinc in lymphocyte function, and their results could be summarized as follows: administration of zinc in incubation media stimulates DNA synthesis of lymphocytes within 6–7 days; at this time, approximately 10% of DNA synthesis in cultured lymphocytes was maximal within a narrow range of zinc concentrations varying between 0.1 and 0.2 mM. Among several cations tested, only zinc and mercury were stimulatory. Zinc must be present in the media for the entire culture period to produce maximal stimulation of [H^3]thymidine incorporation in DNA lymphocytes.

Prasad and Oberleas (1971) reported that thymus may be a zinc-sensitive tissue. Pneumotropic viral infections and secondary bacterial infections (e.g., *Salmonella* species, *Pasteurella,* and pyrogenic bacteria) have been noted to lead to rapid death in many cases of heriditary zinc-deficient Dutch Friesian cattle, probably related to a faulty development of the immune system (Kroneman *et al.,* 1975). Absolute lymphopenia has been noted to occur in patients with cirrhosis of the liver, an example of a conditioned zinc-deficient state, and in some species of animals made zinc-deficient (Prasad, 1966). Whether or not zinc deficiency affects thymus-dependent lymphocytes in man needs to be investigated inasmuch as intercurrent infections are commonly observed in patients with zinc deficiency (Prasad, 1966).

Haas *et al.* (1976) reported that mice immunized with keyhole limpet hemocyanin-P-azophenylarsonate on the first day of beginning a zinc-deficient diet and subsequently at 10-day intervals up to 30 days showed a severe depression in their antibody response to this antigen. These findings have been interpreted to show that the primary immune response may be defective, and that the immune memory response is impaired in zinc-deficient animals. Recent studies by Frost *et al.* (1976) in sickle cell anemia patients, an example of a conditioned zinc-deficiency state, showed that there is a considerable suppression of peripheral T-cell numbers and an increased number of null cells in these patients. Thus, it appears that zinc may have an important role in immune functions, and further studies in this area are warranted.

EFFECTS ON RED CELLS

The interaction of zinc with calcium on the red cell membrane was discovered only recently. A search for a safe antisickling agent led to the possibility that zinc may competitively inhibit calcium leak into the red cells of sickle cell anemia patients, an event considered to be very crucial for the development of irreversible sickle cells.

One *in vitro* model with which to test antisickling agents is filterability. A 3.0-μm Nuclepore filter challenges the deformability of red cells in somewhat the same manner as does a tissue capillary. It was observed that zinc in a concentration as low as 0.3 mM, but not at a lower concentration, improved the filterability of sickle cells at intermediate (15–30 mm Hg) oxygen tensions (Brewer and Oelshlegel, 1974). Assay of zinc in red cells revealed that the amount of additional zinc incorporated after incubation with 0.3 mM zinc under these conditions was equal to a zinc/hemoglobin ratio of less than 0.01. Improvement in filterability at such low concentration suggested that this effect was not directed to the hemoglobin molecule, and the effects of zinc on red cell membrane were investigated with this question in mind (Dash *et al.,* 1974). It was observed that zinc markedly decreased the amount of hemoglobin retention by red cell membrane (Dash *et al.,* 1974). Single-stage red cell ghosts prepared by the hypotonic lysis technique of Hoffman (1958) were studied, with agents incorporated into the membranes during a single 20-min hypotonic exposure. After resealing and repeated washing, the hemoglobin levels of the ghost preparations were measured. Zinc caused a six- to sevenfold reduction in the amount of hemoglobin normally retained by these ghosts (Dash *et al.*, 1974). It was previously shown that calcium increases the amount of hemoglobin retained by single-stage ghosts (Weed *et al.*, 1969; Palek *et al.*, 1971). Zinc partially blocks the hemoglobin-retaining effect of calcium on single-stage ghosts (Dash *et al.*, 1974).

Calcium accumulation in red cells greatly decreased their deformability, and recent studies by Eaton *et al.* (1973) implicated calcium incorporation as a pathogenic event in the formation of irreversibly sickled cells. The effect of zinc on calcium incorporation into intact sickled cells was studied, and it was found that the amount of calcium incorporation is decreased about twofold in the presence of zinc (Brewer and Oelshlegel, 1974).

It is possible that the effect of zinc on calcium-binding or hemoglobin retention, or both, of red cell membranes is involved in the beneficial effect of zinc on the filterability of sickle cells. It is becoming clearer that the process of formation of irreversibly sickled cells involves the membrane of the cells. Calcium or hemoglobin binding, or both, may promote the process of formation of irreversibly sickled cells, thus hindering the filterability of such cells. Zinc may act favorably on the filterability of sickled cells by blocking the proposed binding of calcium or hemoglobin, or both, to the membrane.

ZINC AS A VIRAL INHIBITOR

The trace elements serve a well-known role in biological systems, often as cofactors in enzymes, membranes, and other macromolecular structures. Some of these elements may have a control function, since they readily inhibit certain enzymatic reactions (Vallee and Wacker, 1972). Thus, trace elements could play a significant role in various features of virus replication in susceptible host cells. Little attention has been paid, however, to the effects of trace elements in the replication process of mammalian viruses.

The rhinoviruses, or common-cold viruses, are a large group of very small, simple human parasites. The infectious viruses are composed of a single strand of RNA enclosed in a protein coat or capsid (Korant *et al.*, 1972). They are able to form visible sites of infection on the host cells unless an inhibitor is present. Of nine human rhinoviruses, eight were studied and found to be susceptible to 10^{-4} M zinc ion. One rhinovirus, type 5, was resistant, as were two serotypes of poliovirus (Korant *et al.*, 1972).

From studies reported earlier, it is known that certain of the larger polypeptides are precursors to smaller ones. Zinc in 10^{-4} M concentration rapidly blocks cleavage of some precursors and prevents formation of the capsid polypeptides. Poliovirus, which is able to form plaques in zinc-containing agar, is able to process its precursor proteins as usual at this zinc level, although higher zinc concentrations can also limit proteolysis in polio-infected cells (Butterworth and Korant, 1974).

It has been suggested that zinc ions bind to rhinovirus capsid polypeptides and prevent their nascent cleavage. Whether or not these observations have any clinical significance with respect to viral infections in man remains to be elucidated (Butterworth and Korant, 1974).

METABOLISM

DISTRIBUTION IN THE BODY

Several studies have been published on the distribution of zinc in the tissues. Extensive analyses for trace elements in human tissues by emission spectrophotography were carried out by Tipton and co-workers (Tipton and Cook, 1963; Tipton *et al.*, 1965). About half the subjects had died from accidental causes, but the remainder had died of various diseases. Other investigators have also reported similar data; these data are summarized in Table XV. For comparison, zinc levels of some animal tissues are also included in Table XV.

Liver, kidney, bone, retina, prostate, and muscle appear to be rich in zinc. In man, the zinc content of the testes and skin has not been determined accurately, although it appears clinically that these tissues are sensitive to zinc depletion. In our laboratory, the hair zinc level in normal subjects is 193 ± 18 μg/g (Prasad, 1976). Acute changes in the zinc content of the body due to nutritional or other factors will not be reflected in hair zinc assays.

ZINC IN PLASMA AND RED CELLS

Zinc in serum is 16% higher than in plasma (Foley *et al.*, 1968). The higher content of zinc in serum has been attributed to the liberation of zinc from the platelets during the process of clotting and to invisible hemolysis of red cells, which occurs regularly. Values for the plasma zinc in normal subjects obtained by different investigators using various techniques are with few exceptions in reasonably good agreement. Better methods of avoiding contamination and more precise analytical tools now provide accurate data for plasma zinc. The plasma zinc concentration (mean + S.D.) in normal subjects according to our techniques is 112 ± 12 μg/100 ml (Prasad *et al.*, 1975b).

Table XV. Zinc Concentrations in Human and Animal Tissues (mg/kg dry weight)[a]

Tissue	Human	Rat		Calf		Pig	
		Normal	Zinc-deficient	Normal	Zinc-deficient	Normal	Zinc-deficient
Liver	141–245	101 ± 13	89 ± 12	101	84	150.8 ± 12	96.1 ± 8
Kidney	184–230	91 ± 3	80 ± 3	73	76	97.8 ± 3.0	90.8 ± 4.0
Lung	67–86	81 ± 3	77 ± 9	81	72		
Muscle	197–226	45 ± 5	31 ± 6	86	78		
Pancreas	115–135					139.5 ± 4.0	88.3 ± 4.0
Heart	100	73 ± 16	67 ± 9				
Bone	218	168 ± 8	69 ± 6	78	63	95 ± 1.8	47 ± 1.6
Prostate							
Normal	520						
Hyperplasia	2330						
Cancer	285						
Eye							
Retina	571						
Choroid	562						
Ciliary body	288						
Testis		176 ± 12	132 ± 16	79	70	54 ± 2.0	59 ± 2.0
Esophagus		108 ± 17	88 ± 10			88.1 ± 3.0	97.6 ± 5.0

[a]From Tipton *et al*. 1965). Values are means ± S.D. except human data, which are expressed as the distribution of published mean values.

Plasma zinc levels in the newborn are in the same range as in adults. The levels fall to just below adult level within the first week of life and continue to decline until 3 months, finally reaching the adult level at 4 months of age. Some investigators have shown decreasing plasma zinc values with increasing age over 60 years (Lindeman *et al.*, 1972; Willden and Robinson, 1975; Hallböök and Hedelin, 1977). Whether or not this decrease implies an increased requirement for zinc in the elderly subjects remains to be established.

The binding of zinc to amino acids and serum protein was studied *in vitro* by Prasad and Oberleas (1970a). Following incubation of ^{65}Zn with pooled native human serum *in vitro*, ultrafiltrable zinc was determined to be 2–8% of the total serum zinc, when the zinc/albumin molar ratio was varied from 0.33 to 2.5. Under similar conditions, 0.2–1.2% of zinc was ultrafiltrable when predialyzed serum was used. In physiological concentrations, addition of amino acids to predialyzed serum increased ultrafiltrable ^{65}Zn severalfold (Figs. 13 and 14). Histidine, glutamine, threonine, cystine, and lysine showed the most marked effects in this regard (Figs. 15 and 16). It was suggested that the amino-acid-bound fraction of zinc may have an important role in biological transport of this element. By means of starch-block electrophoresis of predialyzed serum, the stable zinc content was determined to be highest in the albumin fraction, although smaller concentrations of zinc were found in the α-, β-, and γ-globulins as well (Fig. 17). The results obtained by using ^{65}Zn-incubated predialyzed serum, however,

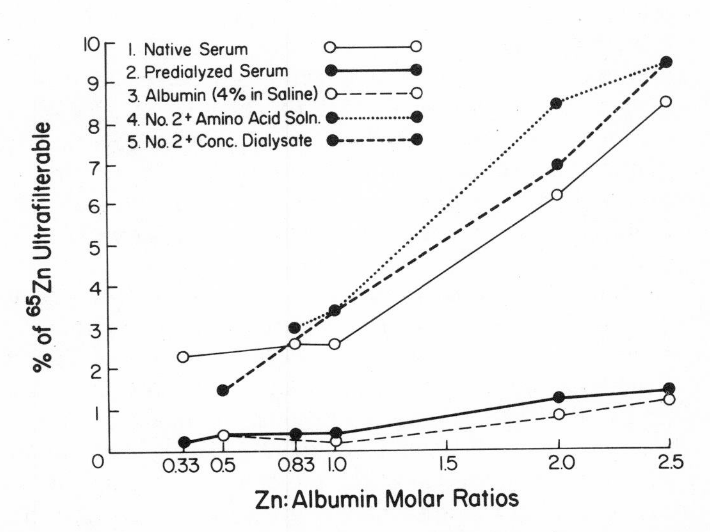

Fig. 13. Percentage of ultrafiltrable ^{65}Zn plotted against zinc albumin molar ratios. From Prasad and Oberleas (1970a).

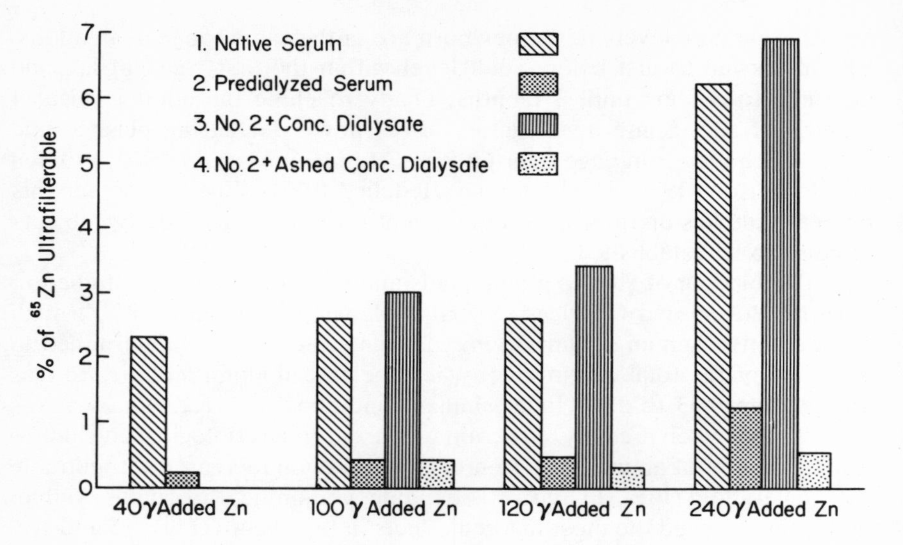

Fig. 14. Percentage of ultrafiltrable ^{65}Zn in native serum, predialyzed serum, predialyzed serum reconstituted with concentrated dialysate, and predialyzed serum reconstituted with ashed concentrated dialysate at different levels of Zn protein molar ratios (0.33, 0.83, 1.0, and 2.0). From Prasad and Oberleas (1970a).

indicated a difference in the behavior of exogenous zinc as compared with the endogenous zinc bound to various serum proteins. *In vitro* studies with the use of predialyzed albumin, haptoglobin, ceruloplasmin, α_2-macroglobin, transferrin, and IgG, incubated with ^{65}Zn, revealed that zinc was bound to all these proteins, and that the binding of zinc to IgG was electrostatic in nature. Whereas amino acids competed effectively with albumin, haptoglobin, transferrin, and IgG for binding of zinc, a similar phenomenon was not observed with respect to ceruloplasmin and α_2-macroglobulin, suggesting that the latter two proteins exhibited a specific binding property of zinc (Fig. 18).

Zinc in red cells has not been measured by many investigators. The reported values in the literature vary from 10 to 14 μg/ml red cells (Prasad, 1966; Mansouri *et al.*, 1970; Ross *et al.*, 1958; McBean and Halsted, 1969). Variations and lack of standardization of techniques are undoubtedly responsible for the widely different results. In our laboratory, normal values (mean + S.D.) for red cell zinc are 42 ± 6μ g/g hemoglobin (Prasad *et al.*, 1975b). The zinc content of the red cells in newborn infants is only one quarter of the normal adult value, rising progressively over the first 12 years of life, when it attains the adult level (Berfenstam, 1952a,b).

Although leukocytes are rich in zinc, only limited data are available in the literature. Technical difficulties are mainly responsible for this lack. With further refinement in techniques, it is hoped that more can be learned from leukocyte zinc analysis in the future.

ABSORPTION OF ZINC

Only a small percentage of ingested dietary zinc is absorbed. Absorption is difficult to ascertain precisely, and intake–output studies are not valid indicators because excretion of zinc is nearly all via the gut. Thus, data indicating an increased absorption may also be interpreted as indicating a decreased excretion and vice verse.

Data on the site or sites of absorption in man and on the mechanism(s) of absorption, whether this be by active, passive, or facultative transport, are meager. Pearson and Reich (1965), using the everted gut sac of the rat,

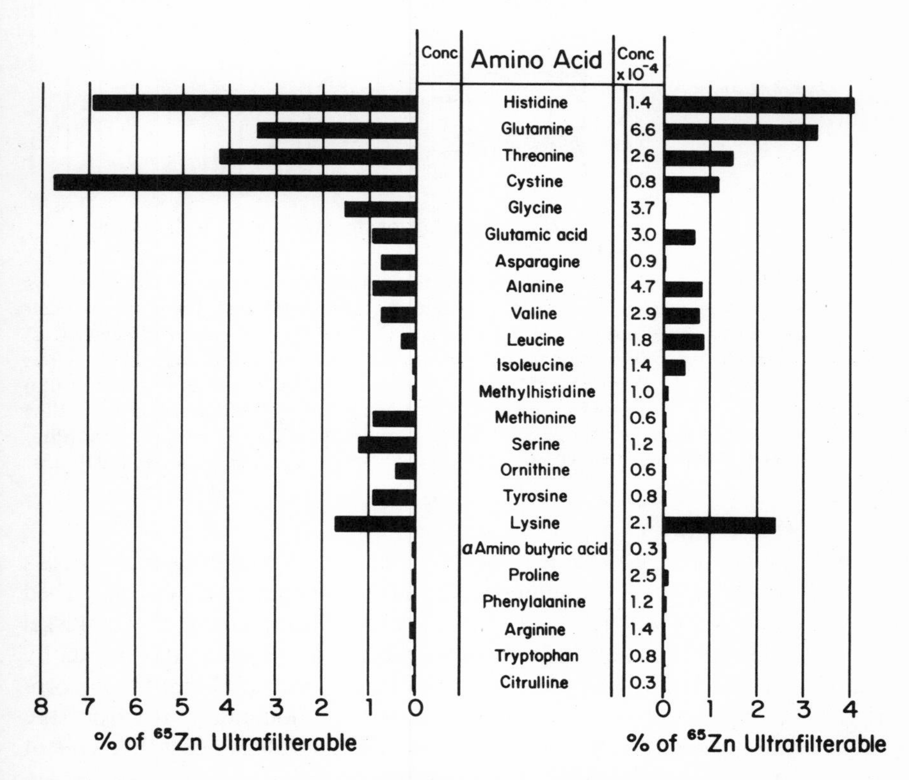

Fig. 15. Effect of addition of single amino acids to predialyzed serum on the percentage of ultrafiltrable ^{65}Zn at Zn/albumin ratio of 2.0. The concentration of amino acids is expressed as $\times\ 10^{\times 4}$ M. From Prasad and Oberleas (1970).

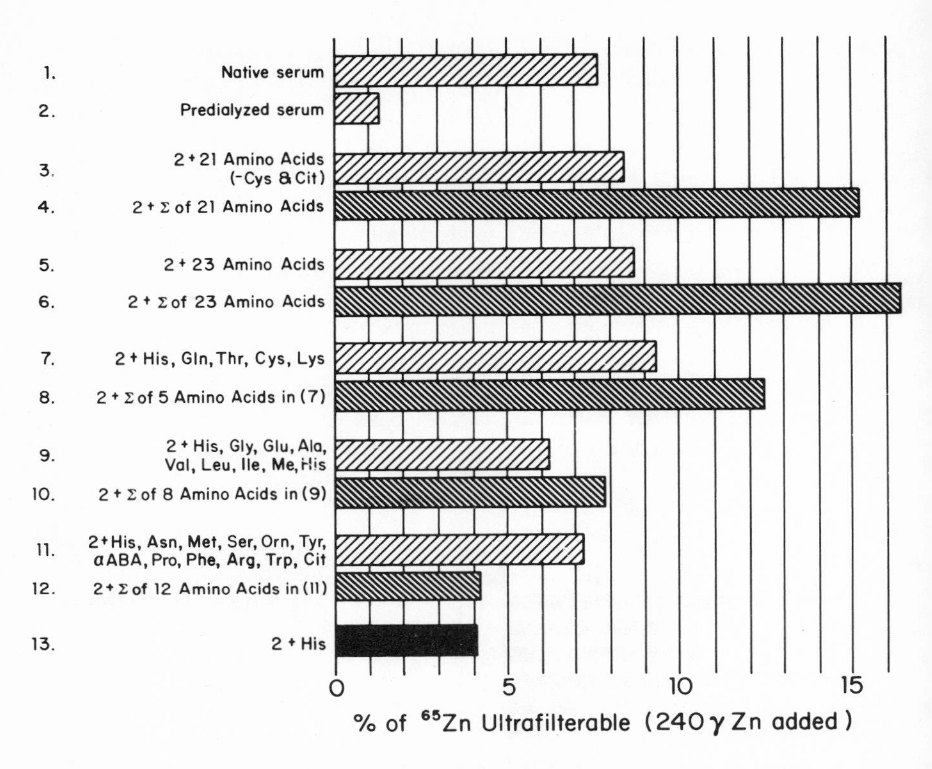

Fig. 16. Effects of additions of physiological concentrations of amino acids in various combinations to samples of predialyzed serum compared with the sum of their individual effects. Zn/albumin molar ratio, 2.0. (Σ) Sum of individual effects; (Cys) cystine; (Cit) citrulline; (His) histidine; (Gln) glutamine; (Thr) threonine; (Lys) lysine; (Gly) glycine; (Glu) glutamic acid; (Ala) alanine; (Val) valine; (Leu) leucine; (Ile) isoleucine; (Me His) 1-methyl histidine; (Asm) asparagine; (Met) methionine; (Ser) serine; (Orn) ornithine; (Tyr) tyrosine; (αABA) α-aminobutyric acid; (Pro) proline; (Phe) phenylalanine; (Arg) arginine; (Trp) tryptophan. From Prasad and Oberleas (1970a).

provided evidence that zinc is actively absorbed into the intestinal mucosa against a concentration gradient. They reported that zinc was absorbed most efficiently from the distal gut segments. More recently, Methfessel and Spencer (1973), using ^{65}Zn, studied specific absorption sites in rats by means of ligated intestinal sacs. These workers concluded that the absorption of ^{65}Zn was significantly greater from the duodenum than from the more distal segments of the small intestines. Their data suggest that sites of zinc absorption may be similar to those of iron.

Becker and Hoekstra (1971) reviewed the available information on intestinal absorption of zinc. They concluded that "zinc absorption is variable in extent and is highly dependent upon a variety of factors." Among the factors that they suggested might affect zinc absorption were body size, the level of zinc in the diet, and the presence in the diet of other potentially interfering substances such as calcium, phytate, other chelating agents, and vitamin D.

Evans (1976) proposed that in the experimental animal, the pancreas secretes a ligand into the duodenum, where zinc is complexed with the molecule. The complexed zinc molecule is transported through the microvillus and into the epithelial cell, where the metal is transferred to binding sites on the basolateral plasma membrane. Metal-free albumin then interacts with the plasma membrane and removes zinc from the receptor sites. The quantity of metal-free albumin available at the basolateral membrane probably determines the amount of zinc removed from the intestinal epithelial cell, and thus regulates the quantity of zinc that enters the body. This hypothesis must be regarded as speculative, and more work is needed in the future to substantiate this.

Recently, a low-molecular-weight zinc-binding ligand was found to occur in human milk. This ligand is not present in cow's milk. It is believed

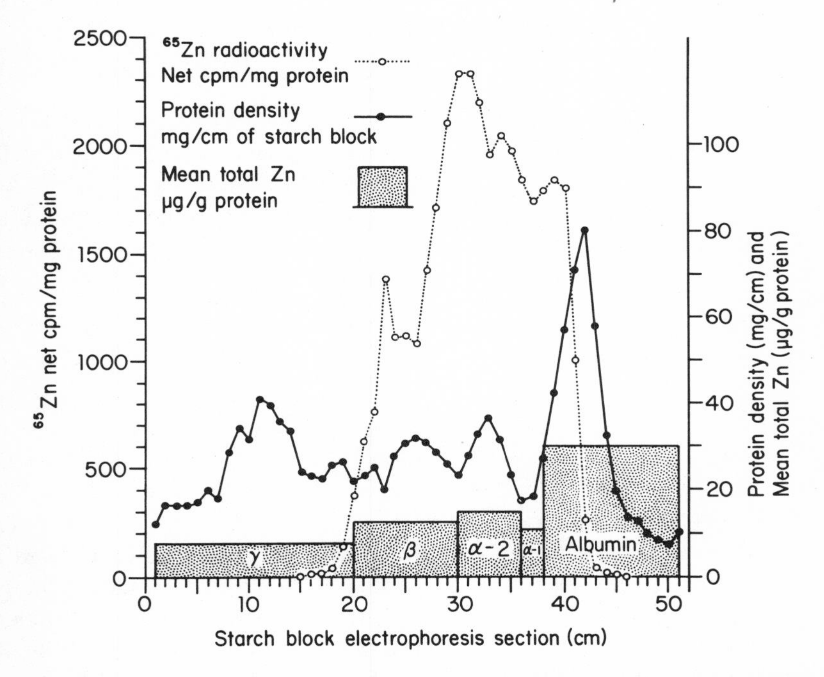

Fig. 17. Distribution of endogenous stable zinc and exogenous ^{65}Zn on starch block, following electrophoresis of predialyzed normal human serum incubated with ^{65}Zn (without carrier zinc). From Prasad and Oberleas (1970a).

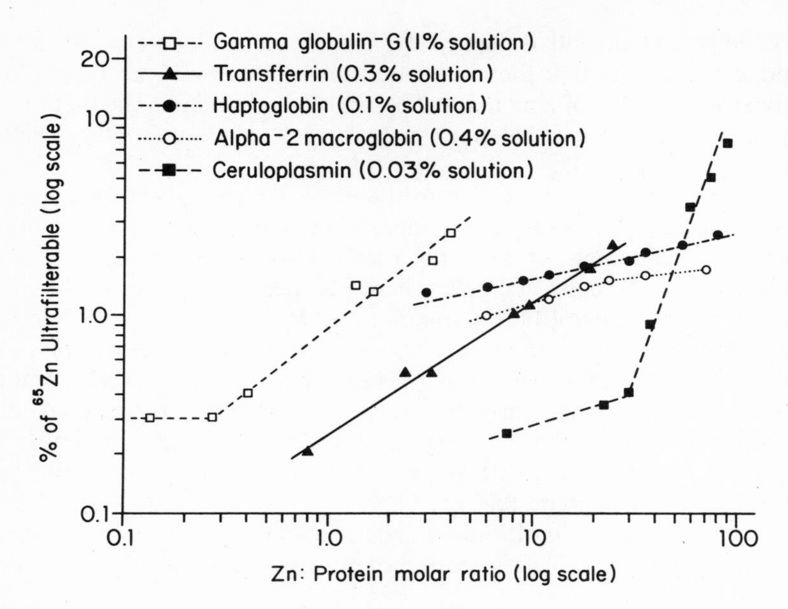

Fig. 18. Changes in percentages of ultrafiltrable ^{65}Zn at different levels of Zn/protein molar ratios for various predialyzed proteins. Data are presented on a log-to-log scale. From Prasad and Oberleas (1970a).

that this zinc-binding ligand of maternal milk may enhance zinc transport in the neonatal period before the development of intestinal mechanisms for zinc absorption (Hurley *et al.,* 1977). This may also explain the therapeutic value of human milk in the treatment of a genetic disorder of zinc metabolism, acrodermatitis enteropathica (see below).

AVAILABILITY OF ZINC

Several factors influence the absorption and retention of zinc and thus its availability from the diet. Phytate (inositol hexaphosphate), which is present in cereal grains, markedly impairs the absorption of zinc. This was first shown in 1960 by O'Dell and Savage (1960). Later, Oberleas *et al.* (1962) showed that phytic acid added to an animal protein diet depressed growth in swine. Using rats, Oberleas and Prasad (1969) demonstrated a close relationship between zinc and the utilization of soybean protein. Without zinc supplementation, rats fed a 12% soybean protein diet gained less than half as much as rats that were supplemented with zinc. Likuski and Forbes (1964) showed that phytic acid depressed the availability of zinc whether the protein source was pure amino acids or casein.

Such studies have a close relationship to zinc in human nutrition because there is strong evidence that phytate exerts a similar effect in man.

Reinhold *et al.* (1976) found that unleavened bread, which is consumed in large amounts by Iranian villagers (often providing the major source of protein), contains significantly more phytate than urban breads, which are leavened and allowed to ferment. Leavening results in destruction of phytate. The omission of the leavening process in Iranian village bread-making is presumably responsible for the high content of phytate. Indeed, zinc deficiency in man was reported by Prasad and co-workers (Prasad *et al.,* 1961; Sandstead *et al.,* 1967) to occur in the Middle East under conditions where unleavened bread was consumed in great amounts, thus supporting the suggestion that phytate enhances the possibility of zinc deficiency in man.

Recent studies indicate that high fiber intake, as is common in subjects consuming high-protein cereals, is detrimental to zinc availability (Reinhold *et al.,* 1976). Binding of the zinc to the fiber of wheat is particularly important because, in contrast to other components, fiber is not degraded by digestive secretions. As a result, zinc remains attached to it and in this state is transported into the large intestine, from which absorption does not occur. Ultimately, it is lost in the feces.

In vitro experiments suggest that binding by phytate may be of secondary importance to binding by fiber of zinc and iron (Reinhold *et al.,* 1976). This conclusion needs confirmation by studies of digestion and additional balance studies in man and other species of animals. Calcium enhances the binding of zinc by phytate, and its adjunctive behavior in the presence of fiber needs to be clarified.

GEOPHAGIA

Minnich *et al.* (1968) found that clay from Turkey inhibited iron absorption in human subjects. Nearly all subjects with severe nutritional dwarfism studied in Iran gave a history of eating large amounts of clay for many years. Since zinc deficiency was the basic cause of this dwarfism syndrome, it was suspected that Iranian clay might hinder zinc absorption. Furthermore, when a solution of ^{65}Zn was mixed with clay, 97% of the radioactivity was removed from the solution. When Iranian clay was fed to zinc-deficient rats, however, it proved to be a life-saving source of zinc (Halsted *et al.,* 1974). It may be speculated that subjects in Iran may have sought zinc through the ingestion of clay. At present, however, no definite conclusions can be drawn with respect to the effect of geophagia on zinc balance in man.

CHELATING AGENTS

Considerable work has been reported on the effect of chelating agents on zinc absorption. Most of these studies were carried out in animals

(Sandstead *et al.,* 1976). Ethylenediaminetetraacetic acid (EDTA) complexes with zinc from dietary sources readily and makes the zinc available for absorption.

INTAKE AND EXCRETION OF ZINC IN MAN

Only meager information was available on the zinc requirement in man up to the recent past. Zinc-balance studies carried out nearly 30 years ago indicated that on dietary zinc intake ranging from 4 to 6 mg/day, the zinc balance was negative in preschool children (Scoular, 1939). In children in the age group 8–12 years, the mean retention of zinc was 4.9 mg/day on a zinc intake ranging from 14 to 18 mg/day (Macy, 1942), indicating a high requirement of zinc during growth and development. In young adults ranging in age from 17 to 27, the retention of zinc was also reported to be very high, 5–8 mg/day, on a zinc intake ranging from 12 to 14 mg/day (Tribble and Scoular, 1954). In a study reported in 1966 in preadolescent girls, about 30% of a dietary zinc intake averaging 7 mg/day was retained (Engle *et al.,* 1966). Variable results have been reported for adults. In early studies, the zinc balance was reported to be in equilibrium in three subjects on a zinc intake of 5 mg/day; however, the retention of zinc was similar in two others receiving twice this amount, while the zinc balance was more positive, ranging up to 2.6 mg/day on a zinc intake of 20 mg/day (McCance and Widdowson, 1942). In a long-term study of two adults receiving a self-selected diet, one subject was in negative zinc balance, −4 mg/day, on a diet containing 11 mg zinc/day, while the other, receiving a dietary zinc intake of 18 mg/day, was in a positive zinc balance of 1 mg/day (Tipton *et al.,* 1969). In a recent zinc-balance study carried out in young women, the zinc balance was in equilibrium on a dietary zinc intake of about 11 mg/day (White and Gynee, 1971), while in a study in young men receiving a synthetic diet having a zinc content of about 20 mg/day, the retention of zinc was high and ranged from 7 to 8 mg/day (Gormican and Catli, 1971).

The protein content of the diet appears to influence the absorption and retention of zinc. The zinc balance of preadolescent girls recieving a zinc intake of about 5 mg/day during a low-protein intake was in equilibrium, the zinc retention ranging from 0.5 to 0.8 mg/day (Price *et al.,* 1970), while on a high-protein intake that had only a slightly higher zinc content, about 7 mg/day, the retention of zinc was about 2 mg/day. The obligatory zinc retention during periods of growth and during stress was caclulated by Sandstead (1973). The zinc retention for growing children, age 11 years, and for yougn adults, age 17 years, was estimated to exceed 0.4 mg/day; for pregnant women, the retention was 0.7 mg/day.

The zinc content of a diet depends on the dietary protein content. A diet containing about 1 g protein/kg body weight for a 70-kg man is expected to contain about 12.5 mg zinc. A diet that is adequate in calories but has a low protein content may contain less than half this amount of zinc, whereas the zinc content of a high-protein diet may be 2–3 times as high as that of the low-protein diet. The main source of the dietary zinc content is meat. However, marked differences in zinc content in different types of meat have been demonstrated, red meat having the highest zinc content (Rose and Willden, 1972). Fish also has a relatively high zinc content. Most other food items that constitute the daily diet have a zinc content of 1 mg or less per 100 g wet weight.

On normal zinc intake of about 12.5 mg/day, the urinary zinc excretion is low, ranging from 0.5 to 0.8 mg/day, while most of the zinc is excreted in the stool (Spencer *et al.,* 1976). The fecal excretion of zinc is due only in part to unabsorbed zinc. The remainder is due to the secretion of zinc from the vascular space into the intestine. Studies of ^{65}Zn administered intravenously in man indicate that the intestinal secretion of ^{65}Zn is as high as 18% of the administered zinc tracer (Spencer *et al.,* 1965a,b).

The zinc balances in adults were in equilibrium on a zinc intake of 12.5 mg/day in one study (Spencer *et al.,* 1976). These balances were quite similar in consecutive study periods. It was also observed, however, that not all subjects are in zinc equilibrium on this intake, and that in some cases, a higher zinc intake of about 15 mg/day is needed to attain equilibrium. All zinc-balance studies in man reported thus far have to be considered as maximal balances, since the loss of zinc in sweat has not been considered and the balances are based only on the zinc intake and the excretion of zinc in the urine and the stool. The loss of zinc in sweat in man was reported to be 1.15 mg/liter for whole sweat and 0.9 mg/liter for cell-free sweat (Prasad *et al.,* 1963d). If these amounts of zinc are lost in sweat, the requirement of 15 mg zinc/day is certainly not excessive.

Persons with a normal body weight who maintain themselves on a low-calorie intake for prolonged periods of time, e.g., patients with chronic alcoholism, show a very high rentention of zinc when given a normal dietary intake. This high zinc retention was observed to continue for several months until the ideal body weight was attained.

When the dietary intake of zinc is completely eliminated, as in total starvation used for weight reduction in marked obesity, the rapid weight loss is associated with a considerable loss of zinc. This zinc loss occurs promptly with onset of the weight loss and is due primarily to a marked increase of the urinary zinc excretion (Spencer *et al.,* 1976).

The high excretion of zinc during starvation resulting in weight loss is most likely due to a catabolic state and breakdown of muscle. Although muscle tissue has a very low concentration of zinc (Mansouri *et al.,* 1970; Spencer *et al.,* 1965a,b), the muscle mass is very large and contains a high percentage of the total body zinc (Schroeder *et al.,* 1967). During weight loss, the loss of muscle tissue is considerable in addition to the loss of fat and water. In studies of zinc metabolism following injury and after surgical procedures, the increased excretion of zinc in urine was related to loss of muscle tissue (Fell *et al.,* 1973; Davies, J. W. L., and Fell, 1974). This finding was supported by the observation that there was a good correlation between the urinary zinc/creatine ratio and the urinary excretion of nitrogen (Fell *et al.,* 1973).

ZINC DEFICIENCY IN MAN

Although the Iranian subjects suffered from severe iron deficiency, it was difficult to explain all the clinical features on the basis of tissue iron deficiency alone. The tissue effects of iron deficiency in animals and human subjects have been well described (Beutler, 1964). Rats and elephants continue to grow on an iron-deficient diet and develop marked anemia during the period of rapid growth (Undritz, 1964). In human subjects, iron deficiency causes changes in the mucosa of the alimentary tract (Beutler, 1964; Darby, 1946). The oral mucosal epithelium is abnormally thin in some patients. Mitoses in the prickle-cell layer were more frequent in iron-deficient than in normal subjects. Melanin deposition is less, and subepithelial inflammation is increased. Changes in the esophagus of iron-deficient patients give rise to "sideropenic dysphagia" (see Chapter 5). Constrictions or webs of the hypopharynx or esophagus result in inability to swallow solid food (Howell and Monto, 1953). Gastric atrophy and achlorhydria are commonly associated with this disorder (Morrison *et al.,* 1937). It is unclear, however, whether these conditions are the result of iron deficiency or whether they are of etiological significance in the development of hyposideremia. Koilonychia also occurs in iron deficiency. It has been suggested that a dietary cystine deficiency may be important in the development of this abnormality (Jalili and Al-Kassab, 1959). Koilonychia and esophageal changes have also been described in zinc-deficient animals (Follis *et al.,* 1941; Nishimura, 1953).

It was considered unlikely that iron deficiency alone could account for all the clinical features noted in the patients described above. The possibility that zinc deficiency may have been present was considered. Zinc deficiency was known to produce retardation of growth in animals, heavy metals may form insoluble complexes with phosphates, one may speculate that some factors responsible for decreased availability of iron in these patients with geophagia may also govern the availability of zinc.

Zinc deficiency in rats results in testicular atrophy. Other manifestations of zinc deficiency in the mouse, rat, and pig include lack of growth and retardation of skeletal maturation. Changes in alkaline phosphatase (widely held to be a zinc-containing enzyme) have also been observed in pigs with zinc deficiency. Increasing activity of this enzyme was noted when zinc-deficient animals received increased amounts of dietary zinc (Luecke *et al.,* 1956, 1957). Thus, in the Iranian subjects, dwarfism, testicular atrophy, retardation of skeletal maturation, and increasing activity of serum alkaline phosphatase following adequate nutritional intake of zinc could have been explained on the basis of zinc deficiency.

Subsequently, in Egypt, similar patients (Fig. 19) were encountered in the villages (Prasad *et al.,* 1963a; Sandstead *et al.,* 1967). The clinical features were similar, except for the following: the Iranian patients exhibited more pronounced hepatosplenomegaly, they gave a history of geophagia, and none had any parasitic infestations, whereas the majority of Egyptian patients had both schistosomiasis and hookworm infestations, and none gave a history of geophagia.

These Egyptian patients were studied in detail. Their dietary history was similar to that of the Iranians. The intake of animal protein was negligible, and their diet consisted mainly of bread and beans *(Vicia fava).*

These subjects were demonstrated to have zinc deficiency. The basis for this conclusion was that (1) the zinc concentrations in plasma, red cells, and hair were decreased; and (2) radioactive ^{65}Zn studies revealed that the plasma zinc turnover rate was greater in the patients, the 24-hr exchangea-

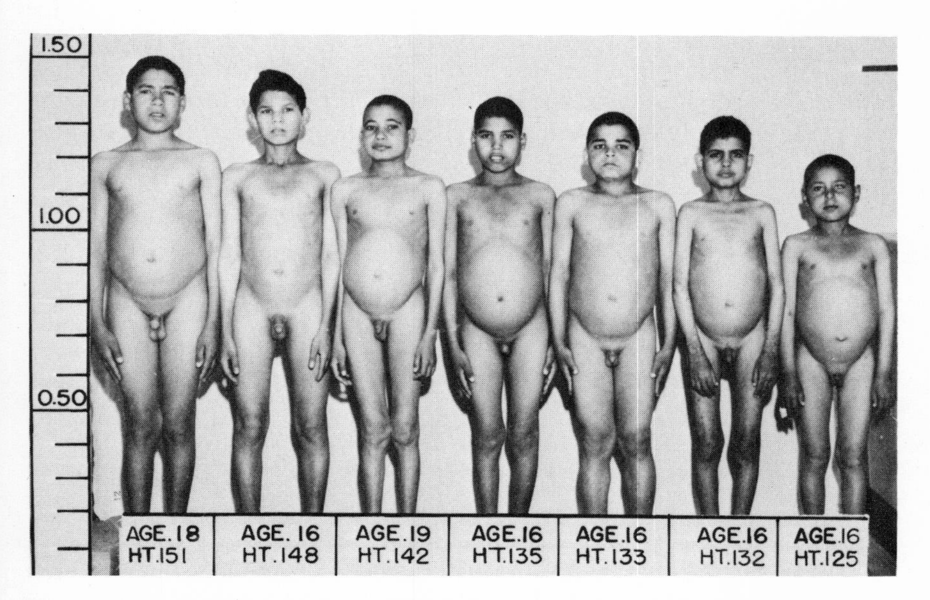

Fig. 19. Seven of the dwarfs from delta villages near Cairo, Egypt. Height is shown in centimeters. From Prasad *et al.* (1963b).

Table XVI. Zinc Content of Plasma, Erythrocytes, and Hair[a]

Subjects	Plasma (μg/100 ml)	RBC (μg/ml)	Hair (μg/g)
Normals	102 ± 13 (19)	12.5 ± 1.2 (15)	99 ± 9 (10)
Dwarfs	67 ± 11 (17)	9.7 ± 1.1 (14)	65 ± 16 (10)

[a]From Prasad (1966). The numbers in parentheses indicate the number of subjects included for each determination. The differences between normals and dwarfs are statistically significant ($p < 0.01$).

ble pool was smaller, and the excretion of ^{65}Zn in the stool and the urine was less than in the control subjects. These data are summarized in Tables XVI and XVII. Zinc deficiency in humans, in the absence of advanced cirrhosis of the liver had not been described before. Liver function tests and biopsy failed to reveal evidence of cirrhosis of the liver in these subjects (Prasad *et al.,* 1963c). Furthermore, in contrast to cirrhotic patients, who excrete abnormally high quantities of zinc in the urine (Vallee *et al.,* 1957), our patients excreted less stable zinc in urine, in comparison with control subjects (Prasad *et al.,* 1963c). These results are presented in Tables XVIII and XIX. Detailed examination of these patients ruled out other chronic debilitating diseases that might possibly have affected the serum zinc levels.

Investigations for other deficiencies were also carried out. Serum iron was decreased, unsaturated-iron-binding capacity was increased, serum copper was slightly increased, and serum magnesium was normal. Analysis of hair for manganese, cobalt, molybdenum, and other elements revealed

Table XVII. Summary of Zinc-65 Studies[a]

Subjects	Turnover rate (mg/kg per day)[b]	24-Hour exchangeable pool (mg/kg)[b]	Urinary excretion (% dose administered in 13 days)[b]	Excretion in stool (% dose administered in 100 g stool)[c]
Normals	1.00 ± 0.09 (9)	7.0 ± 1.6 (8)	2.8 ± 0.56 (7)	0.66 ± 0.19 (7)
Dwarfs	1.50 ± 0.29 (10)	4.6 ± 1.2 (8)	1.6 ± 0.68 (7)	0.42 ± 0.13 (7)

[a]From Prasad (1966). The numbers in parentheses indicate the number of subjects included for each determination.
[b]The differences between normals and dwarfs are statistically significant ($p < 0.01$).
[c]$p < 0.05$.

Table XVIII. Liver Function Studies in Patients with Anemia, Dwarfism, and Hypogonadism[a]

Expt. No.	BSP[b] retention after 45 min (%)	Total serum bilirubin (mg %)	Serum alkaline phosphatase	SGOT units	SGPT units	LDH	Serum total protein (g %)	Albumin (g %)	Thymal turbidity units	Cephalin flocculation—24 hr, 48 hr	Liver biopsy
1	0.3	0.5	8.4 BU	14	7	430	7.9	4.1	4.5	0, 1+	Minimal histological changes
2	0.3	0.4	1.45 SU	18	5	282	6.4	4.3	2.8	1+, 2+	Minimal histological changes
3	4.7	0.33	2.35 SU	16	9	473	7.0	4.1	3.0	2+, 2+	Minimal histological changes
4	0.6	0.33	4.55 SU	33	8	375	7.7	4.6	5.0	1+, 2+	Minimal histological changes
5	2.6	0.4	10.9 BU	32	18	240	7.5	3.9	4.0	2+, 2+	Minimal focal necrosis and periportal infiltrate
6	1.5	0.33	12.8 BU	26	16	325	7.9	4.4	7.7	3+, 4+	Mild focal necrosis and periportal infiltrate
7	0.5	0.33	2.0 SU	33	20	323	8.3	3.8	3.5	2+, 3+	Moderate focal necrosis and periportal infiltrate; granulomas with schistosoma ova
8	0.5	0.25	4.1 SU	29	18	295	8.6	3.9	7.0	2+, 2+	Minimal focal necrosis and periportal infiltrate

[a]From Prasad *et al*. (1963c).
[b](BSP) Bromosulfophthalein.
[c](BU) Bodansky units; (SU) Sigma units (Sigma Technical Bulletin No. 104, August 1961) (normal values: adults 0.8–2.3 SU/ml; children 2.8–6.7 SU/ml).

Table XIX. Plasma, Erythrocyte, and Urinary Zinc in Normals vs. Dwarfs[a]

Subjects[b]	Plasma Zn (μg %)	RBC Zn (μg/ml)	Urinary Zn (μg/day)	Urinary creatinine (g/day)	Urinary creatinine (mg/day per kg)
Normals (9)	108 ± 8	13.4 ± 0.8	613 ± 93	1.42 ± 0.3	22.0 ± 5
Dwarfs (8)	73 ± 6	10.5 ± 0.95	395 ± 46	0.63 ± 0.17	21.9 ± 4

[a]From Prasad (1966). The differences between normals and dwarfs are statistically significant ($P < 0.01$).
[b]The numbers in parentheses indicate the number of subjects included in each group.

no significant decrease in comparison with the normal subjects (Tables XX and XXI).

Investigations for vitamin deficiency in these patients were unrevealing. Serum B_{12}, ascorbic acid, vitamin A, and carotene levels were not abnormally low. Formiminoglutamic acid excretion following histidine loading and xanthurenic acid excretion following tryptophane loading were normal, indicating that folic acid and vitamin B_6 deficiencies were not implicated (Prasad *et al.*, 1963a).

Changes in serum alkaline phosphatase (Fig. 20) similar to those observed in the Iranian patients were again seen in the Egyptian cases (Prasad *et al.*, 1963a–d; Sandstead *et al.*, 1967). Alkaline phosphatase activity in serum increases with administration of growth hormone (Raben, 1962), and many other factors are known to influence its activity. Thus, the increasing activity of this enzyme may be indicative of increased production of growth hormone following treatment. Patients with this syndrome treated with iron and a good diet in Iran developed secondary sexual characteristics and gained in weight and height, the size of the liver and spleen decreased, and their anemia was corrected after adequate treatment (Prasad *et al.*, 1961). Ordinary pharmaceutical preparations of iron contain appreciable quantities of zinc as a contaminant, and thus may supply enough zinc to institute recovery from a deficient state.

Table XX. Trace Elements in Serum[a]

	Normals[b]		Dwarfs[b]	
Copper (μg%)[c]	125 ± 22	(19)	142 ± 24	(17)
Magnesium (meq/liter)	1.92 ± 0.19	(17)	1.82 ± 0.12	(12)
Iron (μg%)[d]	87 ± 14	(19)	35 ± 14	(17)
UIBC (μg%)[d,e]	250–400	(19)	360–650	(17)

[a]From Prasad (1966).
[b]The numbers in parentheses indicate the number of subjects included for each determination.
[c]The difference between normals and dwarfs is statistically significant ($p < 0.05$).
[d]The differences between normals and dwarfs are statistically significant ($p < 0.01$).
[e](UIBC) Unsaturated-iron-binding capacity.

Table XXI. Various Elements in Hair (ppm)[a]

Dwarf No.	Calcium	Copper	Nickel	Manganese	Chromium	Cobalt	Molybdenum	Vanadium
1	1000	25	0.3	1	0.3	0.2	0.2	0.10
2	385	22	8.0	3	0.5	0.2	0.2	0.20
3	1550	24	1.0	1	0.5	0.2	0.3	0.10
4	400	22	1.0	5	0.4	0.2	0.2	0.10
5	440	22	0.6	1	0.4	0.2	0.2	0.05
Range								
1. Egyptian controls (12)	410–1050	22–32	1–6	1–7	0.2–0.3	0.2	0.2	0.08–0.45
2. American[b] (90)	60–400	14–40	0.3–2	0.2–0.7	0.3–0.8	0.2	0.2	0.02–0.13

[a]From Prasad (1966). All hair samples were collected at the same time. Determinations were done by National Spectrographic Laboratories, Inc., Cleveland 3, Ohio.
[b]Strain, W. II. Personal communication.

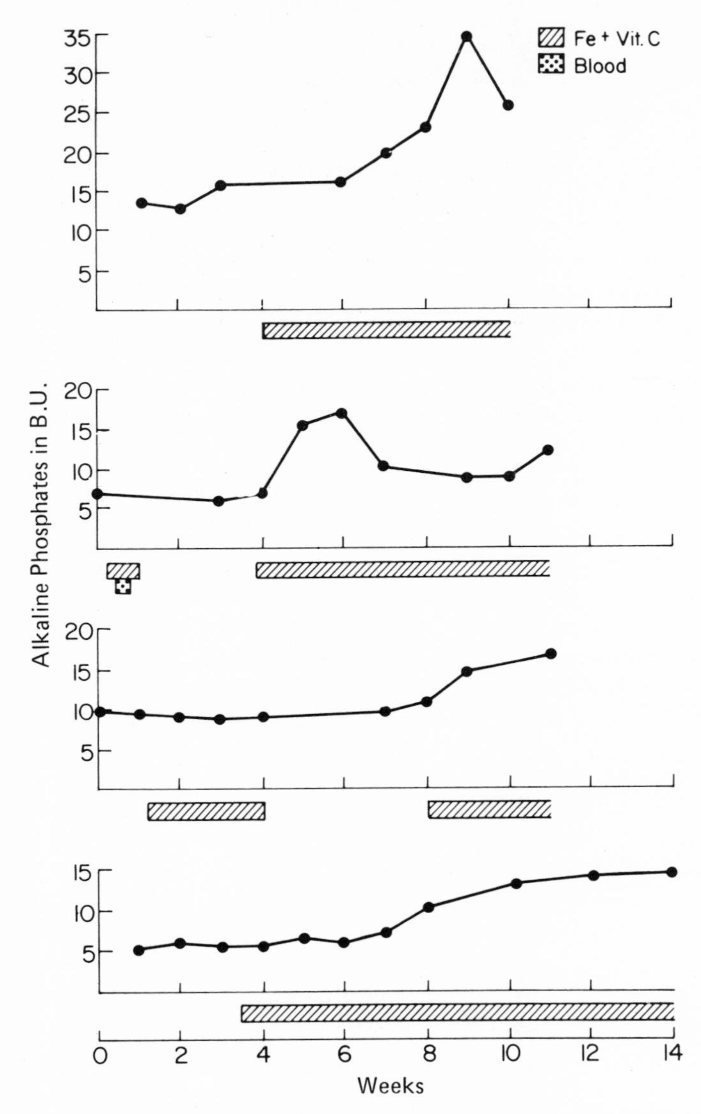

Fig. 20. Changes in alkaline phosphatase in four dwarfs from delta villages of Egypt, following hospitalization. From Prasad *et al.* (1963b).

It is a common belief among medical practitioners in Iran that severe retardation of growth and sexual hypofunction, as noted above, are the results of visceral leishmaniasis and geophagia. In our detailed investigations, no evidence for visceral leishmaniasis was found. The role of geophagia is not entirely clear at present. It is believed that the excess amount of phosphate in the clay may make both dietary iron and zinc unavailable for absorption. The predominantly wheat diet in the Middle East, which has a high content of phytate and fiber, may also reduce the availability of zinc (Oberleas *et al.*, 1962; Reinhold *et al.*, 1976).

The constant finding of hepatosplenomegaly deserves brief comment. As indicated earlier, we were unable to account for this finding on the basis of liver disease. This leaves three possibilities: (1) anemia, (2) zinc deficiency, or (3) a combination of these two. From our studies, no conclusion could be reached as to its pathogenesis at this time. In all cases, however, following treatment with zinc, the size of the liver and spleen decreased markedly.

Our studies in the Middle East included only male subjects. Female patients in villages refused to be examined. Furthermore, our facilities at U.S. Naval Medical Research Unit No. 3 (NAMRU-3), Cairo, Egypt, were such that we could not study any females. Thus, one could not be certain at that time whether this syndrome affected females or not. It is possible, however, that males were more susceptible to zinc deficiency, inasmuch as zinc seems to be concentrated in male genital tracts, whereas in female genital tracts, zinc is not preferentially accumulated. Thus, one could have predicted that zinc deficiency in females manifesting growth retardation was probably prevalent. Later, two zinc-deficient female patients were described by Halsted *et al.* (1972). A similar syndrome affecting females was also described from Turkey (Cavdar and Arcasoy, 1972). The clinical features included growth retardation, hepatosplenomegaly, and facial hyperpigmentation.

The endocrine abnormalities in these patients resembled those of idiopathic hypopituitarism (Prasad *et al.*, 1963b). Growth failure and hypogonadism were the most outstanding features in the male subjects. In addition, in some cases, decreased pituitary adrenocorticotropic hormone reserve and abnormal oral glucose tolerance were found. Hypothyroidism was not present.

Further studies in Egypt showed that the rate of growth was greater in patients who received supplemental zinc than in those who received iron instead or only an animal protein diet that consisted of bread, beans, lamb meat, chicken, eggs, and vegetables daily (Prasad *et al.*, 1963b). Pubic hair appeared in the majority of cases within 7–12 weeks after zinc supplementation was started. Genital size became normal, and secondary sexual characteristics developed within 12–24 weeks after zinc supplementation (Fig. 21). On the other hand, no such changes were observed in a comparable length of time in the iron-supplemented group or in the group on an animal protein diet alone. Thus, the growth retardation and gonadal hypofunction in these subjects were related to a deficiency of zinc. The anemia was due to iron deficiency and responded to oral iron treatment alone.

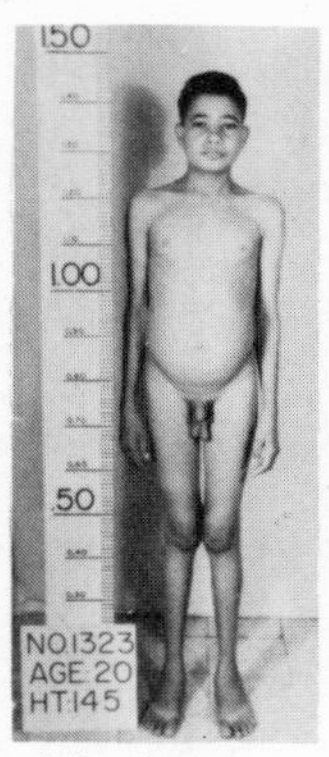

Before treatment.

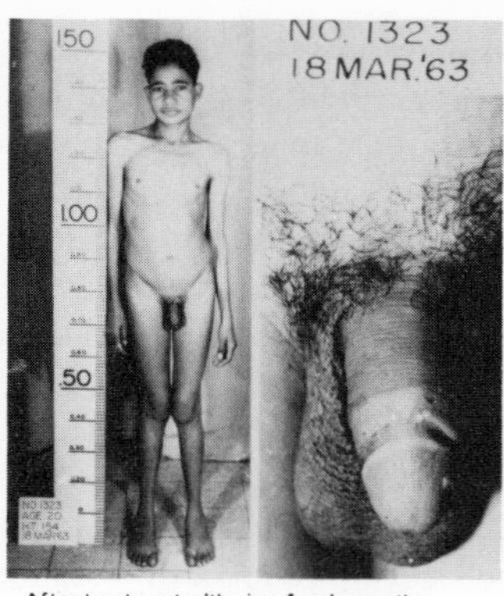

After treatment with zinc for six months.

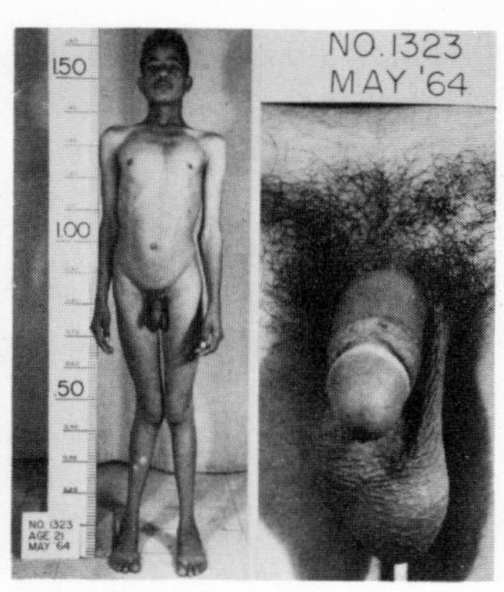

After treatment with zinc for twenty months.

Fig. 21. General appearance of Case 5 before and after zinc treatment. Notice the increase in height, growth of pubic hair, and size of the external genitalia following zinc therapy. The scale is in meters. From Prasad (1966).

Carter *et al.* (1969) administered zinc, iron, or placebo as supplements to different groups of adolescent Egyptian village schoolboys between the ages of 11 and 18 years for 5½ months. No differences in height, weight, or sexual development were observed among the three groups. Their studies were not well designed. The subjects for such a study must be paired according to age, height, and sexual development, inasmuch as the growth rates of children and adolescents normally differ greatly from one age group to another. This was an important factor responsible for their negative results. One other possibility accounting for the negative results in the Cairo study (Carter *et al.,* 1969) should be considered. The supplementation program lasted for a total period of only 5½ months, which under the dietary conditions of the villagers may not have been adequate to see any difference in growth and gonads.

A similar study was carried out in Iran by Ronaghy *et al.* (1969). The subjects were matched according to age, height, and sexual development, prior to supplementation with placebo, iron, or zinc. These boys were between 12 and 14 years of age and received supplements for two 5-month periods with an interval of 7 months during which they received no supplements. In this study, the zinc-supplemented group showed significant sexual development and a significant increase in the cortical thickness of the metacarpal bone, thus providing evidence for the important role of zinc in growth and gonadal development.

A more recent study from Iran employed 50 village schoolboys aged 13 years for supplementation studies (Ronaghy *et al.,* 1974). A high protein–vitamin liquid supplement was used to provide all essential micronutrients.

Group A received placebo. Groups B and C received protein–vitamin liquid supplement. Group C received zinc, 40 mg, whereas Group B received no zinc. This supplementation program was carried out for two 9-month periods, and no supplementation was given during the summer months, since the schools were closed. The zinc-supplemented boys made gains in height and weight that exceeded those of the boys who received identical supplementation minus zinc. Also, the zinc-supplemented boys showed a higher proportion of developed genitalia at the end of the study.

These studies clearly demonstrate that zinc is a principal limiting factor in the nutrition of children when the intake of unleavened wholemeal bread is high. It is also clear that the 25–28 mg zinc supplement used in the previous studies were not adequate, and that 40 mg zinc, as used in the last study (Ronaghy *et al.,* 1974), may also have been marginal, inasmuch as plasma zinc levels were still low at the end of the study period. In contrast, when our subjects in Egypt received only 18 mg supplemental zinc with adequate animal protein and calorie diet, the response to zinc was very rapid and obvious. Thus, requirements of zinc under different dietary conditions must vary widely, and this variation must be considered to correct zinc deficiency in a given population.

Halsted *et al.* (1972) recently published the results of their study in a group of 15 men who were rejected at the Iranian Army Induction Center because of "malnutrition." A unique feature was that all were 19 or 20 years of age. Their clinical features were similar to those of the zinc-deficient dwarfs reported earlier by Prasad and co-workers (Prasad *et al.,* 1963a; Sandstead *et al.,* 1967). They were studied for 6–12 months. One group was given a well-balanced nutritious diet containing ample animal protein plus a placebo capsule. A second group was given the same diet plus a capsule of zinc sulfate containing 27 mg zinc. A third group was given the diet alone without additional medication for 6 months, followed by the diet plus zinc for another 6 months.

The development in subjects receiving the diet alone was slow, and the effect on height increment and onset of sexual function was strikingly enhanced in those receiving zinc. The zinc-supplemented boys gained considerably more height than those receiving only the ample-protein diet. The zinc-supplemented subjects showed evidence for early onset of sexual function, as defined by nocturnal emission in males and menarchy in females (Halsted *et al.,* 1972).

Brief mention should be made regarding the prevalence of zinc deficiency in human populations throughout the world. Clinical pictures similar to those reported by us in zinc-deficient dwarfs have been observed in many countries, such as Turkey, Portugal, and Morocco (Halsted *et al.,* 1974). Also, zinc deficiency should be prevalent in other countries where primarily cereal proteins are consumed by the population. Clinically, it is perhaps not very difficult to recognize extreme examples of zinc-deficient dwarfs in a given population, but it is the marginally deficient subjects who would present great difficulties, and only future studies can provide insight into this problem. It is now becoming clear that not only nutritional deficiency, but also conditioned deficiency, of zinc may complicate many disease states.

Research on the nutritional status of zinc in infants and young children has been very limited. The importance of adequate zinc nutrition in the young is apparent, however, from data on other mammals. Dietary zinc requirements are relatively high in young as compared with those of mature animals of the same species, and the effects of dietary insufficiency are particularly severe.

ZINC DEFICIENCY IN YOUNG CHILDREN

A clinical syndrome similar to that of "adolescent nutritional dwarfism" has been identified in younger children in Iran, though failure of sexual maturation is not evident prior to adolescence. Clinical features included anemia, hepatosplenomegaly, and growth retardation. This syndrome is common in small, rural communities in which there is also a high incidence of adolescent nutritional dwarfism. Eminians *et al.* (1967) found that mean plasma zinc levels of children with this syndrome were significantly lower than those of normal children in the same village, and of normal suburban children of the same age.

The similarities of this syndrome to that of adolescent nutritional dwarfism and the presence of low serum zinc levels suggest that zinc deficiency contributed to the poor growth of these children. Their diets, which contain large quantities of phytate and fiber, are known to have poor availability of zinc. Unfortunately, no studies of dietary zinc supplementation have been reported for these preadolescent children, and the incidence of this syndrome in younger age groups is unknown.

Plasma zinc levels were measured in infants and young children suffering from kwashiorkor in Cairo (Sandstead *et al.,* 1965), Pretoria (Smit and Pretorius, 1964), Cape Town (Hansen and Lehmann, 1969), and Hyderabad (Kumar and Rao, 1973). At the time of hospital admission, plasma zinc levels were very low in all four locations. The hypozincemia could be attributed at least in part to hypoalbuminemia. During the subsequent 8 weeks, plasma zinc levels increased, and in Cape Town and Hyderabad reached normal control levels. In Cairo and Pretoria, however, plasma zinc levels remained significantly below normal at a time of "clinical cure," when total serum protein and serum albumin levels were normal. This persistent hypozincemia suggests that zinc deficiency is associated with kwashiorkor in some geographical locations. The clinical significance of this deficiency has not been defined, but may, for example, have contributed to the growth failure (Sandstead *et al.*, 1965) and to the incidence of skin ulceration in kwashiorkor patients (Hansen and Lehmann, 1969). After recovery from kwashiorkor, children in some areas of the world, including Egypt, are likely to receive a diet inadequate in zinc, and thus a deficiency of this nutrient may persist indefinitely.

In Cape Town, the zinc concentration in the liver, but not in the brain, heart, or muscle, of children dying from kwashiorkor was significantly lower than normal. Plasma zinc levels were also low in marasmic infants.

SECONDARY ZINC DEFICIENCY IN CHILDREN

Though data are limited, some children are at increased risk from zinc deficiency secondary to excessive loss of this element such as is seen in intestinal malabsorption. Hypozincemia was reported in association with celiac disease (Hellwege, 1971), disaccharidase deficiency (MacMahon *et al.*, 1968), and cystic fibrosis (Halsted and Smith, 1970). The incidence of low hair zinc levels (more than 2 S.D. below the normal adult mean) in children with cystic fibrosis is ten times that in normal children. Symptomatic zinc deficiency was detected in patients with regional enteritis (Solomons *et al.*, 1974).

An increased risk of zinc deficiency is associated with the therapeutic use of synthetic oral (Moynahan and Barnes, 1973) and intravenous (Green *et al.*, 1972) diets unless these preparations are zinc-supplemented. A wide range of zinc concentrations have been found in parenteral hyperalimentation solutions even for the same commercial preparation. However, the majority of solutions that have been analyzed (Hambidge and Walravens, 1976) have had zinc concentrations less than 10 μg/100 ml, which is inadequate for the infant and young child maintained on total parenteral hyperalimentation. Administration of an additional 20–40 μg zinc i.v./kg body weight per day is necessary to reverse the hypozincemia resulting from the use of these solutions (Hambidge, 1974).

NUTRITIONAL ZINC DEFICIENCY IN CHILDREN IN THE UNITED STATES

In 1972, a number of Denver children from middle-income families were reported to show evidence of symptomatic zinc deficiency (Hambidge *et al.*, 1972). Of a group of 132 children, aged 4–16 years, 10 had hair zinc concentrations less than 70 μg/g, or more than 3 S.D. below the normal adult mean. Of these 10 children, 8 were found to have heights at or below the 10th percentile on the Iowa Growth Charts, though the children included in this study were not preselected according to height. There was no apparent cause for the relatively poor growth. Most of the children with low hair zinc levels in the original Denver study had a history of poor appetite. In particular, the consumption of meats was very limited despite access to larger quantities. Since animal products are the best source of available zinc, it is quite possible that the dietary zinc intake of these children was inadequate.

Another feature manifested by these children was hypogeusia (impaired taste acuity). Tests were repeated 1–3 months after commencing dietary zinc supplementation (0.2–0.4. mg Zn/kg body weight per day), and taste acuity became normal in every case. This improvement could not be attributed to placebo effect (Schechter *et al.,* 1972). Hair zinc levels increased concurrently with the improvement in taste acuity. The rapid response to small quantities of supplemented zinc provided evidence for a preexisting nutritional deficiency of this metal.

Long considered impossible, it has been calculated recently that substantial sections of the population of the United States are at risk from suboptimal zinc nutrition (Sandstead, 1973). Those at particular risk from a deficiency of this metal include subjects whose zinc requirements are relatively high—e.g., those in periods of rapid growth—and people subsisting on low-income diets. Another study in Denver was carried out in children from low-income families. In 29 young children enrolled in the Denver Head Start program, heights, with only three exceptions, were below the 3rd percentile. The mean hair zinc level of this group was significantly lower than that of children of the same age from middle- and upper-income families, and 43% had hair zinc levels less than 70 μg/g. The mean plasma zinc concentration and the mean rate of zinc secretion in parotid saliva were also significantly lower than normal. Satisfactory measurements of taste acuity were achieved in 6 children, and objective hypogeusia was present in each case.

Serum vitamin A was decreased in 33% of these children (< 20 μg/100 ml). Zinc depletion in the rat prevents normal release of vitamin A from the liver, resulting in low serum levels of this vitamin (Smith *et al.,* 1973); thus, it is conceivable that low serum vitamin A levels were related to hypozincemia in children. These children had received supplemental iron for 3 months prior to this study and were not anemic. Total serum protein and serum albumin levels were normal in each case.

ZINC DEFICIENCY IN INFANTS

Hair and plasma zinc levels are low in infants in the United States in comparison with other age groups including the neonate, older children, and adults (Hambidge *et al.,* 1972; Henkin *et al.,* 1973). In the Denver survey, the mean hair zinc level was only 74 ± 8 μg/g for the 26 apparently normal infants, aged 3–12 months, compared with 174 ± 8 μg/g for neonates and 180 ± 4 μg/g for adults. Of these infants from middle- and upper-income families, 54% had hair zinc levels of less than 70 μg/g. Exceptionally low hair zinc levels were also noted in infants residing in Dayton, Ohio (Strain *et al.,* 1966a,b). It is unlikely that these low levels are normal for this age, since levels are not equally low in other countries where comparable data have been obtained. For example, in Thailand, the mean hair zinc level of 15 infants from upper socioeconomic levels was 202 ± 26 μg/g; no source of external contamination could be identified in Bangkok to account for these higher levels. Hair zinc concentrations of adults in Thailand were closely comparable to those of Denver adults (Hambidge *et al.,* 1974), but age-related differences in the younger children as well as in infants were very different from those in Denver (Fig. 22). These discrepancies indicate that variations with age are not related directly to age, and that the low levels in Denver infants cannot necessarily be accepted as physiological.

Similar considerations apply equally to the low plasma zinc levels reported for infants in this country (Henkin *et al.,* 1973). Plasma zinc concentrations in infants in Sweden (Berfenstam, 1952a,b) and Germany (Hellwege, 1971) were reported to be similar to those for adults in these countries.

Factors such as difficulty in achieving positive zinc balance in early postnatal life (Bergmann and Fomon, 1974; Cavell and Widdowson, 1964) and a "dilutional" effect of rapid growth may contribute to zinc depletion

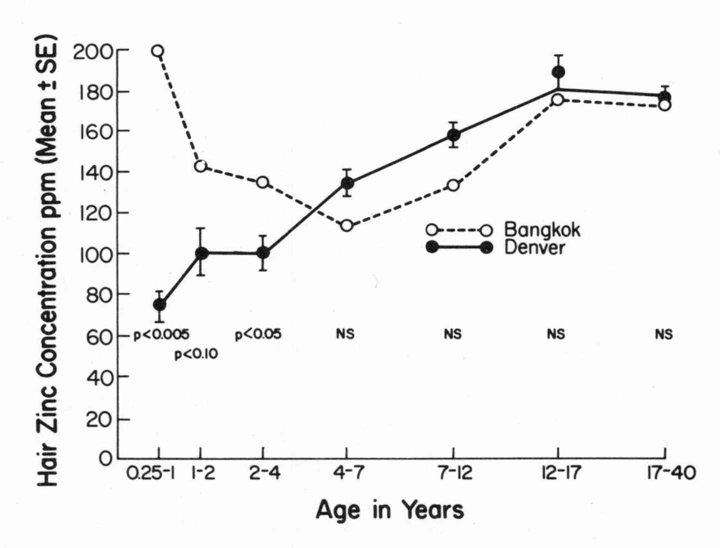

Fig. 22. Mean hair zinc concentrations of normal subjects from middle- and upper-income families in Denver and Bangkok. From Hambidge and Walravens (1976).

in infants. A unique factor in the United States that may contribute to zinc deficiency is the low concentration of this element in certain popular infant milk formulas. Formulas in which the protein content of the original cow's milk is reduced to levels comparable to those of human milk have a parallel reduction in zinc content. Unless supplemented with zinc, these formulas typically have a zinc concentration of less than 2 mg/liter, or approximately half that of cow's milk and of human milk during the first 2 months of lactation. Zinc supplementation of all these formulas has not been routine. It is likely that these formulas will be supplemented with zinc in the near future, following the recent recommendations of the Food and Nutrition Board of the National Academy of Sciences with respect to zinc intake in infants (*Recommended Dietary Allowances,* 1974).

The majority of infants from Denver with low levels of zinc in plasma and hair have not had any detectable signs of zinc deficiency. It appears, however, that those at the lower end of a spectrum of zinc depletion, as manifested by low levels of hair and plasma zinc, and perhaps those who remain moderately depleted for a prolonged period of time, do develop symptomatic zinc deficiency. In the original Denver study, 8 of 93 infants and children aged less than 4 years had hair zinc levels less than 30 ppm, and 6 of these manifested declining growth percentiles and poor appetite (Hambidge *et al.,* 1972). It was noted also that the high percentiles of the older children with hair zinc levels less than 70 μg/g first declined during infancy; thus, if their poor growth resulted from an insufficiency of this nutrient, the latter must have commenced during infancy. It is conceivable that once a deficiency state has been established, the resulting anorexia may tend to perpetuate the deficient state. Experience with a number of infants who have had low levels of zinc in plasma and hair, and who have responded favorably to zinc supplementation, indicates that some cases of failure to thrive in infancy may be caused by zinc deficiency. Anorexia has been a prominent feature in these infants, and one case manifested a bizarre form of pica that improved dramatically following zinc supplementation (Hambidge and Silverman, 1973). Currently, however, there is a lack of controlled studies of dietary zinc supplementation in these infants.

DIAGNOSIS OF ZINC DEFICIENCY IN MAN

The laboratory criteria for the diagnosis of zinc deficiency are not completely well established. The response to therapy with zinc is probably the most reliable index for making a diagnosis of the zinc-deficient state in man.

Low levels of plasma zinc have been observed in patients with many disease states (Table XXII). It is not certain at present whether a low level of plasma zinc is indicative of "zinc deficiency" in all these conditions. It

Table XXII. Possible Causes of Conditioned Zinc Deficiency in Man

1. Nutritional factors—excessive intake: phytate, fiber, alcohol, geophagia, and laundry starch
2. Cirrhosis of the liver
3. Gastrointestinal disorders
   Malabsorption syndrome
4. Chronic renal disease
5. Burns
6. Chronically debilitated states including malignancy
7. Parasitic infestations
   Hookworm
8. Iatrogenic causes
   Antimetabolites and antianabolic agents
   Penicillamine therapy
   Prolonged intravenous therapy
9. Diabetes
10. Collagen diseases
11. Pregnancy and use of oral contraceptive agents
12. Genetic disorders
    Sickle cell disease
    Acrodermatitis enteropathica

seems likely that a low plasma zinc reflects an impaired zinc nutriture in many, while in others it may reflect a shift of zinc from the plasma to another body pool. In acute infections and myocardial infarction, one may see a drop in the plasma zinc level that is most likely related to a shift of zinc from the plasma pool to the tissues.

The concentration of zinc in hair appears to reflect chronic zinc nutriture (Prasad, 1966; Hambidge and Walravens, 1976; Sandstead *et al.*, 1976). Hair zinc, however, does not reflect changes in the status of zinc on an acute basis. Similar remarks apply with respect to zinc in the red cells. Inasmuch as these cells are not turning over rapidly, their zinc content cannot be expected to reflect acute changes taking place in the body as a result of altered zinc nutriture. In terms of the assessment of zinc status in man, perhaps leukocyte or platelet zinc determination may prove to be useful; at present, however, only limited data are available, and more investigation is therefore needed.

Excretion of zinc in the urine decreases as deficiency of zinc progresses (Prasad, 1966). This test, however, requires a complete collection of urine on a 24-hr basis. Although in most cases zinc deficiency in man is associated with hypozincuria, there may be certain exceptions. In cirrhosis of the liver and sickle cell disease, although deficiency of zinc may be present, these conditions are usually associated with hyperzincuria. The mechanism of hyperzincuria in these diseases remains to be elucidated.

Hyperzincuria has also been observed to occur in certain renal diseases and infections and following injury, burns, and acute starvation (Pories *et al.*, 1976; Spencer *et al.*, 1976).

Metabolic balance study and turnover rate and 24-hr exchangeable pool for zinc, as measured by ^{65}Zn may provide additional tools for assessing zinc status in man (Prasad *et al.*, 1963b; Reinhold *et al.*, 1973a,b). Zinc-balance study, though difficult, may provide a good basis for assessment of zinc status, and a positive retention of zinc by human subjects would be indicative of zinc deficiency. By the use of ^{65}Zn, it was shown that in zinc deficiency, plasma zinc turnover was increased, the 24-hr exchangeable pool was decreased, and cummulative excretion of ^{65}Zn in the urine and the stool was low (Sandstead *et al.*, 1967). Unfortunately, the half-life of ^{65}Zn is 245 days, and thus this isotope is not regularly available for clinical use.

Urinary sulfate excretion is enhanced following an injection of [^{35}S]-cystine to zinc-deficient rats, presumably due to their inability to utilize sulfur-containing amino acids for protein synthesis (Hsu, J. M., and Anthony, 1970; Somers and Underwood, 1969a). Whether or not a similar approach will be fruitful in man remains to be tested. Undoubtedly, further work is needed to establish tests that may be considered definitive for making a diagnosis of zinc deficiency in man.

The activities of certain zinc-dependent enzymes may be measured in the plasma. In our experience, a good correlation between zinc status and the activity of ribonuclease (RNase) has been observed (Prasad *et al.*, 1975a). We have also observed an increase in the activity of plasma alkaline phosphatase following zinc supplementation to subjects with zinc deficiency (Prasad *et al.*, 1961, 1963b; Prasad, 1966), which may provide additional evidence retrospectively for making a diagnosis of zinc deficiency in man.

CONDITIONED DEFICIENCY OF ZINC IN MAN

Nutritional Factors

All the conditioned factors listed in Table XXII, with the exception of alcohol, probably influence zinc nutriture by making zinc unavailable for absorption. The formation of insoluble complexes with calcium and phytate in the alkaline intestinal environment has been shown to markedly decrease the availability of zinc for intestinal absorption by experimental animals (Oberleas *et al.*, 1966). Dietary fiber has also been shown to decrease the availability of zinc for intestinal absorption by man (Reinhold *et al.*, 1976). It seems probable that both dietary phytate and fiber may contribute to the occurrence of zinc deficiency in populations that subsist largely on bread and other foods rich in fiber and phytate (Reinhold *et al.,* 1976; Reinhold, 1971).

The effects on human zinc nutriture of EDTA and polyphosphates that may be added to foods during processing are unknown. In the rat, EDTA has a beneficial effect on zinc absorption (Oberleas *et al.,* 1966). However, it also increases excretion of zinc in the urine (Stand *et al.,* 1962). The net effect of EDTA on animals fed zinc-deficient diets containing soybean protein is beneficial rather than harmful (Vohra and Kratzer, 1964).

Geophagia (clay-eating) is known to contribute to the occurrence of dwarfism in Iran (Halsted *et al.,* 1972). Clay probably complexes zinc in much the same manner as it binds iron (Minnich *et al.,* 1968). It is unknown whether clay-eating by pregnant black women in certain areas of the United States has a significant effect on their zinc nutriture. Laundry starch is included in Table XXII because iron deficiency is known to occur in women who consume it in large amounts. Whether zinc deficiency also occurs in such persons is not known, although the probability seems high.

Alcohol induces an increase in the urinary excretion of zinc (Helwig *et al.,* 1966; Sullivan, 1962a). The mechanism is unknown. A direct effect of alcohol on the renal tubular epithelium may be responsible for hyperzincuria. Acute ingestion of alcohol did not induce hyperzincuria in one experiment (Sullivan, 1962b); another group of investigators, however, reported increased urinary zinc excretion following alcohol ingestion (Gudbjarnason and Prasad, 1969).

Liver Disease

Vallee *et al.* (1956, 1957) initially described the abnormal zinc metabolism that occurs in patients with alcoholic cirrhosis. These investigators demonstrated that patients with cirrhosis had low serum zinc, diminished hepatic zinc, and, paradoxically, hyperzincuria. These observations led them to suggest that zinc deficiency in the alcoholic cirrhotic patient may be a conditioned deficiency that is somehow related to alcohol ingestion.

The initial observation that cirrhotic patients had low serum and hepatic zinc levels and hyperzincuria has been corroborated in many laboratories (Sullivan, 1962a,b; Van Peenen and Lucas, 1961; Van Peenen and Patel, 1964; Sullivan and Lankford, 1962, 1965; Sullivan *et al.,* 1969; Sullivan and Heaney, 1970; Kahn *et al.,* 1965; Prasad *et al.,* 1965; Halsted *et al.,* 1968a; Sinha and Gabrielli, 1970; Boyett and Sullivan, 1970). Thus, the initial observations seem to be firmly established, although there is some variance of opinion as to how often such phenomena occur in cirrhosis and other liver diseases. Kahn *et al.* (1965) reported that 4 of 11 patients with viral hepatitis had elevated urinary zinc and 8 of 10 had at least one serum zinc that was above normal levels. Halsted *et al.* (1968a) found that the plasma zinc was decreased in 6 patients with viral hepatitis. Henkin and Smith (1972) studied 19 patients with viral hepatitis and found a significantly decreased serum zinc and a normal serum copper during the early stages of the illness. As the hepatitis subsided, the serum zinc rose to normal levels and the serum copper increased significantly. Initially, patients had hyperzincuria and hypercupruria. Both urinary abnormalities reverted to normal as the hepatitis subsided.

Normal subjects excreted 322 ± 167 μg (mean ± 1 S.D.) urinary zinc/24 hr, and the serum values were 94 ± 11 g/100 ml (Sullivan, 1962a; Sullivan and Lankford, 1965). In 53 of 124 alcoholic patients, the mean normal urinary excretion exceeded 700 μg/24 hr. In 21 of 30 alcoholic patients, serum zinc was less than 70 μg/100 ml (Sullivan and Lankford, 1965). In the majority of the alcoholic patients with hyperzincuria, the abnormal zinc excretion reverted to normal within 1–2 weeks following alcohol abstention and an adequate diet.

The incidence of low serum zinc and hyperzincuria in cirrhosis varies somewhat from one series to the other. Kahn *et al.* (1965) found these abnormalities of zinc metabolism only in the most severely ill cirrhotic patients who were classified as decompensated.

Patek and Haig (1939) showed that some cirrhotic patients had night blindness that did not improve with vitamin A therapy. One may speculate that retinol-binding protein may be zinc-dependent, and that zinc administration may therefore be required to correct night blindness in cirrhotic subjects.

Several interesting studies have been directed at elucidating the role of zinc in the pathogenesis of liver disease. Kahn and Ozeran (1967) chronically injected rats with carbon tetrachloride to produce cirrhosis and found that these cirrhotic animals had low serum zinc and diminished levels of hepatic zinc. In another study, Kahn *et al.* (1968) demonstrated low serum zinc and enhanced uptake of ^{65}Zn by the cirrhotic livers of carbon tetrachloride-treated rats. These studies seemed to indicate a decreased pool size of zinc and thus implied true zinc deficiency. Kinetic studies of ^{65}Zn in ten human cirrhotics also suggested a diminished pool size and a slower turnover of zinc (Sullivan and Heaney, 1970). Voigt and Saldeen (1965), Saldeen and Brunk (1967), Saldeen (1969), and Srinivasan and Balwani (1969) showed that zinc salts protect rat liver from damage by carbon tetrachloride.

Chvapil *et al.* (1972) showed that zinc inhibits lipid peroxidation of membranes and thereby stabilizes them. Such an effect protects hepatic cells and their organelles against injury. Further studies are required to show: (1) whether cellular injury results in the zinc loss from the body or (2) whether zinc loss from the body (and the mechanism for the loss) occurs first, resulting in enhanced lability of the cells to injury.

Gastrointestinal Disorders

Of the variety of mechanisms proposed for zinc deficiency in patients with gastrointestinal disease, steatorrhea may be the most common. In an alkaline environment, zinc would be expected to form insoluble complexes with fat and phosphate analogous to those formed by calcium and magnesium. Thus, fat malabsorption due to any cause should result in an increased loss of zinc in the stool. Zinc deficiency was reported in patients with steatorrhea (MacMahon *et al.,* 1968), and low concentrations of plasma zinc were observed in patients with disease known to cause steatorrhea (Halsted and Smith, 1970). Thus, although metabolic studies have been limited, it seems reasonable to assume that steatorrhea may significantly influence zinc nutrition. In patients with achlorhydria, the formation of zinc soaps and other insoluble zinc chelates may be potentiated.

Another potential cause of impaired absorption of zinc may be a lack of "zinc-binding factor." Recent studies (Evans, 1976) indicate that a zinc-binding ligand is secreted into the intestinal lumen by the pancreas in experimental animals. The ligand appears to facilitate the uptake of zinc by intestinal epithelial cells. At present, it is unknown whether a lack of the zinc-binding ligand in man may have contributed to the occurrence of low plasma zinc concentration in the patients with cystic fibrosis of the pancreas and growth retardation (Halsted and Smith, 1970). Recently, Kowarski *et al.* (1974) isolated from rat jejunal mucosa a soluble zinc-binding protein that is apparently involved in active transport of zinc across the intestinal mucosa. Whether or not such a mechanism for zinc absorption exists in man has not been demonstrated. If indeed a specific protein in the small intestine is needed for zinc absorption in man, one may speculate that a lack of this protein may cause malabsorption of zinc.

Exudation of large amounts of zinc protein complexes into the intestinal lumen may also contribute to the decrease in plasma zinc concentrations that occur in patients with inflammatory disease of the bowel. It seems likely that protein-losing enteropathy due to other causes may also impair zinc homeostasis.

Hyperzincuria and Renal Disease

Increased urinary losses of zinc may occur in some patients with cirrhosis and other types of liver disease (Vallee *et al.,* 1957, 1959; Stand *et al.,* 1962; Sullivan, 1962a; Sullivan and Lankford, 1962), and sickle cell disease (Prasad *et al.,* 1975a). Presumably, the tubular reabsorption of zinc is decreased. One might expect the failure of zinc tubular reabsorption to be mediated by aldosterone. A limited study suggests, however, that aldosterone does not influence zinc excretion (Szadkowski *et al.,* 1969). Patients with cirrhosis and sickle cell disease who excrete large amounts of zinc in their urine may have an increased risk of zinc deficiency, particularly if they consume diets that are limited in animal protein, since the level of dietary zinc is correlated with dietary protein (Schlage and Worberg, 1972; Osis *et al.*, 1972).

The potential causes of conditioned deficiency of zinc in patients with renal disease include proteinuria (Underwood, 1977) and failure of tubular reabsorption. In the former instance, the loss of zinc–protein complexes across the glomerulus is the mechanism. In the latter, an impairment in the metabolic machinery of tubular reabsorption would result in zinc loss.

In patients with renal failure (Halsted and Smith, 1970; Rose and Willden, 1972; Mansouri *et al.*, 1970), the occurrence of conditioned zinc deficiency may be the result of a mixture of factors that are not well defined. If 1,25-dihydroxycholecalciferol plays a role in the intestinal absorption of zinc, an impairment in its formation by the diseased kidney would be expected to result in malabsorption of zinc. It seems likely that plasma and soft tissue concentrations of zinc may not be affected adversely in some persons with renal failure, inasmuch as the dissolution of bone that occurs as a result of increased parathyroid activity in response to low serum calcium would contribute to an increase of zinc in the plasma pool. In experimental animals, calcium deficiency was shown to cause release of zinc from bone (Hurley and Tao, 1972). In some patients who are successfully treated for hyperphosphatemia and hypocalcemia, the plasma zinc concentration may be expected to decline due to the deposition of zinc along with calcium in bone (Heth *et al.*, 1966; Haumont, 1961). Thus, in the latter group, a diet low in protein and high in refined cereal products and fat would be expected to contribute to a conditioned deficiency of zinc. Such a diet would be low in zinc (Schlage and Worberg, 1972; Osis *et al.*, 1972; Schroeder, 1971). The patients reported by Mansouri *et al.* (1970), who were treated with a diet containing 20–30 g protein daily and who had low plasma concentrations of zinc, appear to represent such a clinical instance. Presumably, the patients of Halsted and Smith (1970) were similarly restricted in dietary protein. In other patients with renal failure whose dietary protein was not restricted, plasma zinc concentrations were not decreased (Rose and Willden, 1972). Patients on dialysis had higher levels of plasma zinc, particularly following dialysis. Apparently, zinc deficiency may not be a problem in patients on dialysis if their dietary consumption of protein is not restricted.

Burns and Skin Disorders

The causes of zinc deficiency in patients with burns include losses in exudates (Henzel *et al.*, 1970; Cohen, I. K., *et al.*, 1973; Nielsen and Jemec, 1968; Cuthbertson *et al.*, 1972). Starvation of patients with burns is a well-recognized cause of morbidity and mortality. The contribution of conditioned zinc deficiency to the morbidity of burned patients is not defined. Limited studies indicate that epithelialization of burns may be improved by treatment with zinc (Henzel *et al.,* 1970; Nielsen and Jemec, 1968; Sandstead *et al.,* 1970a). Such a finding is consistent with the beneficial effect of zinc on the treatment of leg ulcers (Husain, 1969; Serjeant *et al.,* 1970; Greaves, 1972a; Haeger *et al.,* 1972; Oberleas *et al.,* 1971), and with the well-defined requirement of zinc for collagen synthesis (Fernandez-Madrid *et al.,* 1973).

In psoriasis, the loss of large numbers of skin cells may result in zinc depletion. The skin contains approximately 20% of the body zinc. Thus, if the loss of epithelial cells is great enough, it is conceivable that the massive formation of new cells by the skin could lead to conditioned deficiency. Low levels of plasma zinc were reported in some patients with extensive psoriasis (Greaves and Boyde, 1967; Greaves, 1972a); however, others were not able to confirm these findings (Portnoy and Molokhia, 1971, 1972).

Impaired Wound Healing in Chronically Diseased Subjects

In 1966, Pories and collaborators (Pories *et al.,* 1967a,b; Pories and Strain, 1966) reported that oral administration of zinc sulfate to military personnel with marsupialized pilonidal sinuses was attended by a twofold increase in the rate of reepithelialization. The authors' conclusion that zinc can promote the healing of cutaneous sores and wounds has been controversial during the past several years. As summarized in Table XXIII, clinical investigations by C. Cohen (1968), Husain (1969), Greaves and Skillen (1970), and Serjeant *et al.* (1970) substantiated the beneficial effects of zinc on wound healing, whereas studies by Barcia (1970), Myers and Cherry (1970), Clayton (1972), and Greaves and Ive (1972) failed to demonstrate any therapeutic benefit. Hallböök and Lanner (1972) found that the reepithelialization rate of venous leg ulcers was enhanced by zinc in patients who initially had diminished concentrations of serum zinc, but they did not find any benefit in patients whose initial measurements of serum zinc were within the normal range. On the other hand, Husain *et al.* (1970) did not observe any relationship between response to zinc treatment of venous leg ulcers and the initial level of plasma zinc.

Studies in experimental animals demonstrated that (1) healing of incised wounds is impaired in rats with dietary zinc deficiency (Oberleas *et al.,* 1971; Rahmat *et al.,* 1974; Sandstead *et al.,* 1970b; Sandstead and Shepard, 1968); (2) collagen and noncollagen proteins are reduced in skin and connective tissues from rats with dietary zinc deficiency (Fernandez-Madrid *et al.,* 1973; McClain *et al.,* 1973; Stephan and Hsu, 1973); (3) zinc supplementation does *not* augment wound healing in normal rats (Groundwater and MacLeod, 1970; Lee and Green, 1972); and (4) zinc supplemen-

Table XXIII. Clinical Trials of Oral $ZnSO_4$ in Healing of Sores[a]

Investigator	Lesions	Number of patients		Observation on reepithelialization rate
		Controls	Treated	
Pories *et al.* (1967a,b)	Pilonidal sinus	10	10	Twofold increase vs. controls
C. Cohen (1968)	Bedsores	0	6	Improvement
Husain (1969)	Leg ulcers	52	52[b]	Twofold increase vs. controls
Barcia (1970)	Pilonidal sinus	10	10	No influence vs. controls
Greaves and Skillen (1970)	Leg ulcers	0	18	Complete healing in 11 patients; partial healing in 7 patients
Serjeant *et al.* (1970)	Leg ulcers	17	17[b]	Threefold increase vs. controls
Myers and Cherry (1970)	Leg ulcers	16	16[b]	No influence vs. controls
Clayton (1972)	Leg ulcers	5	5[b]	Slower in treated vs. controls
Greaves and Ive (1972)	Leg ulcers	18	18[b]	No influence vs. controls
Hallböök and Lanner (1972)	Leg ulcers	14	13	Fourfold increase vs. controls in patients with low serum Zn; no influence vs. controls in patients with normal serum Zn

[a] $ZnSO_4$, 220 mg three times daily.
[b] Double-blind study.

tation *does* augment wound healing in chronically ill rats (Elias and Chvapil, 1973). These data provide evidence that zinc supplementation may promote wound healing in zinc-deficient patients.

Neoplastic Disease

The occurrence of conditioned deficiency of zinc in patients with neoplastic disease will obviously depend on the nature of the neoplasm (Davies, I. J. T., 1972; Gul'ko, 1961). Anorexia and starvation (Henzel *et al.*, 1970), plus avoidance of foods rich in available zinc, are probably important conditioning factors. An increased excretion of zinc subsequent to its mobilization by leukocyte endogenous mediator (LEM) (Pekarek *et al.*, 1972) in response to tissue necrosis may be another factor (Lindeman *et al.*, 1972).

Parasitic Infestations

Parasitic diseases that cause blood loss may contribute to conditioned deficiency of zinc. Such appears to have been the case in the zinc-responsive "dwarfs" reported from Egypt (Prasad *et al.*, 1963a,b). Since red blood cells contain 12–14 μg zinc/ml, infections with hookworm that are severe enough to cause iron deficiency will probably contribute to the occurrence of zinc deficiency.

Iatrogenic Causes

Possible iatrogenic causes of conditioned deficiency of zinc include use of antimetabolites and antianabolic drugs (Flynn *et al.,* 1971). Treatment with some of these drugs makes patients feel ill. They become anorectic and may starve. With catabolism of body mass, urinary excretion of zinc is increased (Cuthbertson *et al.,* 1972). Commonly used intravenous fluids are relatively zinc-free. Thus, under usual circumstances, a negative zinc balance should occur in patients who are given antimetabolites, antianabolic agents, or prolonged intravenous therapy.

Failure to include zinc in fluids for total intravenous feeding (TPN) is another example of iatrogenically induced conditioned deficiency of zinc. A decline of plasma zinc was observed in some patients given TPN fluids containing less than 1.25 mg zinc daily (Sandstead *et al.,* 1976). A recent report indicates that excessive losses of urinary zinc (up to 24 mg/day) during intravenous alimentation may occur (Van Rij *et al.,* 1975). This loss may be related to hyperaminoaciduria, inasmuch as several amino acids have great affinity for binding of zinc (Prasad and Oberleas, 1970a).

Zinc deficiency occurring in a patient following penicillamine therapy for Wilson's disease was reported recently (Klingberg *et al.,* 1976). The manifestations consisted of parakeratosis, ''dead'' hair and alopecia, keratitis, and centrocecal scotoma. Following supplementation with zinc, several clinical manifestations were reversed.

Diabetes

Some patients with diabetes mellitus have been found to have increased urinary losses of zinc (Tarui, 1963; Pidduck *et al.,* 1970). The mechanism is unknown. Perhaps the failure of some diabetics to heal ulcers of their feet and elsewhere is related to zinc deficiency. Healing of such ulcers in diabetes was reported subsequent to zinc therapy (Henzel *et al.,* 1970). Further studies are needed to establish zinc deficiency in diabetes and the role of zinc in therapy of leg ulcers in diabetic patients.

Collagen Diseases

In patients with inflammation such as rheumatoid arthritis, lupus erythematosus (McCall *et al.,* 1971), infection, or injury, two factors may lead to zinc deficiency. The loss of zinc from catabolized tissue (Cuthbertson *et al.*, 1972) and mobilization of zinc by LEM (Pekarek *et al.*, 1972) to the liver and its subsequent excretion in the urine may account for conditioned zinc deficiency in such cases. Detailed investigations of zinc metabolism in such patients are lacking at present. Recently, Simkin (1977) showed that administration of zinc to rheumatoid arthritis patients was beneficial with respect to inflammatory manifestations of this disease. Further studies must be carried out in the future to establish a therapeutic role of zinc in this disease.

Pregnancy and Oral Contraceptives

The plasma concentration of zinc decreases in human pregnancy (Henkin *et al.*, 1971). Presumably, the decrease reflects in part the uptake of zinc by the fetus and the other products of conception. It has been estimated that a pregnant woman must retain approximately 750 μg zinc/day for growth of the products of conception during the last two thirds of pregnancy (Sandstead, 1973). Thus, when zinc deficiency occurs in pregnancy, a conditioning factor is the demand of the fetus for zinc. Studies in the rat suggest that the placenta actively provides zinc to the fetus (Sandstead *et al.*, 1970a). If the diet of the pregnant woman does not include liberal amounts of animal protein, the likelihood of conditioned deficiency of zinc is increased, since zinc is probably less available from cereal proteins (O'Dell *et al.*, 1972).

The possible importance of zinc deficiency in human pregnancy is implied by the observations reported by Hurley (1976), Caldwell *et al.* (1970), and Halas *et al.* (1976). Zinc deficiency in pregnant rats was shown to cause fetal abnormalities, behavioral impairment in the offspring, and difficulty in parturition in the mother (Hurley, 1976, 1977; Caldwell *et al.*, 1970; Halas *et al.*, 1976). Caldwell *et al.* (1970) were the first to show that in both prenatal and postnatal nutrition, even a mild zinc deficiency in rats had a profound influence on behavior potential despite an apparently adequate protein level in the diet. Zinc deficiency in fetal and suckling rats results in adverse biochemical effects in the brain (Halas *et al.*, 1976). The adverse effects on the brains of the suckling rats are apparently not readily reversible, since behavioral testing of nutritionally rehabilitated 60 to 80-day-old male rats showed that they performed poorly on a Tolman–Honzik maze (Lokken *et al.*, 1973) in comparison with pair-fed and ad-libitum-fed control rats. These findings suggested that zinc deficiency during the critical development period of the rat brain induces poorly reversible abnormalities that are manifested by impaired behavioral development.

Hurley and co-workers (Hurley, 1976) showed that short-term depletion of zinc in maternal rats results in a wide variety of congenital anomalies in the offspring. In view of the important role of zinc in nucleic acid metabolism, Hurley and Shrader (1972) proposed that impaired DNA synthesis in zinc-deprived embryos prolongs the mitotic cycle and reduces the number of normal neural cells, leading to malformations of the central nervous system. It is tempting to speculate that the exceptionally high rates of congenital malformations of the central nervous system as reported from the Middle East (Damyanov and Dutz, 1971) might be caused by maternal zinc deficiency.

Human amniotic fluid was shown to contain an inorganic bacterial inhibitory component that was identified as zinc (Schlievert *et al.*, 1976a,b). The average zinc concentration in amniotic fluid was found to be 0.44 μg/ml. The phosphate concentration of amniotic fluid appeared to determine the expression of zinc inhibitory activity. The average phosphate concentration was found to be 92 μg/ml. For 22 fluids tested, a phosphate/zinc ratio of 100 or less predicted a bactericidal fluid. A ratio between 100 and 200 predicted a bacteriostatic fluid, whereas a ratio greater than 200 was noninhibitory. These observations may have clinical significance if indeed maternal zinc nutrition affects the concentration of zinc in the amniotic fluid.

Plasma zinc is known to decrease following use of oral contraceptive agents (Prasad *et al.*, 1975c; Halsted *et al.*, 1968b; O'Leary and Spellacy, 1969). Our recent data indicate that whereas the plasma zinc may decline, the zinc content of the red blood cells increases as a result of administration of oral contraceptive agents. This phenomenon may merely mean a redistribution of zinc from the plasma pool to the red cells. Alternatively, oral contraceptive agents may enhance synthesis of carbonic anhydrase (a zinc metalloenzyme), thus increasing the red-cell zinc content.

Genetic Disorders

Sickle Cell Disease. Recently, deficiency of zinc in sickle cell disease was recognized (Prasad *et al.*, 1975a). Certain clinical features are common to some sickle cell anemia patients and zinc-deficient patients, the latter as reported from the Middle East (Prasad, 1966; Prasad *et al.*, 1975a). These features include delayed onset of puberty and hypogonadism in the male, characterized by decreased facial, pubic, and axillary hair; short stature and low body weight; rough skin; and poor appetite (Fig. 23). Inasmuch as zinc is an important constituent of erythrocytes, it appeared possible that long-continued hemolysis in patients with sickle cell disease might lead to a zinc-deficient state, which could account for some of the clinical manifestations mentioned above. Delayed healing of leg ulcers and the reported beneficial effect of zinc therapy on leg ulcers in sickle cell anemia patients would also appear to be consistent with this hypothesis (Fig. 23).

In a study reported by Prasad *et al.* (1975a), zinc in plasma, erythro-

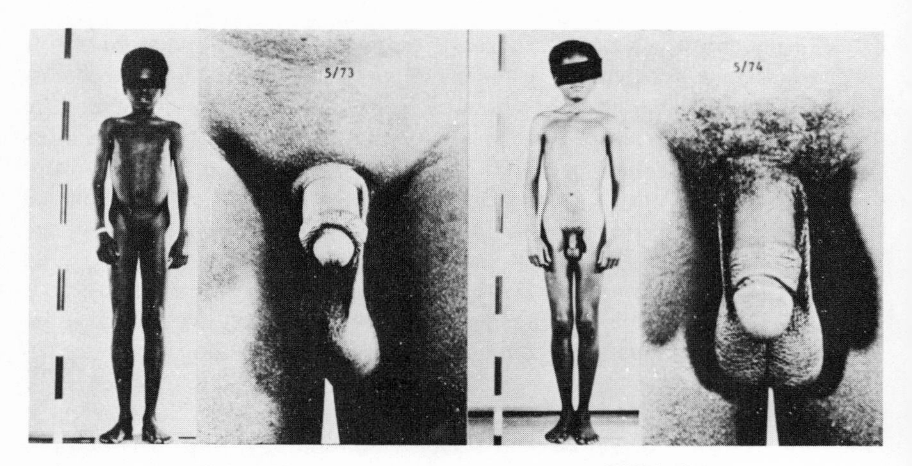

MAY 1973
144 cm.

BEFORE Zn THERAPY

MAY 1974
149 cm.

AFTER Zn THERAPY

Fig. 23. A sickle cell anemia patient, before and after zinc therapy. Changes in external genitalia and growth of pubic hair as a result of therapy are evident. From Prasad *et al.* (1975a).

cytes, and hair was decreased and urinary zinc excretion was increased in sickle cell anemia patients as compared with controls (Table XXIV). Erythrocyte zinc and daily urinary zinc excretion were inversely correlated in the anemia patients ($r = -0.71$, $p < 0.05$), suggesting that hyperzincuria may have caused zinc deficiency in these patients (Fig. 24). Carbonic anhydrase, a zinc metalloenzyme, correlated significantly with erythrocyte zinc ($r = +0.94$, $p < 0.001$) (Fig. 25). Plasma RNase activity was signifi-

Table XXIV. Zinc in Plasma, Erythrocyte, Hair, and Urine, and RNase Activity in Plasma of Sickle Cell Anemia Patients and Controls[a]

	Zinc in:				
	Plasma (μg/100 ml)	Erythrocytes (μg/g Hb)	Hair (μg/g)	Urine (μg/g creatinine)	Plasma RNase (ΔA/min per ml)
Controls	112 ± 2.5 (23)	41.7 ± 1.2 (23)	193 ± 4.3 (17)	495 ± 35 (10)	0.310 ± 0.001 (16)
Patients	102 ± 2.7 (32)	35.2 ± 1.6 (27)	149 ± 10.3 (21)	739 ± 60 (12)	0.435 ± 0.002 (31)
P	< 0.025	< 0.01	< 0.01	< 0.01	< 0.001

[a]From Prasad *et al.* (1975a). Values are means ± S.E. The numbers in parentheses are the numbers of subjects. At least three 24-hr urines were collected from each subject.

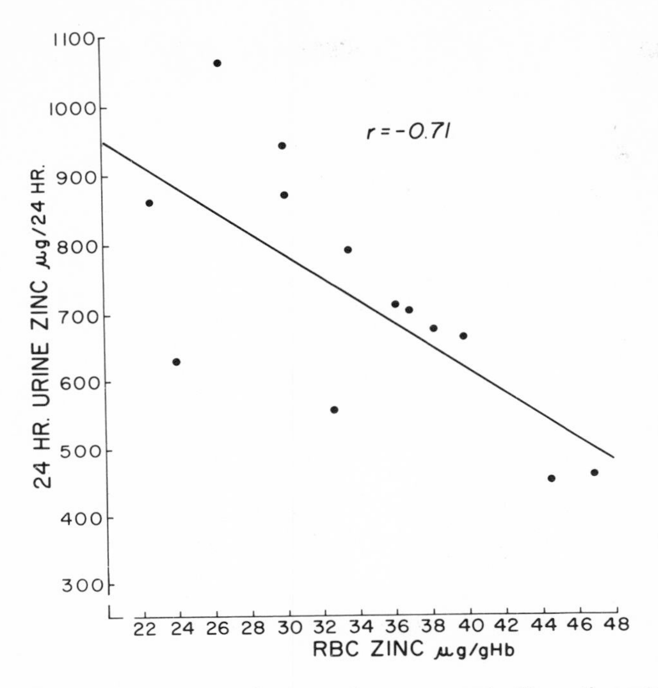

Fig. 24. Twenty-four-hour urinary zinc excretion compared with erythrocyte zinc content of sickle cell disease patients. From Prasad *et al.* (1975a).

cantly greater in anemia subjects than in controls, consistent with the hypothesis that sickle cell anemia patients were zinc-deficient. Zinc sulfate (660 mg/day) was administered orally to seven men and two women with sickle cell disease. Two 17-year-old males gained 10 cm in height during 18 months of therapy. All but one patient gained weight (Fig. 26). Five of the males showed increased growth of pubic, axillary, facial, and body hair, and in one, a leg ulcer healed in 6 weeks on zinc, and in two others, some benefit of zinc therapy on healing of ulcers was noted (Table XXV).

In a recent study by Abbasi *et al.* (1976), it was established that androgen deficiency in sickle cell anemia patients is a result of primary rather than secondary hypogonadism. As judged by the levels of FSH, LH, and testosterone following administration of gonadotropin-releasing hormone, it was concluded that the functions of the anterior pituitary and hypothalamus were intact. The erythrocyte and hair zinc concentrations were significantly decreased, and there was positive correlation between erythrocyte zinc and serum testosterone ($r = 0.61$, $p < 0.01$) in sickle cell anemia. Furthermore, these hormonal data in sickle cell anemia subjects were very similar to those described for zinc-deficient rats, in that in

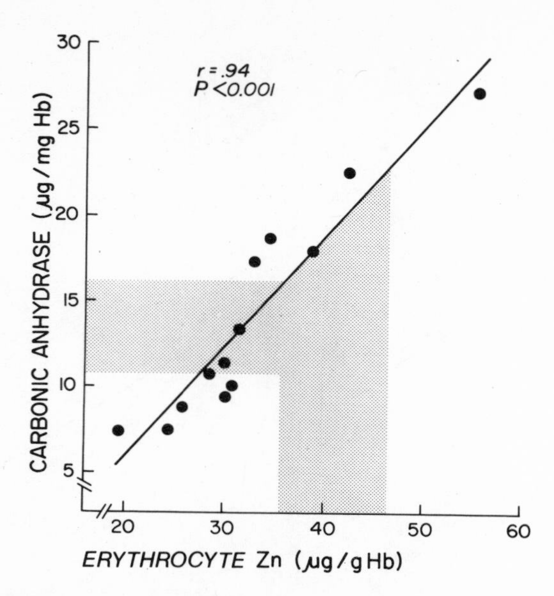

Fig. 25. Carbonic anhydrase protein and zinc content of erythrocytes in sickle cell disease patients. Shaded areas indicate mean ± SaDn for erythrocyte zinc (*vertical*) and erythrocyte carbonic anhydrase protein (*horizontal*). From Prasad *et al.* (1975a).

experimental zinc deficiency, a primary testicular failure results (Lei *et al.*, 1976).

These data show that some sickle cell anemia patients are zinc-deficient, although the severity varied considerably from one patient to another in this group. Despite the tissue zinc depletion in sickle cell anemia patients, the mean urinary excretion of zinc was higher than in the controls. This may have been directly a result of increased filtration of zinc by the glomeruli owing to continued hemolysis, or there may have been a defect in tubular reabsorption of zinc somehow related to sickle cell anemia—a possibility that cannot be excluded at present. Continued hyperzincuria may have been responsible for tissue depletion of zinc, as suggested by a significant negative correlation between values for 24-hr urinary zinc excretion and erythrocyte zinc. At this stage, however, one cannot rule out additional factors such as predominant dietary use of cereal protein and other nutritional factors that affect zinc availability adversely, thus accounting for zinc deficiency. Further work is warranted for proper elucidation of the pathogenesis of zinc deficiency in sickle cell anemia.

Recent studies have demonstrated a potential beneficial effect of zinc on the sickling process, *in vitro,* mediated by its effect on the oxygen dissocation curve (Oelshlegel *et al,* 1973, 1974) and the erythrocyte membrane (Brewer *et al.*, 1975). Zinc-bound hemoglobin has increased oxygen affinity, a normal Bohr effect, and a decreased Hill coefficient (Oelshlegel *et al.*, 1974). Theoretically, increased oxygen affinity of S hemoglobin should be beneficial to sickle cell disease patients inasmuch as this hemoglobin sickles on deoxygenation. Whether or not this zinc effect on S hemoglobin can be achieved *in vivo* remains to be seen. It is conceivable that the zinc-binding residue could be one involved with the α_1–β_2 (or α_2–β_1) contact points, which might result in decreasing the stability of the contact and favor the oxy form of hemoglobin (Oelshlegel *et al.*, 1974). More definitive studies, such as X-ray diffraction, are needed before the exact zinc-binding residue and oxygen-affinity mechanism are defined with certainty.

It has been proposed that binding of hemoglobin to the inside of the sickled red cell membrane is an important aspect of the development of the so-called irreversibly sickled cell. Calcium facilitates the binding of hemoglobin particles to the cell membrane, which leads to increased stiffness and rigidity. Zinc protects against these changes by partially blocking the

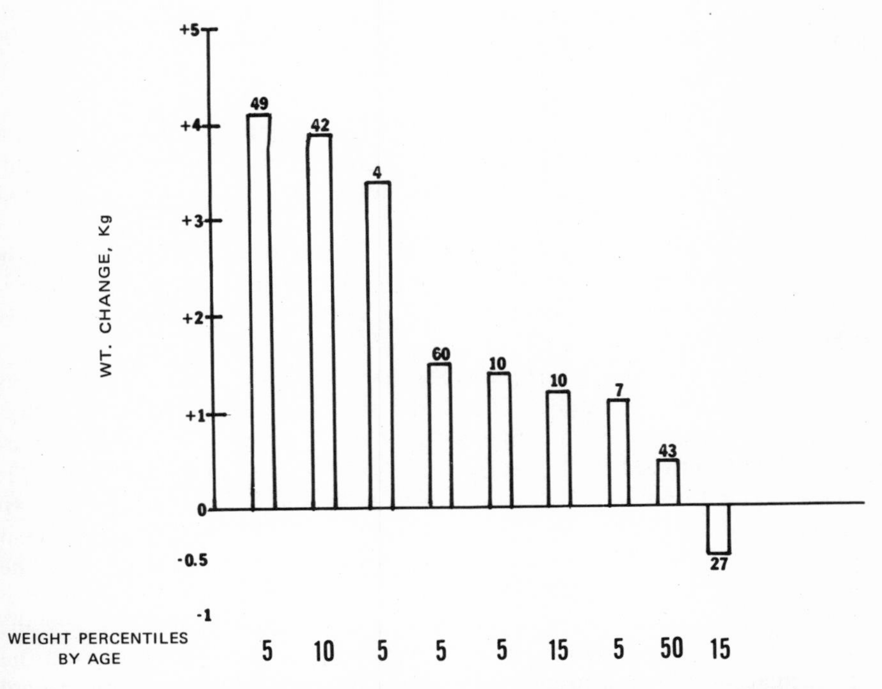

Fig. 26. Changes in body weight of sickle cell anemia patients during zinc therapy. Number of weeks each patient had been on zinc therapy is given at top of columns. From Prasad *et al.* (1975a).

Table XXV. Growth of Body Hair in Seven Sickle Cell Anemia Male Patients on Zinc Therapy[a]

Patient No.	Pubic	Axillary	Facial	Abdominal	Chest	Weeks on Zn therapy
1	0	0	0	0	0	49
	3+	1+	0	0	0	
2	2+	0	0	0	0	42
	3+	2+	1+	0	0	
3	3+	2+	1+	0	0	60
	4+	3+	3+	3+	3+	
4	3+	2+	0	0	0	10
	3+	3+	2+	2+	1+	
5	3+	2+	1+	0	0	7
	3+	2+	1+	2+	1+	
6	3+	2+	1+	0	0	43
	3+	2+	1+	0	0	
7	3+	2+	0	1	0	4
	3+	2+	0	1	0	

[a]From Prasad *et al.* (1975a). The top line of data in each set is for pretreatment; the bottom line is after the indicated number of weeks of therapy. (0) None; (1+) fine hair; (2+) definite; (3+) definite and bushy; (4+) adultlike.

binding of hemoglobin to the membrane either directly or by an interaction with calcium, and as a result, less hemoglobin is bound to the membrane in the presence of zinc, and the deformability of the cell is thereby protected (Brewer *et al.,* 1975).

In limited uncontrolled studies, zinc appears to have been effective in decreasing symptoms and crisis of sickle cell anemia patients. Undoubtedly, more thorough evaluation of zinc therapy in sickle cell disease is needed in the future.

Acrodermatitis Enteropathica. Acrodermatitis enteropathica was described in 1942 by Danbolt and Closs (1942), and the clinical and pathological features have been delineated by numerous investigators (Aguilera-Diaz, 1971; Entwisle, 1965; Freier *et al.,* 1973; Juljulian and Kurban, 1971; Perry, 1974; Robin and Goldman, 1969; Wells and Winkelmann, 1961). In brief, acrodermatitis enteropathica is a lethal, autosomal, recessive trait that usually occurs in infants of Italian, Armenian, or Iranian lineage. The disease is not present at birth, but typically develops in the early months of life, soon after weaning from breast-feeding. Dermatological manifestations include progressive bullous–pustular dermatitis of the extremities and the oral, anal, and genital areas, combined with paronychia and generalized alopecia. Infection with *Candida albicans* is a frequent complication.

Ophthalmic signs include blepharitis, conjunctivitis, photophobia, and corneal opacities. Gastrointestinal disturbances are usually severe, including chronic diarrhea, malabsorption, steatorrhea, and lactose intolerance. Neuropsychiatric signs include irritability, emotional disorders, tremor, and occasional cerebellar ataxia. The patients generally have retarded growth and hypogonadism. Prior to the serendipitous discovery of diiodohydroxyquinolone therapy in 1953 by Dillaha *et al.* (1953), patients with acrodermatitis enteropathica invariably died from cachexia, usually with terminal respiratory infection. Although diiodohydroxyquinolone has been used successfully for the therapy of this condition for 20 years, the mechanism of drug action has never been elucidated. It now seems possible that the efficacy of diiodohydroxyquinolone might be related to the formation of an absorbable zinc-chelate, inasmuch as diiodohydroxyquinolone is a derivative of 8-hydroxyquinolone, a chelating agent (Moynahan, 1966).

In 1973, Barnes and Moynahan (Moynahan and Barnes, 1973; Barnes and Moynahan, 1973) studied a 2-year-old girl with severe acrodermatitis enteropathica who was being treated with diiodohydroxyquinolone and a lactose-deficient synthetic diet. The clinical response to this therapy was not satisfactory, and the physicians sought to identify contributory factors. They found that the concentration of zinc in the patient's serum was profoundly reduced, and therefore they administered oral zinc sulfate. The skin lesions and gastrointestinal symptoms cleared completely, and the patient was discharged from the hospital. When zinc was inadvertently omitted from the child's regimen, she suffered a relapse that responded promptly to oral zinc sulfate administration. In their initial reports, Barnes and Moynahan (Mornahan and Barnes, 1973; Barnes and Moynahan, 1973) attributed zinc deficiency in this patient to the synthetic diet.

It was later appreciated that zinc might be fundamental to the pathogenesis of this rare inherited disorder, and that the clinical improvement reflected improvement in zinc status. Support for the zinc-deficiency hypothesis came from the observation that a close resemblance between the symptoms of zinc deficiency in animals and man as reported earlier (Prasad, 1966) and in subjects with acrodermatitis enteropathica existed, particularly with respect to skin lesions, growth pattern, and gastrointestinal symptoms.

Zinc supplementation for these patients led to complete clearance of skin lesions and restoration of normal bowel function, which had previously resisted various dietary and drug regimens. This original observation was quickly confirmed in other cases with equally good results (Hambidge and Walravens, 1976). The underlying mechanism of the zinc deficiency in these patients is most likely malabsorption. The cause of poor absorption is obscure, but an abnormality of Paneth's cells may be involved.

Miscellaneous Genetic Disorders. Low plasma zinc levels were noted in patients with mongolism (Halsted and Smith, 1970). The mechanism is unknown. Congenital hypoplasia of the thymus gland in cattle may be an example of zinc deficiency on a genetic basis (Brummerstedt *et al.*, 1971). It is unknown whether thymus hypoplasia in man is in some way related to zinc deficiency.

Acute Zinc Deficiency

Kay and Tasman-Jones (1975) used the term "acute zinc deficiency" in man to describe clinical features of zinc deficiency noted to occur as a result of hyperalimentation. The clinical features are very similar to those observed in patients with acrodermatitis enteropathica and in one patient with Wilson's disease who received penicillamine therapy and subsequently became zinc-deficient (Klingberg *et al.*, 1976). It appears that in all likelihood, severe dermatological manifestations of zinc deficiency are a result of the severity of depletion rather than the rapidity with which the body store of zinc is being depleted. This being the case, perhaps a clinical distinction between acute and chronic zinc deficiency may not be entirely correct.

HYPERZINCEMIA

A high level of plasma zinc was found to occur in five of seven members of one family and in two of three second-generation individuals, indicating that hyperzincemia may be genetically determined (Smith *et al.*, 1976). The increased level of plasma zinc was not accompanied by any adverse clinical features. The metabolic or absorptive defect accounting for this phenomenon remains unresolved at present.

ZINC TOXICITY

In man, three types of toxic reactions to zinc have been reported. First, "metal fume fever," characterized by pulmonary manifestations, fever, chills, and gastroenteritis, was observed to occur in industrial workers who are exposed to fumes (Papp, 1968). In the second type, toxicity was observed in a 16-year-old male who ingested 12 g zinc sulfate over a 2-day period. The toxicity was characterized by drowsiness, lethargy, and increased serum lipase and amylase levels (Murphy, 1970). The third type of acute zinc toxicity was observed in a patient with renal failure following hemodialysis. The water for hemodialysis was stored in a galvanized tank.

The patient suffered from nausea, vomiting, fever, and severe anemia (Gallery *et al.,* 1972).

In comparison with other trace elements such as lead, cadmium, arsenic, and antimony, zinc is relatively nontoxic. Many of the toxic effects attributed to zinc by early investigators may actually be due to other contaminating elements such as lead, cadmium, or arsenic (Heller and Burke, 1927). Zinc is noncommulative, and the proportion absorbed is thought to be inversely related to the amount ingested (Furchner and Richmond, 1962). Vomiting, a protective mechanism, occurs after ingestion of large quantities of zinc, and in fact 2 g zinc sulfate has been recommended as an emetic (*Merck Index,* 1960).

In addition to vomiting, the symptoms of zinc toxicity in humans include dehydration, electrolyte imbalance, abdominal pain, nausea, lethargy, dizziness, and muscular incoordination. Acute renal failure caused by zinc chloride poisoning was reported by Csata *et al.* (1968). The symptoms occurred within hours after large quantities of zinc were ingested. Death is reported to have occurred after ingestion of 45 g zinc sulfate (Osol *et al.,* 1955). This dose would be considered very massive, since the daily requirement of zinc for man is considered to be in the range of 15–30 mg.

In patients with sickle cell disease in a limited trial, 660 mg zinc sulfate was administered orally for nearly 2 years without adverse effects. On a longer-term basis, the side effects of zinc administration for therapeutic purposes remain to be elucidated. Physicians must remain cautious in the use of zinc salts for prolonged periods.

Numerous studies have examined zinc toxicity in experimental animals. These studies were reviewed by Van Reen (1966). In rats, ingestion of 0.5–1.0% zinc results in reduced growth, anemia, poor reproduction, and decreased activity of liver catalase and cytochrome oxidase. The latter could be reversed by copper administration, thus indicating that excessive intake of zinc may cause copper deficiency.

In view of the long-term clinical usage of zinc in therapeutic dosages in man for wound healing and sickle cell disease, one must remain on guard for toxic effects. It is well known that zinc and copper compete with each other for similar protein binding sites, and it is conceivable that one may induce copper deficiency in subjects receiving high amounts of zinc for several months. There may be other side effects of zinc administration in high dosage for long periods of time, but they are not recognized at present.

REFERENCES

Abbasi, A. A., Prasad, A. S., Ortega, J., Congco, E., and Oberleas, D. 1976. Gonadal function abnormalities in sickle cell anemia. *Ann. Intern. Med.* **85,** 601–605.

Aguilera-Diaz, L. F. 1971. Un nouveau symptome dans l'acrodermatite entéropathique: la demarche ataxique. *Bull. Soc. Fr. Dermatol. Syphiligr.* **78,** 259–260.

Alford, R. H. 1970. Metal cation requirements for phytohemaglutinin-induced transformation of human peripheral blood leukocytes. *J. Immunol.* **104,** 698–703.

Barcia, P. J. 1970. Lack of acceleration of healing with zinc sulfate. *Ann. Surg.* **172,** 1048–1050.

Barnes, P. M., and Moynahan, E. J. 1973. Zinc deficiency in acrodermatitis enteropathica: Multiple dietary intolerance treated with synthetic diet. *Proc. R. Soc. Med.* **66,** 327–329.

Becker, W. M., and Hoekstra, W. G. 1971. The intestinal absorption of zinc. In: *Intestinal Absorption of Metal Ions, Trace Elements and Radionuclides* (S. C. Skoryma and D. Waldron-Edward, eds.). Pergamon Press, New York, pp. 229–256.

Berfenstam, R. 1952a. Studies on blood zinc. *Acta Paediatr.* **41,** 389–391.

Berfenstam, R. 1952b. A clinical and experimental investigation into the zinc content of plasma and blood corpuscles with special reference to infancy. *Acta Paediatr.* **41,** 3–97.

Berger, N. A., and Skinner, A. M. 1974. Characterization of lymphocyte transformation induced by zinc ions. *J. Cell Biol.* **61,** 45–55.

Bergman, K. E., and Fomon, S. J. 1974. Trace minerals. In: *Infant Nutrition* (S. J. Fomon, ed.). W. B. Saunders Co., Philadelphia, pp. 320–337.

Bertrand, G., and Javillier, M. 1911. Influence du zinc et du manganese sur la composition minerale de *L'aspergillus niger. C. R. Acad Sci. (Paris)* **152,** 1337–1342.

Beutler, E. 1964. Tissue effects of iron deficiency. In: *Iron Metabolism* (F. Gross, ed.). Springer-Verlag, Berlin—Göttingen—Heidelberg, pp. 256–272.

Blamberg, D. L., Blackwood, U. B., Supplee, W. C., and Combs, G. F. 1960. Effect of zinc deficiency in hens on hatchability and embryonic development. *Proc. Soc. Exp. Biol. Med.* **104,** 217–220.

Boquist, L. 1967. Some aspects of the blood glucose regulation and the glutathione content of the non-diabetic adult Chinese hamsters *Cricetulus griseus. Acta Soc. Med. Ups.* **72,** 358–375.

Boquist, L. 1968. Alloxan administration in the Chinese hamster. I. Blood glucose variations, glucose tolerance, and light microscopical changes in pancreatic islets and other tissues. *Virchows Arch. B:* **1,** 157–168.

Boquist, L., and Lernmark, A. 1969. Effects of the endocrine pancreas in Chinese hamsters fed zinc-deficient diets. *Acta Pathol. Microbiol. Scand.* **76,** 215–228.

Boyett, J. D., and Sullivan, J. F. 1970. Zinc and collagen content of cirrhotic liver. *Amer. J. Dig. Dis.* **15,** 797–802.

Brewer, G. J., and Oelshlegel, F. J., Jr. 1974. Antisickling effects of zinc. *Biochem. Biophys. Res. Commun.* **58,** 854–861.

Brewer, G. J., Oelshlegel, F. J., Jr., and Prasad, A. S. 1975. Zinc in sickle cell anemia. In: *Erythrocyte Structure and Function (Progress in Clinical and Biological Research),* Vol. I (G. J. Brewer, ed.). Alan R. Liss, New York, pp. 417–435.

Brummerstedt, E., Flagstad, T., Basse, A., and Andresen, E. 1971. The effect of zinc on calves with hereditary thymus hypoplasia (lethal trait A 46). *Acta Pathol. Microbiol. Scand. Sect. A:* **79,** 686–687.

Butterworth, B. E., and Korant, B. D. 1974. Characterization of the large picornaviral polypeptides produced in the presence of zinc ion. *J. Virol.* **14,** 282–291.

Caldwell, D. F., Oberleas, D., Clancy, J. J., and Prasad, A. S. 1970. Behavioral impairment in adult rats following acute zinc deficiency. *Proc. Soc. Exp. Biol. Med.* **133,** 1417–1421.

Carpenter, F. H., and Vahl, J. M. 1973. Leucine aminopeptidase (bovine lens): Mechanism of activation by Mg^{2+} and Mn^{2+} of the zinc metalloenzyme, amino acid composition, and sulfhydryl content. *J. Biol. Chem.* **248,** 294–304.

Carter, J. P., Grivetti, L. E., Davis, J. T., Nasiff, S., Mansouri, A., Mousa, W. A., Atta, A.,

Patwardhan, V. N., Moneim, M. A., Abdou, I. A., and Darby, W. J. 1969. Growth and sexual development of adolescent Egyptian village boys: Effects of zinc, iron, and placebo supplementation. *Amer. J. Clin. Nutr.* **22,** 59–78.

Cavdar, A. O., and Arcasoy, A. 1972. Hematologic and biochemical studies of Turkish children with pica. *Clin. Pediatr.* **11,** 215–223.

Cavell, P. A. and Widdowson, E. M. 1964. Intakes and excretions of iron, copper, and zinc in the neonatal period. *Arch. Dis. Child.* **39,** 496–501.

Chesters, J. K. 1972. The role of zinc ions in the transformation of lymphocytes by phytohaemaglutinin. *Biochem. J.* **130,** 133–139.

Chen, R. W., Vasey, E. J., and Whanger, P. D. 1977. Accumulation and depletion of zinc in rat liver and kidney metallothioneins. *J. Nutr.* **107,** 805–813.

Chvapil, M., and Walsh, D. 1972. *Excerpta Med. Found. Int. Congr. Ser.* **264,** 226–228.

Chvapil, M., Ryan, J. N., and Zukowski, C. F. 1972. The effect of zinc on lipid peroxidation in liver microsomes and mitochondria. *Proc. Soc. Exp. Biol. Med.* **141,** 150–153.

Chvapil, M., Zukowski, C. F., Hattler, B. G., Stankova, L., Montgomery, D., Carlson, E. C., and Ludwig, J. C. 1976. Zinc and activity of cell membranes. In: *Trace Elements in Human Health and Disease* (A. S. Prasad, ed.). Academic Press, New York, pp. 269–281.

Clayton, R. J. 1972. Double-blind trial of oral zinc sulphate in patients with leg ulcers. *Brit. J. Clin. Pract.* **26,** 368–370.

Cohen, C. 1968. Zinc sulfate and bed sores. *Brit. Med. J.* **2,** 561.

Cohen, I. K., Schecter, P. J., and Henkin, R. I. 1973. Hypogeusia, anorexia, and altered zinc metabolism following thermal burn. *J. Amer. Med. Assoc.* **223,** 914–916.

Cox, R. P., and Ruckenstein, A. 1971. Studies on the mechanism of hormonal stimulation of zinc uptake in human cell cultures: Hormone–cell interactions and characteristics of zinc accumulation. *J. Cell. Physiol.* **77,** 71–82.

Csata, S., Gallays, F., and Toth, M. 1968. Akute Niereninsuffizienz als Folge einer Zinkchloridvergiftung. *Z. Urol.* **61,** 327–330.

Cuthbertson, D. P., Fell, G. S., Smith, C. M., and Tilstone, W. J. 1972. Metabolism after injury. I. Effects of severity, nutrition, and environmental temperature on protein, potassium, zinc, and creatine. *Brit. J. Surg.* **59,** 926–931.

Damyanov, I., and Dutz, W. 1971. Anencephaly in Shiraz, Iran. *Lancet* **1,** 82.

Danbolt, N., and Closs, K. 1942. Akrodermatitis enteropathica. *Acta Derm-Venereol.* **23,** 127.

Darby, W. J. 1946. The oral manifestations of iron deficiency. *J. Amer. Med. Assoc.* **130,** 830–835.

Dash, S., Brewer, G. J., and Oelshlegel, F. J., Jr. 1974. Effect of zinc on haemoglobin binding by red blood cell membranes. *Nature (London)* **250,** 251–252.

Davies, I. J. T. 1972. Plasma-zinc concentration in patients with bronchogenic carcinoma. *Lancet* **1,** 149.

Davies, J. W. L., and Fell, G. S. 1974. Tissue catabolism in patients with burns. *Clin. Chim. Acta* **51,** 83–92.

Davies, M. J., and Motzok, J. 1971. Zinc deficiency in the chick: Effect on tissue alkaline phosphatases. *Comp. Biochem. Physiol.* **40B,** 129–137.

Day, H. G., and McCollum, E. V. 1940. Effects of acute dietary zinc deficiency in the rat. *Proc. Soc. Exp. Biol. Med.* **45,** 282–284.

Dillaha, C. J., Lorincz, A. L., and Aavick, O. R. 1953. Acrodermatitis enteropathica. *J. Amer. Med. Assoc.* **152,** 509–512.

Donaldson, J., St-Pierre, T., Minich, J., and Barbeau, A. 1971. Seizures in rats associated with divalent cation inhibition of Na^+–K^+–ATPase. *Canad. J. Biochem.* **49,** 1217–1224.

Dreosti, I. E., and Hurley, L. S. 1975. Depressed thymidine kinase activity in zinc-deficient rat embryos. *Proc. Soc. Exp. Biol. Med.* **150,** 161–165.

Dreosti, I. E., Grey, P. C., and Wilkins, P. J. 1972. Deoxyribonucleic acid synthesis, protein synthesis, and teratogenesis in zinc-deficient rats. *S. Afr. Med. J.* **46,** 1585–1588.

Drum, D. E., Harrison, J. H. Li, T.-K., Bethune, J. L., and Vallee, B. L. 1967. Structural and functional zinc in horse liver alcohol dehydrogenase. *Proc. Natl. Acad. Sci. U.S.A.* **57,** 1434–1440.

Eaton, J. W., Skelton, T. D., Swofford, H. A., Kolpin, C. E., and Jacob, H. S. 1973. Elevated erythrocyte calcium in sickle cell disease. *Nature (London)* **246,** 105–106.

Elias, S., and Chvapil, M. 1973. Zinc and wound healing in normal and chronically ill rats. *J. Surg. Res.* **15,** 59–66.

Eminians, J., Reinhold, J. G., Kfoury, G. A., Amirhakimi, G. H., Sharif, H., and Ziai, M. 1967. Zinc nutrition of children in Fars Province of Iran. *Amer. J. Clin. Nutr.* **20,** 734–742.

Engel, R. W., Miller, R. F., and Price, N. O. 1966. Metabolic patterns in preadolescent children. XIII. Zinc balance. In: *Zinc Metabolism* (A. S. Prasad, ed.). Charles C. Thomas, Springfield, Illinois, pp. 326–338.

Engelbart, K., and Kief, H. 1970. Über das funktionelle Verhalten von Zink und Insulin in den β-Zellen das Rattenpankreas. *Virchows Arch. B:* **4,** 294–302.

Entwisle, B. R. 1965. Acrodermatitis enteropathica: Report of a case in a twin with dramatic response to expressed human milk. *Aust. J. Dermatol.* **8,** 13–21.

Evans, G. W. 1976. Absorption and transport of zinc. In: *Trace Elements in Human Health and Disease* (A. S. Prasad, ed.). Academic Press, New York, pp. 181–187.

Fasel, J., Hadjikhani, M. D. H., and Felder, J. P. 1970. The insulin secretory effect of the human duodenal mucosa. *Gastroenterology* **59,** 109–113.

Fell, G. S., Fleck, A., Cuthbertson, D. P., Queen, K., Morrison, C., Bessent, R. G., and Husain, S. L. 1973. Urinary zinc levels as an indication of muscle catabolism. *Lancet* **1,** 280–282.

Fernandez-Madrid, F., Prasad, A. S., and Oberleas, D. 1973. Effect of zinc deficiency on nucleic acids, collagen, and noncollagenous protein of the connective tissue. *J. Lab. Clin. Med.* **82,** 951–961.

Flynn, A., Pories, W. J., Strain, W. H., Hill, O. A., Jr., and Fratianne, R. B. 1971. Rapid serum-zinc depletion associated with corticosteroid therapy. *Lancet* **2,** 1169–1172.

Foley, B., Johnson, S. A., Hackley, B., Smith, J. C., Jr., and Halsted, J. A. 1968. Zinc content of human platelets. *Proc. Soc. Exp. Biol. Med.* **128,** 265–269.

Follis, R. H., Jr., Day, H. G., and McCollum, E. V. 1941. Histologic studies of tissues of rats fed a diet extremely low in zinc. *J. Nutr.* **22,** 223–237.

Fox, M. R. S., and Harrison, B. N. 1964. Use of Japanese quail for the study of zinc deficiency. *Proc. Soc. Exp. Biol. Med.* **116,** 256–259.

Fox, M. R. S., and Harrison, B. N. 1965. Effects of zinc deficiency on plasma proteins of young Japanese quail. *J. Nutr.* **86,** 89–92.

Freier, M. B., Faber, J., Goldstein, R., and Mayer, M. 1973. Treatment of acrodermatitis enteropathica by intravenous amino acid hydrolysate. *J. Pediatr.* **82,** 109–112.

Frost, P., Chen, J. C., Amjad, H., and Prasad, A. S. 1976. The "null lymphoid" cells in sickle cell disease: An elevation of null cells. *Clin. Res.* **24,** 570A.

Furchner, J. E., and Richmond, C. R. 1962. Effect of dietary zinc on the absorption of orally administered Zn^{65}. *Health Phys.* **8,** 35–40.

Gallery, E. D. M., Blomfield, J., and Dixon, S. R. 1972. Acute zinc toxicity in hemodialysis. *Brit. Med. J.* **4,** 331–333.

Gombe, S., Apgar, J., and Hansel, W. 1973. Effect of zinc deficiency and restricted food intake on plasma and pituitary LH and hypothalmic LRF in female rats. *Biol. Reprod.* **9,** 415–419.

Gormican, A., and Catli, E. 1971. Mineral balance in young men fed a fortified milk-base formula. *Nutr. Metab.* **13,** 364–377.

Greaves, M. W. 1972a. Zinc in cutaneous ulceration due to vascular insufficiency. *Amer. Heart J.* **83,** 716–717.

Greaves, M. W. 1972b. Zinc and copper in psoriasis. *Brit. J. Dermatol.* **86,** 439–440.

Greaves, M. W., and Boyde, T. R. C. 1967. Plasma zinc concentrations in patients with psoriasis, other dermatoses and venous leg ulceration. *Lancet* **2,** 1019–1020.

Greaves, M. W., and Ive, F. A. 1972. Double-blind trial of zinc sulphate in the treatment of chronic venous leg ulceration. *Brit. J. Dermatol.* **87,** 632–634.

Greaves, M. W., and Skillen, A. W. 1970. Effects of long-continued ingestion of zinc sulphate in patients with venous leg ulceration. *Lancet* **2,** 889–391.

Green, H. L., Hambidge, K. M., and Herman, Y. F. 1972. Trace elements and vitamins. In: *Parenteral Nutrition in Infancy and Childhood* (H. H. Bode and J. B. Warshaw, eds.). Plenum Press, New York, pp. 131–145.

Grey, P. C., and Dreosti, I. E. 1972. Deoxyribonucleic acid and protein metabolism in zinc-deficient rats. *J. Comp. Pathol.* **82,** 223–228.

Groundwater, W., and MacLeod, I. B. 1970. The effects of systemic zinc supplements on tbe strength of healing incised wounds in normal rats. *Brit. J. Surg.* **57,** 222–225.

Gudbjarnason, S., and Prasad, A. S. 1969. Cardiac metabolism in experimental alcoholism. In: *Biochemical and Clincal Aspects of Alcohol Metabolism* (V. M. Sardesai, ed.). Charles C. Thomas, Springfield, Illinois, pp. 266–277.

Gul'ko, I. S. 1961. The content of zinc, copper, manganese, cadmium, cobalt, and nickel in the blood, organs, and tumors of cancer patients. *Vopr. Onkol.* **7**(9), 46–51.

Haas, S., Fraker, P., and Luecke, R. W. 1976. The effect of zinc deficiency on the immuno responses of A/J mice. *Fed. Proc. Fed. Amer. Soc. Exp. Biol.* **35,** 659.

Haeger, K., Lanner, E., and Magnusson, P. O. 1972. Oral zinc sulfate in the treatment of venous leg ulcers. *Vasa* **1,** 62–69.

Halas, E. S., Rowe, M. C., Johnson, O. R., McKenzie, J. M., and Sandstead, H. H. 1976. Effects of intra-uterine zinc deficiency on subsequent behavior. In: *Trace Elements in Human Health and Disease* (A. S. Prasad, ed.). Academic Press, New York, pp. 327–343.

Hallböök, T., and Hedelin, H. 1977. Zinc metabolism and surgical trauma. *Brit. J. Surg.* **64,** 271–273.

Hallböök, T., and Lanner, E. 1972. Serum-zinc and healing of venous leg ulcers. *Lancet* **2,** 780–782.

Halsted, J. A., and Smith, J. C., Jr. 1970. Plasma-zinc in health and disease. *Lancet* **1,** 322–324.

Halsted, J. A., Hackley, B., Rudzki, C., and Smith J. C. 1968a. Plasma zinc concentrations in liver disease. *Gastroenterology* **64,** 1098–1105.

Halsted, J. A., Hackley, B. M., and Smith, J. C., Jr. 1968b. Plasma-zinc and copper in pregnancy and after oral contraceptives. *Lancet* **2,** 278–279.

Halsted, J. A. Ronaghy, H. A., Abadi, P., Haghshenass, M., Amirhakemi, G. H., Barakat, R. H., and Reinhold, J. C. 1972. Zinc deficiency in man: The Shiraz experiment. *Amer. J. Med.* **53,** 277–284.

Halsted, J. A., Smith, J. C., Jr., and Irwin, M. I. 1974. A conspectus of research on zinc requirements of man. *J. Nutr.* **104,** 345–378.

Hambidge, K. M. 1974. Zinc deficiency in children. In: *Trace Element Metabolism in Animals, Proceedings of the 2nd International Symposium* (W. G. Hoekstra, ed.). University Park Press, New York, pp. 171–183.

Hambidge, K. M., and Silverman, A. 1973. Pica with rapid improvement after dietary zinc supplementation. *Arch. Dis. Child.* **48,** 567–568.

Hambidge, K. M., and Walravens, P. A. 1976. Zinc deficiency in infants and pre-adolescent children. In: *Trace Elements in Human Health and Disease* (A. S. Prasad, ed.). Academic Press, New York, pp. 21–32.

Hambidge, K. M., Hambidge, C., Jacobs, M., and Baum, J. D. 1972. Low levels of zinc in hair, anorexia, poor growth, and hypogeusia in children. *Pediatr. Res.* **6,** 868–874.

Hambidge, K. M., Walravens, P. A., Kumar, V., and Tuchinda, C. 1974. Chromium, zinc, manganese, copper, nickel, iron and cadmium concentrations in the hair of residents of Chandigarh, India and Bangkok, Thailand. In: *Trace Substances in Environmental Health, Proceeding of the 8th Annual Conference,* (D. Hemphill, ed.). University of Missouri, pp. 39–44.

Hansen, J. D. L., and Lehmann, B. H. 1969. Serum zinc and copper concentrations in children with protein–calorie malnutrition. *S. Afr. Med. J.* **43,** 1248–1251.

Haumont, S. 1961. Distribution of zinc in bone tissue. *J. Histochem. Cytochem.* **9,** 141–145.

Heller, V. G., and Burke, A. D. 1927. Toxicity of zinc. *J. Biol. Chem.* **74,** 85–93.

Hellwege, H. H. 1971. Der Serumzinkspiegel und Veränderungen bei einigen Krankheiten im Kindesalter. *Monatsschr. Kinderheilkd.* **119,** 37–41.

Helwig, H. L., Hoffer, E. M., Thielen, W. C., Alcocer, A. E., Hotelling, D. R., Rogers, W. H., and Lench, J. 1966. Urinary and serum zinc levels in chronic alcoholism. *Amer. J. Clin. Pathol.* **45,** 156–159.

Hendricks, D. G., and Mahoney, A. W. 1972. Glucose tolerance in zinc-deficient rats. *J. Nutr.* **102,** 1079–1084.

Henkin, R. I., and Smith, F. R. 1972. Zinc and copper metabolism in acute viral hepatitis. *Amer. J. Med. Sci.* **264,** 401–409.

Henkin, R. I., Marshall, J. R., and Meret, S. 1971. Maternal–fetal metabolism of copper and zinc at term. *Amer. J. Obstet. Gynecol.* **110,** 131–134.

Henkin, R. I., Schulman, J. D., Schulman, C. B., and Bronzert, D. A. 1973. Changes in total, nondiffusible, and diffusible plasma zinc and copper during infancy. *J. Pediatr.* **82,** 831–837.

Henzel, J. H., DeWeese, M. S., and Lichti, E. L. 1970. Zinc concentrations within healing wounds. *Arch. Surg.* **100,** 349–357.

Heth, D. A., Becker, W. M., and Hoekstra, W. G. 1966. Effect of calcium, phosphorus, and zinc on zinc-65 absorption and turnover in rats fed semi-purified diets. *J. Nutr.* **88,** 331–337.

Hill, C. H., Matrone, G., Payne, W. L., and Barber, C. W. 1963. *In vivo* interactions of cadmium with copper, zinc and iron. *J. Nutr.* **80,** 227–235.

Hoffman, J. F. 1958. Physiological characteristics of human red blood cell ghosts. *J. Gen. Physiol.* **42,** 9–28.

Homan, J. D. H., Overbeek, G. A., Neutlings, J. P. J., Booiy, L. J., and Van der Vies, J. 1954. Corticotrophin zinc phosphate and hydroxide: Long acting aqueous preparations. *Lancet* **1,** 541–543.

Hove, E., Elvehjem, C. A., and Hart, E. B. 1937. The physiology of zinc in the nutrition of the rat. *Amer. J. Physiol.* **119,** 768–775.

Howell, J. T., and Monto, R. W. 1953. Syndrome of anemia, dysphagia and glossitis (Plummer–Vinson syndrome). *N. Engl. J. Med.* **249,** 1009–1012.

Hsu, J. M. 1976. Zinc as related to cystine metabolism. In: *Trace Elements in Human Health and Disease,* Vol. I (A. S. Prasad, ed.). Academic Press, New York, pp. 295–309.

Hsu, J. M., and Anthony, W. L. 1970. Zinc deficiency and urinary excretion of taurine-^{35}S and inorganic sulfate-^{35}S following cystine-^{35}S injection in rats. *J. Nutr.* **100,** 1189–1196.

Hsu, J. M., Anilane, J. K., and Scanlan, D. E. 1966. Pancreatic carboxypetidase: Activities in zinc-deficient rats. *Science* **153,** 882–883.

Hsu, J. M., Anthony, W. L., and Buchanan, P. J. 1968. Incorporation of glycine-1-^{14}C into liver glutathione in zinc deficient rats. *Proc. Soc. Exp. Biol. Med.* **127,** 1048–1051.

Hsu, J. M., Anthony, W. L., and Buchanan, P. J. 1970. Zinc deficiency and the metabolism of labeled cystine in rats. In: *The Proceedings of the First International Symposium on*

Trace Element Metabolism in Animals (C. F. Mills, ed.). E. and S. Livingstone, Edinburg, pp. 151–158.

Hsu, T. H. S., and Hsu, J. M. 1972. Zinc deficiency and epithelial wound repair: An autoradiographic study of ^{3}H-thymidine incorporation. *Proc. Soc. Exp. Biol. Med.* **140,** 157–160.

Huber, A. M., and Gershoff, S. N. 1973a. Effects of dietary zinc on the enzymes in the rat. *J. Nutr.* **103,** 1175–1181.

Huber, A. M., and Gershoff, S. N. 1973b. Effect of zinc-deficiency in rats of insulin release from the pancreas. *J. Nutr.* **103,** 1739–1744.

Hurley, L. S. 1976. Perinatal effects of trace element deficiencies. In: *Trace Elements in Human Health and Disease,* Vol. II (A. S. Prasad, ed.). Academic Press, New York, pp. 301–314.

Hurley, L. S. 1977. Zinc deficiency in prenatal and neonatal development. In: *Zinc Metabolism: Current Aspects in Health and Disease* (G. J. Brewer and A. S. Prasad, eds.). Alan R. Liss, New York, pp. 47–58.

Hurley, L. S., and Shrader, R. E. 1972. Congenital malformations of the nervous system of zinc deficient rats. *Int. Rev. Neurobiol. Suppl.* **1,** 7–51.

Hurley, L. S., and Tao, S. H. 1972. Alleviation of teratogenic effects of zinc deficiency by simultaneous lack of calcium. *Amer. J. Physiol.* **222,** 322–325.

Hurley, L. S., Duncan, J. R., Sloan, M. V., and Eckhert, C. D. 1977. Zinc-binding ligands in milk and intestine: A role in neonatal nutrition. *Proc. Natl. Acad. Sci. U.S.A.* **74,** 3547–3549.

Husain, S. L., Fell, G. S., and Scott, R. 1970. Zinc and healing. *Lancet* **2,** 1361–1362.

Husain, S. L. 1969. Oral zinc sulfate in leg ulcers. *Lancet* **1,** 1069–1071.

Iqbal, M. 1971. Activity of alkaline phosphatase and carbonic anhydrase in male and female zinc-deficient rats. *Enzyme* **12,** 33–40.

Jalili, M. A., and Al-Kassab, S. 1959. Koilonychia and cystine content of nails. *Lancet* **2,** 108.

Juljulian, H. H., and Kurban, A. K. 1971. Acantholysis: A feature of acrodermatitis enteropathica. *Arch. Dermatol.* **103,** 105–106.

Kahn, A. M., and Ozeran, R. S. 1967. Liver and serum zinc abnormalities in rats with cirrhosis. *Gastroenterology* **53,** 193–197.

Kahn, A. M., Helwig, H. L., Redecker, A. G., and Reynolds, T. B. 1965. Urine and serum zinc abnormalities in disease of the liver. *Amer. J. Clin. Pathol.* **44,** 426–435.

Kahn, A. M., Rizer, J. G., Thomas, P. B., Ponchita, T. B., and Gordon, E. H. 1968. Metabolism of zinc-65 in cirrhosis. *Surgery* **63,** 678–682.

Karl, L., Chvapil, M., and Zukoski, C. F. 1973. Effect of zinc on the viability and phagocytic capacity of peritoneal macrophages. *Proc. Soc. Exp. Biol. Med.* **142,** 1123–1127.

Kay, R. G., and Tasman-Jones, C. 1975. Acute zinc deficiency in man during intravenous alimentation. *Aust. N. Z. J. Surg.* **45,** 325–330.

Keilin, D., and Mann, J. 1940. Carbonic anhydrase: Purification and nature of the enzyme. *Biochem. J.* **34,** 1163–1176.

Kessler, B., and Monselise, S. P. 1959. Studies on ribonuclease, ribonucleic acid, and protein synthesis in healthy and zinc-deficient citrus leaves. *Physiol. Plant.* **12,** 1–7.

Kfoury, G. A., Reinhold, J. G., and Simonian, S. J. 1968. Enzyme activities in tissues of zinc-deficient rats. *J. Nutr.* **95,** 102–110.

Kirchgessner, M., and Roth, H. P. 1975a. Beziehungem zwischen klinischen Mangelsmptomen und Enzymaktivitäten bei Zinkmangel. *Zentralbl. Veterinaermed. Reihe A* **22,** 14–26.

Kirchgessner, M., and Roth, H. P. 1975b. Zur Bestimmung der Verfügbarkeit von Zink in Stoffwechsel sowie zur Ermittlung des Zinkbedarfs mittels Aktivitäsänderungen von Zn-Metallo-enzymen. *Arch. Tierernaehr.* **25,** 83–92.

Kirchgessner, M., Roth, H. P., and Weigand, E. 1976. Biochemical changes in zinc deficiency. In: *Trace Elements in Human Health and Disease,* Vol. I (A. S. Prasad, ed.). Academic Press, New York, pp. 189–219.

Klingberg, W. G., Prasad, A. S., and Oberleas, D. 1976. Zinc deficiency following penicillamine therapy. In: *Trace Elements in Human Health and Disease,* Vol. I (A. S. Prasad, ed.). Academic Press, New York, pp. 51–65.

Korant, B. D., Lonberg-Holm, K. K., Noble, J., and Stasny, J. T. 1972. Naturally occurring and artificially produced components of three rhinoviruses. *Virology* **48,** 71–86.

Kowarski, S., Blair-Stanek, C. S., and Schachter, D. 1974. Active transport of zinc and identification of zinc-binding protein in rat jejunal mucosa. *Amer. J. Physiol.* **226,** 401–407.

Kroneman, J., Mey, G. J. W., and Helder, A. 1975. Hereditary zinc deficiency of Dutch Friesian cattle. *Zentralbl. Veterinaered. A:* **22,** 201–208.

Ku, P. K. 1971. Nucleic acid and protein metabolism in the zinc-deficient pig. *Diss. Abstr. Int. B:* **31,** 6717.

Ku, P. K., Ullery, D. E., and Miller, E. R. 1970. Zinc deficiency and tissue nucleic acid and protein concentration. In: *Trace Element Metabolism in Animals* (C. F. Mills, ed.). Livingstone, Edinburgh and London, pp. 158–164.

Kulonen, E. 1970. Studies on experimental granuloma. In: *Chemistry and Molecular Biology of the Intracellular Matrix,* Vol. 3 (E. A. Balazs, ed.). Academic Press, New York, pp. 1811–1818.

Kumar, S., and Rao, K. S. J. 1973. Plasma and erythrocyte zinc levels in protein–calorie malnutrition. *Nutr. Metab.* **15,** 364–371.

Lee, P. W. R., and Green, M. A. 1972. Zinc and wound healing. *Lancet* **2,** 1089.

Lei, K. Y., Abbasi, A., and Prasad, A. S. 1976. Function of pituitary–gonadal axis in zinc deficient rats. *Amer. J. Physiol.* **230,** 1730–1732.

Lemann, I. I. 1910. A study of the type of infantilism in hookworm disease. *Arch. Intern. Med.* **6,** 139–146.

Lieberman, I., Abrams, R., Hunt, N., and Ove, P. 1963. Levels of enzyme activity and deoxyribonucleic acid synthesis in mammalian cells cultured from the animal. *J. Biol. Chem.* **238,** 3955–3962.

Likuski, H. J. A., and Forbes, R. M. 1964. Effect of phytic acid on the availability of zinc in amino acid and casein diets fed to chicks. *J. Nutr.* **84,** 145–148.

Lindeman, R. D., Bottomley, R. G., Cornelison, R. L., Jr., and Jacobs, L. A. 1972. Influence of acute tissue injury on zinc metabolism in man. *J. Lab. Clin. Med.* **79,** 452–460.

Lokken, P. M., Halas, E. S., and Sandstead, H. H. 1973. Influence of zinc deficiency on behavior. *Proc. Soc. Exp. Biol. Med.* **144,** 680–682.

Luecke, R. W., and Baltzer, B. V. 1968. The effect of dietary intake on the activity of intestinal alkaline phosphatase in the zinc-deficient rat. *Fed. Proc. Fed. Amer. Soc. Exp. Biol. Med.* **27,** 483.

Luecke, R. W., Hoefer, J. A., Brammell, W. S., and Thorp, F., Jr., 1956. Mineral interrelationships in parakeratosis of swine. *J. Anim. Sci.* **15,** 347–351.

Luecke, R. W., Hoefer, J. A., Brammell, W. S., and Schmidt, D. A. 1957. Calcium and zinc in parakeratosis in swine. *J. Anim. Sci.* **16,** 3–11.

Luecke, R. W., Olman, M. E., and Baltzer, B. V. 1968. Zinc deficiency in the rat: Effect on serum and intestinal alkaline phosphatase activities. *J. Nutr.* **94,** 344–350.

Macapinlac, M. P., Pearson, W. N., and Darby, W. J. 1966. Some characteristics of zinc deficiency in the albino rat. In: *Zinc Metabolism* (A. S. Prasad, ed.). Charles C Thomas, Springfield, Illinois, pp. 142–166.

Macapinlac, M. P., Pearson, W. N., Barney, G. H., and Darby, W. J. 1968. Protein and nucleic acid metabolism in the testes of zinc-deficient rats. *J. Nutr.* **95,** 569–577.

MacMahon, R. A., Parker, M. L., and McKinnon, M. C. 1968. Zinc treatment in malabsorption. *Med. J. Aust.* **2,** 210–212.

Macy, I. G. 1942. Nutrition and chemical growth in childhood. In: *Evaluation,* Vol. 1. Charles C Thomas, Springfield, Illinois, pp. 198–202.

Magee, A. C., and Matrone, G. 1960. Studies on growth, copper metabolism and iron metabolism of rats fed high levels of zinc. *J. Nutr.* **72,** 233–242.

Mansouri, K., Halsted, J., and Gombos, E. A. 1970. Zinc, copper, magnesium and calcium in dialyzed and nondialyzed uremic patients. *Arch. Intern. Med.* **125,** 88–93.

Margoshes, M., and Vallee, B. L. 1957. A cadmium protein from equine kidney cortex. *J. Amer. Chem. Soc.* **79,** 4813–1814.

McBean, L. D., and Halsted, J. A. 1969. Fasting versus postprandial plasma zinc levels, *J. Clin. Pathol.* **22,** 623.

McCall, J. T., Goldstein, N. P., and Smith, L. H. 1971. Implications of trace metals in human disease. *Fed. Proc. Fed. Amer. Soc. Exp. Biol.* **30,** 1011–1015.

McCance, R. A., and Widdowson, E. M. 1942. The absorption and excretion of zinc. *Biochem. J.* **36,** 692–696.

McClain, P. E., Wiley, E. R., Beecher, G. R., Anthony, W. L., and Hsu, J. M. 1973. Influence of zinc deficiency on synthesis and crosslinking of rat-skin collagen. *Biochim. Biophys. Acta* **304,** 457–465.

McIntyre, N., Holdsworth, C. D., and Turner, D. S. 1965. Intestinal factors in the control of insulin secretion. *J. Clin. Endocrinol. Metab.* **25,** 1317–1324.

Merck Index, 7th ed. 1960. Merck and Co., Rahway, New Jersey, p. 1118.

Methfessel, A. H., and Spencer, H. 1973. Zinc metabolism in the rat. II. Secretion of zinc into intestine. *J. Appl. Physiol.* **34,** 63–67.

Millar, M. J., Elcoate, P. V., Fischer, M. I., and Mawson, C. A. 1960. Effect of testosterone and gonadotrophin injections on the sex organ development of zinc-deficient male rats. *Canad. J. Biochem. Physiol.* **38,** 1457–1466.

Miller, E. R., Luecke, R. W., Ullrey, D. E., Baltzer, B. V., Bradley, B. L., and Hoefer, J. A. 1968. Biochemical, skeletal, and allometric changes due to zinc deficiency in the baby pig. *J. Nutr.* **95,** 278–286.

Miller, J. K., and Miller, W. J. 1960. Development of zinc deficiency in holstein calves fed a purified diet. *J. Dairy Sci.* **43,** 1854–1856.

Miller, J. K., and Miller, W. J. 1962. Experimental zinc deficiency and recovery of calves. *J. Nutr.* **76,** 467–474.

Mills, C. F., Quarterman, J., Williams, R. B., Dalgarno, A. C., and Panic, B. 1967. The effects of zinc defiency on pancreatic carboxypeptidase activity and protein digestion and absorption in the rat. *Biochem. J.* **102,** 712–718.

Mills, C. F., Quarterman, J., Chesters, J. K., Williams, R. G., and Dalgarno, A. C. 1969. Metabolic role of zinc. *Amer. J. Clin. Nutr.* **22,** 1240–1249.

Minnich, V., Okevogla, A., Tarcon, Y., Arcasoy, A., Cin, S., Yorukoglu, O., Renda, F., and Demirag, B. 1968. Pica II in Turkey: Effect of clay upon iron absorption. *Amer. J. Clin. Nutr.* **21,** 78–86.

Morrison, L. M., Swalm, W. A., and Jackson, C. L. 1937. Syndrome of hypochromic anemia, achlorhydria and atrophic gastritis. *J. Amer. Med. Assoc.* **109,** 108–111.

Moynahan, E. J. 1966. Acrodermatitis enteropathica with secondary lactose intolerance and tertiary deficiency state, probably due to chelation of essential nutrients by di-iodohydroxyquinolone. *Proc. R. Soc. Med.* **59,** 445–447.

Moynahan, E. J., and Barnes, P. M. 1973. Zinc deficiency and a synthetic diet for lactose intolerance. *Lancet* **1,** 676–677.

Murphy, J. V. 1970. Intoxication following ingestion of elemental zinc. *J. Amer. Med. Assoc.* **212,** 2119–2120.

Mustafa, M. G., Cross, C. E., and Hardie, J. A. 1970. Localization of Na^+-K^+, Mg^{++} adenosinetriphosphatase activity in pulmonary alveolar macrophase subcellular fractions. *Life Sci.* **9**(1), 947–954.

Mustafa, M. G., Cross, C. E., Munn, R. J., and Hardie, J. A. 1971. Effects of divalent metal ions on alveolar macrophage membrane adenosine triphosphatase activity. *J. Lab. Clin. Med.* **77**, 563–567.

Myers, M. B., and Cherry, G. 1970. Zinc and the healing of chronic leg ulcers. *Amer. J. Surg.* **120**, 77–81.

Nielsen, S. P., and Jemec, B. 1968. Zinc metabolism in patients with severe burns. *Scand. J. Plast. Reconstr. Surg.* **2**, 47–52.

Nikolson, V. J., and Veldstra, H. 1972. The influence of various cations on the binding of colchicine by rat brain homogenates: Stabilization of intact neurotubules by zinc and calcium ions. *FEBS Lett.* **23**, 309–313.

Nishimura, H. 1953. Zinc deficiency in suckling mice deprived of colostrum. *J. Nutr.* **49**, 79–97.

Oberleas, D., and Prasad, A. S. 1969. Growth as affected by zinc and protein nutrition: Symposium on zinc metabolism. *Amer. J. Clin. Nutr.* **22**, 1304–1314.

Oberleas, D., Muhrer, M. E., and O'Dell, B. L. 1962. Some effects of phytic acid on zinc availability and physiology of swine. *J. Anim. Sci.* **21**, 57–61.

Oberleas, D., Muhrer, M. E., and O'Dell, B. L. 1966. Dietary metal complexing agents and zinc availability in the rat. *J. Nutr.* **90**, 56–62.

Oberleas, D., Seymour, J. K., Lenaghan, R., Hovanesian, J., Wilson, R. F., and Prasad, A. S. 1971. Effect of zinc deficiency on wound healing in rats. *Amer. J. Surg.* **121**, 566–568.

O'Dell, B. L., and Savage, J. E. 1957. Potassium, zinc and distillers dried solubles as supplement to a purified diet. *Poult. Sci.* **36**, 459–460.

O'Dell, B. L., and Savage, J. E. 1960. Effect of phytic acid on zinc availability. *Proc. Soc. Exp. Biol. Med.* **103**, 304–306.

O'Dell, B. L., Newberne, P. M., and Savage, J. E. 1958. Significance of dietary zinc for the growing chicken. *J. Nutr.* **65**, 503–518.

O'Dell, B. L., Burpo, C. E., and Savage, J. E. 1972. Evaluation of zinc availability in foodstuffs of plant and animal origin. *J. Nutr.* **102**, 653–660.

Oelshlegel, F. J., Jr., Brewer, G. J., Prasad, A. S., Knutsen, C., and Schoomaker, E. B. 1973. Effect of zinc on increasing oxygen affinity of sickle and normal red blood cells. *Biochem. Biophys. Res. Commun.* **53**, 560–566.

Oelshlegel, F. J., Jr., Brewer, G. J., Knutsen, C., Prasad, A. S., and Schoomaker, E. B. 1974. Studies on the interaction of zinc with human hemoglobin. *Arch. Biochem. Biophys.* **163**, 742–748.

Ohtaka, Y., Uchida, K., and Sakai, T. 1963. Purification and properties of ribonuclease from yeast. *J. Biochem. (Tokyo)* **54**, 322–327.

O'Leary, J. A., and Spellacy, W. N. 1969. Zinc and copper levels in pregnant women and those taking oral contraceptives: A preliminary report. *Amer. J. Obstet. Gynecol.* **102**, 131–132.

O'Neal, R. M., Pla, G. W., Fox, M. R. S., Gibson, F. S., and Fry, B. E. 1970. Effect of zinc deficiency and restricted feeding on protein and ribonucleic acid metabolism of rat brain. *J. Nutr.* **100**, 491–497.

Osis, D., Kramer, L., Wiatrowski, E., and Spencer, H. 1972. Dietary zinc intake in man. *Amer. J. Clin. Nutr.* **25**, 582–588.

Osol, A., Farrar, G. E., Jr., and Pratt, R. 1955. *Dispensatory of the U.S.*, 25th ed. Lippincott, Philadelphia, pp. 1520–1521.

Ott, E. A., Smith, W. H., Stob, M., Parker, H. E., Harrington, R. B., and Beeson, W. M. 1965. Zinc requirement of the growing lamb fed a purified diet. *J. Nutr.* **87**, 459–463.

Palik, J., Curby, W. A., and Lionetti, F. J. 1971. Effects of calcium and adenosine triphosphate on volume of human red cell ghosts. *Amer. J. Physiol.* **220,** 19–26.

Papp, J. P. 1968. Metal fume fever. *Postgrad. Med.* **43,** 160–163.

Parisi, A. F., and Vallee, B. L. 1969. Zinc metalloenzymes: Characteristics and significance in biology and medicine. *Amer. J. Nutr.* **22,** 1222–1239.

Patek, A. J., and Haig, C. 1939. The occurrence of abnormal dark adaption and its relation to vitamin A metabolism in patients with cirrhosis of the liver. *J. Clin. Invest.* **18,** 609–616.

Pearson, W. N., and Reich, M. 1965. *In vitro* studies of Fe^{59} absorption by everted intestinal sacs of the rat. *J. Nutr.* **87,** 117–124.

Pekarek, R. S., Wannemacher, R. W., and Beisel, W. R. 1972. The effect of leukocyte endogenous mediator (LEM) on the tissue distribution of zinc and iron. *Proc. Soc. Exp. Biol. Med.* **140,** 685–688.

Perry, H. O. 1974. Acrodermatitis enteropathica. In: *Clinical Dermatology,* Vol. 1 (D. J. Demis, R. G. Crounse, R. L. Dobson, and J. McGuire, eds.). Harper and Row, New York, p. 1.

Pidduck, H. G., Wren, P. J. J., and Evans, D. A. 1970. Plasma zinc and copper in diabetes mellitus. *Diabetes* **19,** 234–239.

Pories, W. J., and Strain, W. H. 1966. Zinc and wound healing. In: *Zinc Metabolism* (A. S. Prasad, ed.). Charles C Thomas, Springfield, Illinois, pp. 378–394.

Pories, W. J., Henzel, J. H., Rob, C. G., and Strain, W. H. 1967a. Acceleration of wound healing with zinc sulfate. *Ann. Surg.* **165,** 432–436.

Pories, W. J., Henzel, J. H., Rob, C. G., and Strain, W. H. 1967b. Acceleration of wound healing in man with zinc sulfate given by mouth. *Lancet* **1,** 121–124.

Pories, W. J., Mansouri, E. G., Plecha, F. R., Flynn, A., and Strain, W. H. 1976. Metabolic factors affecting zinc metabolism in the surgical patient. In: *Trace Elements in Human Health and Disease,* Vol. I (A. S. Prasad, ed.). Academic Press, New York, pp. 115–141.

Portnoy, B., and Molokhia, M. 1971. Zinc and copper in psoriasis. *Brit. J. Dermatol.* **85,** 597.

Portnoy, B., and Molokhia, M. M. 1972. Zinc and copper in psoriasis. *Brit. J. Dermatol.* **86,** 205.

Prasad, A. S. 1966. Metabolism of zinc and its deficiency in human subjects. In: *Zinc Metabolism* (A. S. Prasad, ed.). Charles C Thomas, Springfield, Illinois, Chapter 15, pp. 250–302.

Prasad, A. S. 1976. Deficiency of zinc in man and its toxicity. In: *Trace Elements in Human Health and Disease* (A. S. Prasad, ed.). Academic Press, New York, pp. 1–20.

Prasad, A. S., and Oberleas, D. 1970a. Binding of zinc to amino acids and serum proteins *in vitro. J. Lab. Clin. Med.* **76,** 416–425.

Prasad, A. S., and Oberleas, D. 1970b. Zinc: Human nutrition and metabolic effects. *Ann. Intern. Med.* **73,** 631–636.

Prasad, A. S., and Oberleas, D. 1971. Changes in activity of zinc-dependent enzymes in zinc-deficient tissues of rats. *J. Appl. Physiol.* **31,** 842–846.

Prasad, A. S., and Oberleas, D. 1973. Ribonuclease and deoxyribonuclease activities in zinc-deficient tissues. *J. Lab. Clin. Med.* **82,** 461–466.

Prasad, A. S., and Oberleas, D. 1974. Thymidine kinase activity and incorporation of thymidine into DNA in zinc-deficient tissue. *J. Lab. Clin. Med.* **83,** 634–639.

Prasad, A. S., Halsted, J. A., and Nadimi, M. 1961. Syndrome of iron deficiency anemia, hepatosplenomegaly, hypogonadism, dwarfism and geophagia. *Amer. J. Med.* **31,** 532–546.

Prasad, A. S., Miale, A., Jr., Farid, Z., Sandstead, H. H., and Darby, W. J. 1963a. Biochemical studies on dwarfism, hypogonadism and anemia. *AMA Arch. Intern. Med.* **111,** 407–428.

Prasad, A. S., Miale, A., Jr., Farid, A., Schulert, A., and Sandstead, H. H. 1963b. Zinc metabolism in patients with the syndrome of iron deficiency anemia, hypogonadism and dwarfism. *J. Lab. Clin. Med.* **61,** 537–549.

Prasad, A. S., Sandstead, H. H., Schulert, A. R., and El Rooby, A. S. 1963c. Urinary excretion of zinc in patients with the syndrome of anemia, hepatosplenomegaly, dwarfism and hypogonadism. *J. Lab. Clin. Med.* **62,** 591–599.

Prasad, A. S., Schulert, A. R., Sandstead, H. H., Miale, A., Jr., and Farid, Z. 1963d. Zinc, iron, and nitrogen content of sweat in normal and deficient subjects. *J. Lab. Clin. Med.* **62,** 84–89.

Prasad, A. S., Oberleas, D., and Halsted, J. A. 1965. Determination of zinc in biological fluids by atomic absorption spectrophotometry in normal and cirrhotic subjects. *J. Lab. Clin. Med.* **66,** 508–516.

Prasad, A. S., Oberleas, D., Wolf, P., and Horwitz, J. P. 1967. Studies of zinc deficiency: Changes in trace elements and enzyme activities in tissues of zinc-deficient rats. *J. Clin. Invest.* **46,** 549–557.

Prasad, A. S., Oberleas, D., Wolf, P., Horwitz, J. P., Miller, E. R., and Luecke, R. W. 1969a. Changes in trace elements and enzyme activities in tissues of zinc-deficient pigs. *Amer. J. Clin. Nutr.* **22,** 628–637.

Prasad, A. S., Oberleas, D., Wolf, P., and Horwitz, J. P. 1969b. Effect of growth hormone on non-hypophysectomized zinc-deficient rats and zinc on hypophysectomized rats. *J. Lab. Clin. Med.* **73,** 486–494.

Prasad, A. S. Oberleas, D., Miller, E. R., and Luecke, R. W. 1971. Biochemical effects of zinc deficiency: Changes in activities of zinc-dependent enzymes and ribonucleic acid and deoxyribonucleic acid content of tissues. *J. Lab. Clin. Med.* **77,** 144–152.

Prasad, A. S., Schoomaker, E. B., Ortega, J., Brewer, G. J., Oberleas, D., and Oelshlegel, F. J. 1975a. Zinc deficiency in sickle cell disease. *Clin. Chem.* **21,** 582–587.

Prasad, A. S., Schoomaker, E. B., Ortega, J., Brewer, G. J., Oberleas, D., and Oelshlegel, F. 1975b. Role of zinc in man and its deficiency in sickle cell disease. In: *Erythrocyte Structure and Function (Progress in Clinical and Biological Research),* Vol. 1 (G. J. Brewer, ed.). Alan R. Liss, New York, pp. 603–619.

Prasad, A. S., Oberleas, D., Lei, K. Y., Moghissi, K. S., and Stryker, J. C. 1975c. Effect of oral contraceptive agents on nutrients. I. Minerals. *Amer. J. Clin. Nutr.* **28,** 377–384.

Price, N. O., Bunce, G. E., and Engel, R. W. 1970. Copper, manganese, and zinc balance in preadolescent girls. *Amer. J. Clin. Nutr.* **23,** 258–260.

Pulido, P., Kagi, J. H. R., and Vallee, B. L. 1966. Isolation and some properties of human metallothionein. *Biochemistry* **5,** 1768–1777.

Quarterman, J., and Florence, E. 1972. Observations on glucose tolerance and plasma levels of free fatty acids and insulin in the zinc-deficient rat. *Brit. J. Nutr.* **28,** 75–79.

Quarterman, J., Mills, C. F., and Humphries, W. R. 1966. The reduced secretion of and sensitivity to insulin in zinc-deficient rats. *Biochem. Biophys. Res. Commun.* **25,** 354–358.

Raben, M. S. 1962. Growth hormone. I. Physiologic aspects. *N. Engl. J. Med.* **266,** 31–35.

Rahmat, A., Norman, J. N., and Smith, G. 1974. The effect of zinc deficiency on wound healing. *Brit. J. Surg.* **61,** 271–273.

Raulin, J. 1869. Ëtudes cliniques sur la vëgëtation. *Ann. Sci. Nat. Bot. Biol. Veg.* **11,** 93.

Recommended Dietary Allowances, 8th ed. 1974. National Academy of Sciences, Washington, D.C.

Reimann, F. 1955. Wachstumsanomalien und Missbildungen bei Eisenmangelzuständen (Asiderosen). *Proc. 5th Kongr. Eur. Gesellschaft Haematol.,* pp. 546–550.

Reinhold, J. G. 1971. High phytate content of rural Iranian bread: A possible cause of human zinc deficiency. *Amer. J. Clin. Nutr.* **24,** 1204–1206.

Reinhold, J. G., and Kfoury, G. A. 1969. Zinc-dependent enzyme in zinc-depleted rats: Intestinal alkaline phosphatase. *Amer. J. Clin. Nutr.* **22,** 1250–1263.

Reinhold, J. G., Hedayati, H., Lahimgarzadeh, A., and Nasr, K. 1973a. Zinc, calcium, phosphorus, and nitrogen balances of Iranian villagers following a change from phytate-rich to phytate-poor diets. *Ecol. Food Nutr.* **2,** 157–162.

Reinhold, J. G., Nasr, K., Lahimgarzadeh, A., and Hedayati, H. 1973b. Effects of purified phytate and phytate-rich bread upon metabolism of zinc, calcium, phosphorus, and nitrogen in man. *Lancet* **1,** 283–288.

Reinhold, J. G., Faradji, B., Abadi, P., and Ismail-Beigi, F. 1976. Binding of zinc to fiber and other solids of wholemeal bread, with a preliminary examination of the effects of cellulose consumption upon the metabolism of zinc, calcium and phosphorus in man. In: *Trace Elements in Human Health and Disease,* Vol. I (A. S. Prasad, ed.). Academic Press, New York, pp. 163–180.

Richards, M. P., and Cousins, R. J. 1975a. Influence of parenteral zinc and actinomycin D on tissue zinc uptake and the synthesis of a zinc-binding protein. *Biol. Inorg. Chem.* **4,** 215–224.

Richards, M. P., and Cousins, R. J. 1975b. Mammalian zinc homeostasis: Requirement for RNA and metallothionein synthesis. *Biochem. Biophys. Res. Commun.* **64,** 1215–1223.

Richards, M. P., and Cousins, R. J. 1976. Zinc-binding protein: Relationship to short term changes in zinc metabolism. *Proc. Soc. Exp. Biol. Med.* **153,** 52–56.

Riordan, J. F., and Vallee, B. L. 1976. Structure and function of zinc metalloenzymes. In: *Trace Elements in Human Health and Disease,* Vol. I (A. S. Prasad, ed.). Academic Press, New York, pp. 227–251.

Robertson, B. T., and Burns, M. J. 1963. Zinc metabolism and the zinc deficiency syndrome in the dog. *Amer. J. Vet. Res.* **24,** 997–1002.

Robin, A. E., and Goldman, A. S. 1969. Autopsy findings in acrodermatitis enteropathica. *Amer. J. Clin. Pathol.* **51,** 315.

Robinson, J. D. 1972. Divalent cations as allosteric modifiers of the (Na^+ + K^+)-dependent ATPase. *Biochim. Biophys. Acta* **226,** 97–102.

Romeo, D., Zabucchi, G., Soranzo, M. R., and Rossi, F. 1971. Macrophage metabolism: Activation of NADPH oxidation by phagocytosis. *Biochem. Biophys. Res. Commun.* **45,** 1056–1062.

Ronaghy, H., Fox, M. R. S., Garn, S. M., Isral, H., Harp, A., Moe, P. G., and Halsted, J. A. 1969. Controlled zinc supplementation for malnourished school boys: A pilot experiment. *Amer. J. Clin. Nutr.* **22,** 1279–1289.

Ronaghy, H. A., Reinhold, J. G., Mahloudji, M., Ghavami, P., Fox, M. R. S., and Halsted, J. A. 1974. Zinc supplementation of malnourished school-boys in Iran: Increased growth and other effects. *Amer. J. Clin. Nutr.* **27,** 112–121.

Rose, G. A., and Willden, E. G. 1972. Whole blood, red cell, and plasma total and ultrafilterable zinc levels in normal subjects and in patients with chronic renal failure with and without hemodialysis. *Brit. J. Urol.* **44,** 281–286.

Rosenbusch, J. P., and Weber, K. 1971. Localization of the zinc binding site of aspartate transcarbamylase in the regulatory submit. *Proc. Natl. Acad. Sci. U.S.A.* **68,** 1019–1023.

Ross, J. F., Ebaugh, R. G., Jr., and Talbot, T. R., Jr. 1958. Radioisotopic studies of zinc metabolism in human subjects. *Trans. Assoc. Amer. Physicians* **71,** 322–336.

Roth, H. P., and Kirchgessner, M. 1974a. Aktivitätsveränderungen verschiedener Dehydrogenasen und der alkalischen Phosphatase in Serum bei Zn-Depletion und -Repletion. *A. Tierphysiol. Tierernaehr. Futtermittelkd.* **32,** 289–296.

Roth, H. P., and Kirchgessner, M. 1974b. Zur Aktivität der Pankreas-Carboxypeptidase A and B bei Zink-Depletion und -Repletion. *Z. Tierphysiol. Tierernaehr. Futtermittelkd.* **33,** 62–67.

Roth, H. P., and Kirchgessner, M. 1974c. Zur Aktivität der Blut-Carbonanhydrase bei Zn-Mangel wachsender Ratten. *Z. Tierphysiol. Tierernaehr. Futtermittelkd.* **32,** 296–300.

Roth, H. P., and Kirchgessner, M. 1974d. Zum Aktivitätsverlauf verschiedener Dehydrogenasen in der Rattenleber bei unterschleidlicher Zinkversorgung. *Z. Tierphysiol. Tierernaehr. Futtermittelkd.* **33,** 1–9.

Roth, H. P., and Kirchgessner, M. 1974e. Zur Enzymaktivität von Dehydrogenasen in Rattenmuskel bei Zinkmangel. *Z. Tierphysiol. Tierernaehr. Futtermittelkd.* **33,** 67–71.

Roth, H. P., and Kirchgessner, M. 1975. Insulingehalte in Serum bzw. Plasma von Zinkmangelratten vor und nach Glucosestimulierung. *Inst. J. Vit. Nutr. Res.* **45,** 202–208.

Rubin, H. 1972. Inhibition of DNA synthesis in animal cells by ethylene diamine tetraacetate and its reversal by zinc. *Proc. Natl. Acad. Sci. U.S.A.* **69,** 712–716.

Rubin, H., and Koide, T. 1973. Inhibition of DNA synthesis in chick embryo cultures by deprivation of either serum or zinc. *J. Cell Biol.* **56,** 777–786.

Ruhl, H., Kirchner, H., and Bochert, G. 1971. Kinetics of the Zn^{2+} stimulation of human peripheral lymphocytes *in vitro*. *Proc. Soc. Exp. Biol. Med.* **137,** 1089–1092.

Sacchetti, G., Gibelli, A., Bellani, D., and Montanari, C. 1974. Effect of manganese ions on human platelet aggregation *in vitro*. *Experientia* **30,** 374–375.

Saldeen, T. 1969. On the protective action of zinc against experimental liver damage due to choline free diet or carbon tetrachloride. *Z. Gesante. Exp. Med.* **150,** 251–259.

Saldeen, T., and Brunk, U. 1967. Enzyme histochemical investigations of the inhibitory effect of zinc on the injurious action of carbon tetrachloride on the liver. *Frankf. Z. Pathol.* **76,** 419–426.

Sandstead, H. H. 1973. Zinc nutrition in the United States. *Amer. J. Clin. Nutr.* **26,** 1251–1280.

Sandstead, H. H., and Rinaldi, R. A. 1969. Impairment of deoxyribonucleic acid synthesis by dietary zinc deficiency in the rat. *J. Cell. Physiol.* **73,** 81–83.

Sandstead, H. H., and Shepard, G. H. 1968. The effect of zinc deficiency on the tensile strength of healing surgical incisions in the integument of the rat. *Proc. Soc. Exp. Biol. Med.* **128,** 687–689.

Sandstead, H. H., Shukry, A. S., Prasad, A. S., Gabr, M. K., Hefney, A. E., Mokhtar, N., and Darby, W. J. 1965. Kwashiorkor in Egypt. I. Clinical and biochemical studies, with special reference to plasma zinc and serum lactic dehydrogenase. *Amer. J. Clin. Nutr.* **17,** 15–26.

Sandstead, H. H., Prasad, A. S., Schulert, A. R., Farid, Z., Miale, A., Jr., Bassilly, S., and Darby, W. J. 1967. Human zinc deficiency, endocrine manifestations and response to treatment. *Amer. J. Clin. Nutr.* **20,** 422–442.

Sandstead, H. H., Glassner, S. R., and Gillespie, D. D. 1970a. Zinc deficiency: Effect on fetal growth, zinc concentration, and zinc-65 uptake. *Fed. Proc. Fed. Amer. Soc. Exp. Biol.* **29,** 297.

Sandstead, H. H., Burk, R. F., Booth, G. H., and Darby, W. J. 1970b. Current concepts on trace minerals: Clinical considerations. *Med. Clin. North Amer.* **54,** 1509–1531.

Sandstead, H. H., Hollaway, W. L., and Baum, V. 1971a. Zinc deficiency: Effect on polysomes. *Fed. Proc. Fed. Amer. Soc. Exp. Biol.* **30,** 517.

Sandstead, H. H., Terhune, M., Brady, R. N., Gillespie, D., and Hollaway, W. L. 1971b. Zinc deficiency: Brain DNA, protein and lipids and liver ribosomes and RNA polymerase. *Clin. Res.* **19,** 83.

Sandstead, H. H., Gillespie, D. D., and Brady, R. N. 1972. Zinc deficiency: Effect on brain of the suckling rat. *Pediatr. Res.* **6,** 119–125.

Sandstead, H. H., Vo-Khactu, K. P., and Solomons, N. 1976. Conditioned zinc deficiencies. In: *Trace Elements in Human Health and Disease,* Vol. I (A. S. Prasad, ed.). Academic Press, New York. pp. 33–49.

Sbarra, A. J., Paul, B. B., Jacobs, A. A., Straus, R. R., and Mitchell, G. W., Jr. 1972.

Biochemical aspects of phagocytic cells as related to bactericidal function. *J. Reticuloendothel. Soc.* **11,** 492–502.

Schechter, P. J. Friedewald, W. T., Bronzert, D. A., Raff, M. S., and Henkin, R. I. 1972. Idiopathic hypogeusia: A description of the syndrome and a single-blind study with zinc sulfate. *Int. Rev. Neurobiol. Suppl.* **1,** 125–140.

Schlage, C., and Worberg, B. 1972. Zinc in the diet of healthy preschool and school children. *Acta Pediatr. Scand.* **61,** 421–425.

Schlievert, P. S., Johnson, W., and Galask, R. P. 1976a. Bacterial growth inhibition by amniotic fluid. V. Phosphate to zinc ratio as a predictor of bacterial inhibitory activity. *Amer. J. Obstet. Gynecol.* **125,** 899–905.

Schlievert, P., Johnson, W., and Galask, R. P. 1976b. Bacterial growth inhibition by amniotic fluid. VI. Evidence for a zinc peptide antibacterial system. *Amer. J. Obstet. Gynecol.* **125,** 906–910.

Schneider, E., and Price, C. A. 1962. Decreased ribonucleic acid levels: A possible cause of growth inhibition in zinc deficiency. *Biochim. Biophys. Acta* **55,** 406–408.

Schroeder, H. A. 1971. Losses of vitamins and trace minerals resulting from processing and preservation of foods. *Amer. J. Clin. Nutr.* **24,** 562–573.

Schroeder, H. A., Nason, A. P., Tipton, I. H., and Balassa, J. J. 1967. Essential trace metals in man. Zinc: Relation to environmental cadmium. *J. Chron. Dis.* **20,** 179–210.

Scott, D. A. 1934. Crystalline insulin. *Biochem. J.* **28,** 1592–1602.

Scoular, F. L. 1939. A quantitative study, by means of spectrographic analysis, of zinc in nutrition. *J. Nutr.* **17,** 103–113.

Scrutton, M. C., Wu, C. W., and Goldthwait, D. A. 1971. The presence and possible role of zinc in RNA polymerase obtained from *Escherichia coli*. *Proc. Natl. Acad. Sci. U.S.A.* **68,** 2497–2501.

Serjeant, G. R., Galloway, R. E., and Gueri, M. C. 1970. Oral zinc and sulphate in sickle-cell ulcers. *Lancet* **2,** 891–892.

Shrader, R. E., and Hurley, L. S. 1972. Enzyme histochemistry of peripheral blood and bone marrow in zinc-deficient rats. *Lab. Invest.* **26,** 566–571.

Simkin, P. A. 1977. Zinc sulphate in rheumatoid arthritis. In: *Zinc Metabolism: Current Aspects in Health and Disease* (G. J. Brewer and A. S. Prasad, eds.). Alan R. Liss, New York, pp. 343–351.

Sinha, S. N., and Gabrielli, E. R. 1970. Serum copper and zinc levels in various pathological conditions. *Amer. J. Clin. Pathol.* **54,** 570–577.

Slater, J. P., Mildvan, A. S., and Loeb, L. A. 1971. Zinc in DNA polymerases. *Biochem. Biophys. Res. Commun.* **44,** 37–43.

Smith, Z. M., and Pretorius, P. J. 1964. Studies in metabolism of zinc. Part 2. Serum zinc levels and urinary zinc excretions in South African Bantu kwashiorkor patients. *J. Trop. Pediatr.* **9,** 105–112.

Smith, J. C., Jr., McDaniel, E. G., Fan, F. F., and Halsted, J. A. 1973. Zinc: A trace element essential in vitamin A metabolism. *Science* **181,** 954–955.

Smith, J. C., Jr., Zeller, J. A., Brown, E. D., and Ong, S. C. 1976. Elevated plasma zinc: A heritable anomaly. *Science* **193,** 496–498.

Solomons, N. W., Khactu, K. V., Sandstead, H. H., and Rosenberg, I. H. 1974. Zinc nutrition in regional enteritis (RE). *Amer. J. Clin. Nutr.* **27,** 438.

Somers, M., and Underwood, E. J. 1969a. Ribonuclease activity and nucleic acid and protein metabolism in the testes of zinc-deficient rats. *Aust. J. Biol. Sci.* **22,** 1277–1282.

Somers, M., and Underwood, E. J. 1969b. Studies of zinc nutrition in sheep. II. The influence of zinc deficiency in ram lambs upon the digestibility of the dry matter and the utilization of the nitrogen and sulphur of the diet. *Aust. J. Agric. Res.* **20,** 899–903.

Sommer, A. L. 1928. Further evidence of the essential nature of zinc for the growth of higher green plants: The search for elements essential in only small amounts for plant growth. *Science* **66,** 482–484.

Sommer, A. L., and Lipman, C. B. 1926. Evidence on indispensable nature of zinc and boron for higher green plants. *Plant Physiol.* **1,** 231–249.

Spencer, H., Rosoff, B., Feldstein, A., Cohn, S. H., and Gusamano, E. 1965a. Metabolism of zinc-65 in man. *Radiat. Res.* **24,** 432–445.

Spencer, H. Vankinscott, V., Lewin, I., and Samachson, J. 1965b. Zinc-65 metabolism during low and high calcium intake in man. *J. Nutr.* **86,** 169–177.

Spencer, H., Osis, D., Kramer, L., and Norris, C. 1976. Intake, excretion and retention of zinc in man. In: *Trace Elements in Human Health and Disease* (A. S. Prasad, ed.). Academic Press, New York, pp. 345–361.

Springgate, C. F., Mildvan, A. S., and Loeb, L. A. 1973. Studies on the role of zinc in DNA polymerase. *Fed. Proc. Fed. Amer. Soc. Exp. Biol.* **32,** 541.

Squibb, K. S., and Cousins, R. J. 1977. Synthesis of metallothionein in a polysomal cell-free system. *Biochem. Biophys. Res. Commun.* **75,** 806–812.

Squibb, K. S., Cousins, R. J., and Feldman, S. L. 1977. Control of zinc-thionein synthesis in rat liver. *Biochem. J.* **164,** 223–228.

Srinivasan, S., and Balwani, J. H. 1969. Effect of zinc sulfate on carbon tetrachloride hepatoxicity. *Acta Pharmacol. (Copenhagen)* **27,** 424–428.

Stand, F., Rosoff, B., Williams, G. L., and Spencer, H. 1962. Tissue distribution studies of ionic and chelated 65-zinc in mice. *J. Pharmacol. Exp. Ther.* **138,** 399–404.

Stephan, J. K., and Hsu, J. M. 1973. Effect of zinc deficiency and wounding on DNA synthesis in the rat skin. *J. Nutr.* **103,** 548–552.

Strain, W. H., Steadman, L. T., Lankau, C. A., Jr., Berliner, W. P., and Pories, W. J. 1966a. Analysis of zinc levels in hair for the diagnosis of zinc deficiency in man. *J. Lab. Clin. Med.* **68,** 244–249.

Strain, W. H., Lascari, A., and Pories, W. J. 1966b. Zinc deficiency in babies. *Proceedings of the 7th International Congress on Nutrition,* Vol. 5, pp. 759–765. Sullivan, J. F. 1962a. Effect of alcohol on urinary zinc excretion. *Q. J. Stud. Alcohol.* **23,** 216.

Sullivan, J. F. 1962b. The relation of zincuria to water and electrolyte excretion in patients with hepatic cirrhosis. *Gastroenterology* **42,** 439–442.

Sullivan, J. F., and Heaney, R. P. 1970. Zinc metabolism in alcoholic liver disease. *Amer. J. Clin. Nutr.* **23,** 170–177.

Sullivan, J. F., and Lankford, H. G. 1962. Urinary excretion of zinc in alcoholism and post alcoholic cirrhosis. *Amer. J. Clin. Nutr.* **10,** 153–157.

Sullivan, J. F., and Lankford, H. G. 1965. Zinc metabolism and chronic alcoholism. *Amer. J. Clin. Nutr.* **17,** 57–63.

Sullivan, J. F., Parker, M. M., and Boyett, J. D. 1969. Incidence of low serum zinc in noncirrhotic patients. *Proc. Soc. Exp. Biol. Med.* **130,** 591–594.

Swenerton, H. R. 1971. The role of zinc in the mammalian development. *Diss. Abstr. Int. B:* **31,** 5443.

Swenerton, H., and Hurley, L. S. 1968. Severe zinc deficiency in male and female rats. *J. Nutr.* **95,** 8–18.

Swenerton, H., Shrader, R., and Hurley, L. S. 1969. Zinc-deficient embryos: Reduced thymidine incorporation. *Science* **166,** 1014–1015.

Swenerton, H., Shrader, R., and Hurley, L. S. 1972. Lactic and malic dehydrogenases in testes of zinc-deficient rats. *Proc. Soc. Exp. Biol. Med.* **141,** 283–286.

Szadkowski, D., Weimershaus, E., Lindner, K., Schaller, K. H., and Lehnert, G. 1969. Einfluss von Aldosteron auf den Interflux und Efflux arbeitsmedizinisch relevanter Mineralien und Spurenelemente des menschlichen Organismus. *Int. Z. Angew. Physiol.* **27,** 99–109.

Tal, M. 1969. Metal ions and ribosomal conformation. *Biochim. Biophys. Acta* **195,** 76–86.

Tao, S., and Hurley, L. S. 1971. Changes in plasma proteins in zinc-deficient rats. *Proc. Soc. Exp. Biol. Med.* **136,** 165.

Tarui, S. 1963. Studies on zinc metabolism. III. Effects of the diabetic state on zinc metabolism: A clinical aspect. *Endocrinol. Jpn.* **10,** 9–15.

Terhune, M. W., and Sandstead, H. H. 1972. Decreased RNA polymerase activity in mammalian zinc deficiency. *Science* **177,** 68–69.

Theuer, R. C., and Hoekstra, W. G. 1966. Oxidation of ^{14}C-labeled carbohydrate, fat and amino acid substrates by zinc-deficient rats. *J. Nutr.* **89,** 448–454.

Tipton, I. H., and Cook, M. J. 1963. Trace elements in human tissue. Part II. Adult subjects from the United States. *Health Phys.* **9,** 103–145.

Tipton, I. H., Schroeder, H. A., Perry, H. M., Jr., and Cook, M. J. 1965. Trace elements in human tissue. Part III. Subjects from Africa, the Near and Far East and Europe. *Health Phys.* **11,** 403–451.

Tipton, I. H., Stewart, P. L., and Dickson, J. 1969. Patterns of elemental excretion in long term balance studies. *Health Phys* **16,** 455–462.

Todd, W. R., Elvehjem, C. A., and Hart, E. B. 1934. Zinc in the nutrition of the rat. *Amer. J. Physiol.* **107,** 146–156.

Tribble, H. M., and Scoular, F. I. 1954. Zinc metabolism of young college women on self-selected diets. *J. Nutr.* **52,** 209–216.

Tucker, H. F., and Salmon, W. D. 1955. Parakeratosis or zinc deficiency disease in pigs. *Proc. Soc. Exp. Biol. Med.* **88,** 613–616.

Underwood, E. J. 1977. *Trace Elements in Human and Animal Nutrition,* 4th ed. Academic Press, New York, pp. 196–242.

Undritz, E. 1964. Oral treatment of iron deficiency. In: *Iron Metabolism* (F. Gross, ed.). Springer-Verlag, Berlin—Göttingen—Heidelberg, pp. 406–425.

Vallee, B. L. 1955. Zinc and metalloenzymes. *Adv. Protein Chem.* **10,** 317–384.

Vallee, B. L. 1959. Biochemistry, physiology and pathology of zinc. *Physiol. Rev.* **39,** 443–490.

Vallee, B. L., and Wacker, W. E. C. 1970. Metalloproteins. In: *The Proteins: Composition, Structure and Function,* 2nd ed., Vol. 5 (H. Neurath, ed.). Academic Press, New York, pp. 1–192.

Vallee, B. L., and Wacker, W. E. C. 1972. The metalloproteins. In: *The Proteins,* Vol. 5 (H. Neurath, ed.). Academic Press, New York, pp. 143–146.

Vallee, B. L., Wacker, W. E. C., Bartholomay, A. F., and Robin, E. D. 1956. Zinc metabolism in hepatic dysfunction. I. Serum zinc concentrations in Laënnec's cirrhosis and their validation by sequential analysis. *N. Engl. J. Med.* **255,** 403–408.

Vallee, B. L., Wacker, W. E. C., Bartholomay, A. F., and Hoch, F. L. 1957. Zinc metabolism in hepatic dysfunction. II. Correlation of metabolic patterns with biochemical findings. *N. Engl. J. Med.* **257,** 1055–1065.

Vallee, B. L., Wacker, W. E. C., Bartholomay, A. F., and Hoch, F. L. 1959. Zinc metabolism in hepatic dysfunction. *Ann. Intern. Med.* **50,** 1077–1091.

Van Campen, D. R. 1966. Effects of zinc, cadmium, silver and mercury on the absorption and distribution of copper-64 in rats. *J. Nutr.* **88,** 125–130.

Van Peenen, H. J., and Lucas, F. V. 1961. Zinc in liver disease. *Arch. Pathol.* **72,** 700–702.

Van Peenen, H. J., and Patel, A. 1964. Tissue zinc and calcium in chronic disease. *Arch. Pathol.* **77,** 53–56.

Van Reen, R. 1966. Zinc toxicity in man and experimental species. In: *Zinc Metabolism* (A. S. Prasad, ed.). Charles C. Thomas, Springfield, Illinois, pp. 411–426.

Van Rij, A. M., McKenzie, J. M., and Dunckley, J. V. 1975. Excessive urinary zinc losses and aminoaciduria during intravenous alimentation. *Proc. Univ. Utag. Med. Sch. (New Zealand)* **53,** 77–78.

Vohra, P., and Kratzer, F. H. 1964. Influence of various chelating agents on the availability of zinc. *J. Nutr.* **82,** 249–256.

Voigt, G. E., and Saldeen, T. 1965. Über den Schutzeffekt des Zinks gegenüber Mangansulfat- oder Kohlenstofftetrachloridinduzierten Leberschäden. *Frankf. Z. Pathol.* **74,** 572–578.

Wacker, W. E. C. 1962. Nucleic acid and metals. III. Changes in nucleic acid, protein, and metal content as a consequence of zinc deficiency in *Euglena gracilis*. *Biochemistry* **1,** 859–865.

Wacker, W. E. C., and Vallee, B. L. 1959. Nucleic acids and metals. I. Chromium, manganese, nickel, iron, and other metals in ribonucleic acid from diverse biological sources. *J. Biol. Chem.* **234,** 3257–3262.

Warren, L., Glick, M., and Nass, M. 1966. Membranes of animal cells. I. Methods of isolation of the surface membrane. *J. Cell. Physiol.* **68,** 269–288.

Waters, M. D., Moore, R. D., Amato, J. J., and Houck, J. C. 1971. Zinc sulfate failure as an accelerator of collagen biosynthesis and fibroblast proliferation. *Proc. Soc. Exp. Biol. Med.* **138,** 373–377.

Weed, R. I., LaCelle, P. L., and Merrile, E. W. 1969. Metabolic dependence of red cell deformability. *J. Clin. Invest.* **48,** 795–809.

Wegener, W. S., and Romano, A. H. 1963. Zinc stimulation of RNA and protein synthesis in *Rhizopus nigricans*. *Science* **142,** 1669–1670.

Wegener, W. S., and Romano, A. H. 1964. Control of isocitratase formation in *Rhizopus nigricans*. *J. Bacteriol.* **87,** 156–161.

Wells, B. T., and Winkelmann, R. K. 1961. Acrodermatitis enteropathica: Report of 6 Cases. *Arch Dermatol.* **84,** 40–52.

Weser, U., Seeber, S., and Warnecke, P. 1969a. Reactivity of Zn^{2+} on nuclear DNA and RNA biosynthesis of regeneration in rat liver. *Biochim Biophys. Acta* **179,** 422–428.

Weser, U., Seeber, S., and Warnecke, P. 1969b. Effect of Zn^{2+} on nuclear RNA and protein-biosynthesis in rat liver. *Z. Naturforsch. B:* **24,** 866–869.

Weser, U., Hübner, L., and Jung, H. 1970. Zn^{2+}-induced stimulation of nuclear RNA synthesis in rat liver. *FEBS Lett.* **7,** 356–358.

White, H. S., and Gynee, T. N. 1971. Utilization of inorganic elements by young women eating iron-fortified foods. *J. Amer. Diet. Assoc.* **59,** 27–33.

Willden, E. G., and Robinson, M. R. G. 1975. Plasma zinc levels in prostatic disease. *Brit. J. Urol.* **47,** 295–299.

Williams, R. B. 1972, Intestinal alkaline phosphatase and inorganic pyrophosphatase activities in the zinc-deficient rat. *Brit. J. Nutr.* **27,** 121–130.

Williams, R. B., and Chesters, J. K. 1970a. Effects of zinc deficiency on nucleic acid synthesis in the rat. In: *Trace Element Metabolism in Animals* (C. F. Mills, ed.). Livingstone, Edinburgh and London, pp. 164–166.

Williams, R. B., and Chesters, J. K. 1970b. The effects of early Zn deficiency on DNA and protein synthesis in the rat. *Brit. J. Nutr.* **24,** 1053–1059.

Williams, R. B., Mills, C. F. Quarterman, J., and Dalgarno, A. C. 1965. The effect of zinc deficiency on the *in vivo* incorporation of ^{32}P into rat-liver nucleotides. *Biochem J.* **95**(2), 29 pp.

Woessner, J. F., Jr., and Boucek, R. J. 1961. Connective tissue development in subcutaneously implanted polyvinyl sponge. I. Biochemical changes during development. *Arch Biochem. Biophys.* **93,** 85–94.

TOXIC ELEMENTS

CHAPTER 11

CADMIUM

INTRODUCTION

No overt disease due to cadmium exposure has occurred so far in the United States. In Japan, a severe and painful disease, itai itai byo, has been related to prolonged ingestion of food and water containing high concentrations of cadmium. The total daily intake of cadmium was approximately ten times greater than that typical in most parts of the world. The sensitive population group consisted of postmenopausal women who had borne several children. Cadmium has no known essential function, so at this time its presence in any cell must be regarded as undesirable (Fox, 1976).

BIOCHEMISTRY AND METABOLISM

In the gastrointestinal tract during digestion, many types of metal-binding ligands are released, some of which may bind cadmium, typically in competition with other divalent elements. Cadmium and zinc are usually found together in geological and biological systems. Of the two, zinc binds more firmly to nitrogen and oxygen ligands, whereas cadmium binds more firmly to mercapto groups (Fox, 1976).

Cadmium concentrates to a marked extent in the small intestinal wall, presumably in the absorptive mucosal cells. At dietary levels below 10 mg cadmium/kg diet, the duodenums of young Japanese quail accumulated cadmium to concentrations (micrograms per gram fresh weight) 10–20 times greater than the concentration in the dry purified diet (Harland *et al.*, 1973). Other investigators have found that concentrations of cadmium in the liver and kidney are related to the oral dose of cadmium under given conditions (Decker *et al.*, 1958; Anwar *et al.*, 1961; Harland *et al.*, 1973; Cousins *et al.*, 1973; Doyle *et al.*, 1974a). These data suggest that a control mechanism exists at the gut level for absorption and transport of cadmium; however, the exact nature of this regulation is not known (Fox, 1976).

Due to the rapid turnover of intestinal mucosal cells, most of the cadmium is lost from the body when the cells are sloughed from the villi tips. The extent to which cadmium from these shed cells is taken up by mucosal cells lower down in the gastrointestinal tract is unknown. An enteropathy has been observed in patients with itai itai disease (Murata *et al.,* 1970) and in experimental animals fed cadmium (Wilson *et al.,* 1941; Yoshikawa *et al.,* 1960; Stowe *et al.,* 1972; Richardson *et al.,* 1974). It appears that under given conditions, a critical cadmium concentration in the mucosal cell produces structural damage that is probably accompanied by marked changes in absorption of cadmium and other dietary components (Fox, 1976).

The concentration of cadmium in blood is very small, less than 1 μg/100 ml whole blood in persons not exposed to high amounts of cadmium. This small amount is difficult to assay accurately (Fox, 1976).

The liver and kidney are the principal storage sites in the body. It has not been possible to determine the biological half-life of dietary cadmium accurately for either organs or the whole body; it is likely, however, that the half-life is a matter of years for man. From estimates of intake and cross-sectional age data on organ concentrations, estimates of half-life in man range from 16 to 33 years (Fox, 1976; Kjellstroöm, 1971; Tsuchiya and Sugita, 1971).

The critical organ in man with respect to cadmium metabolism appears to be the kidney (Friberg *et al.,* 1971). Friberg *et al.* (1971) postulated that when the concentration of cadmium reaches a critical level (200 μg/g fresh weight) in the renal cortex, renal tubular damage occurs. A variety of compounds have been used in an attempt to flush cadmium from the tissues; however, no method is entirely satisfactory (Fox, 1976).

The placenta and the mammary gland have been shown to act as barriers to cadmium transport into the fetus and newborn, respectively (Lucis *et al.,* 1972). Concentrations of cadmium in the human newborn are extremely small (Fox, 1976; Henke *et al.,* 1970; Chaube *et al.,* 1973).

A protein containing large amounts of cadmium was first isolated from equine renal cortex (Kägi and Vallee, 1960), and later from human renal cortex (Pulido *et al.,* 1966). This protein was named "metallothionein," and the metal-free protein was designated "thionein." Metallothionein has now been characterized by several investigators. The metal content may vary somewhat with different preparations. Typical values are: cadmium, 6%; zinc, 2.2%; small amounts of copper, iron, and mercury; sulfur, 8%, from cysteinyl residues; 20 mercapto groups with 3 mercapto groups per atom of zinc or cadmium; and no aromatic amino acids. The molecular weight is 7000. The cadmium mercaptide is a chromophore with an absorption maximum at 250 nm (Fox, 1976).

Nordberg *et al.* (1972) injected large amounts of cadmium into rabbits. By isoelectric focusing, they were able to resolve metallothionein into two main protein peaks that differed in amino acid content. Both proteins contained cadmium, but only one contained significant amounts of zinc. Other evidence for two forms of cadmium-binding protein in liver and kidney has been reported (Fox, 1976; Shaikh and Lucis, 1971, 1972).

Nordberg *et al.* (1971) reported that soon after injection, cadmium was bound in the liver to high-molecular-weight proteins. By 24 hr after injection, the cadmium was bound entirely to low-molecular-weight proteins. It has also been shown that with repeated injection of cadmium, there is a marked increase in the amount of low-molecular-weight cadmium-binding protein present in the liver (Fox, 1976; Wiśniewska-Knypl and Jabłońska, 1970; Winge and Rajagopalan, 1972).

A low-molecular-weight protein similar to metallothionein that binds copper was isolated from the duodenum of the chick (Starcher, 1969) and from bovine duodenum and liver (Evans *et al.,* 1970). Evidence presented so far indicates that cadmium and zinc could displace copper from that protein (Fox, 1976).

Vallee and Ulmer (1972) reviewed the biochemical effects of cadmium. The biochemistry of cadmium toxicity is not well understood at present. Several *in vitro* studies have shown that cadmium can replace zinc in many of its metalloenzymes, with resultant changes in activity. As noted above, cadmium binds readily to mercapto groups, and these groups are frequently important in enzyme systems. Cadmium also binds to phospholipids and nucleic acids, and has been shown to uncouple oxidative phosphorylation (Fox, 1976).

In general, cadmium can compete with some of the essential divalent elements for ligands. The displacement of the essential element may affect its transport, storage, or function at the active site of an enzyme, or effect a change in the conformation of proteins or nucleic acids required for normal function (Fox, 1976).

In a study conducted by the U.S. Food and Drug Administration concerning intake of dietary cadmium, the annual mean for food composites in certain geographical areas ranged between 0.01 and 0.03 μg/g (Fox, 1976). Higher values in some areas were obtained for dairy products, potatoes, and leafy vegetables. The single highest value was 0.2 μg/g for leafy vegetables (Fox, 1976).

From these calculations, grain and cereals probably supplied the largest amount, 14 μg cadmium/day. Potatoes supplied 7 μg, and amounts between 4 and 5 μg were supplied by each of the following food groups: beverages, leafy vegetables, dairy products, fruits and meats, fish and poultry. The remaining food groups each supplied 1–2 μg/day. From these data, it is estimated that the average daily cadmium intake in the United States is approximately 50 μg. The total daily intake of cadmium in Canada was recently estimated to be 67 μg, based on analysis of foods sampled during 1970–1971 (Fox, 1976; Kirkpatrick and Coffin, 1974).

Oysters, liver, and kidney are known to contain amounts of cadmium that may be appreciably higher than in most foods. It is estimated that single servings of these foods could supply the following amounts of cadmium: beef liver, 20 μg; beef kidney, 40 μg; and oysters, 50 μg. The food composites assayed by the Food and Drug Administration contained liver but no kidneys and oysters (Fox, 1976).

According to the Joint FAO/WHO Expert Committee on Food Additives (Cheftel *et al.,* 1972), a "provisional tolerable weekly intake" of dietary cadmium for a 60-kg man is 400–500 μg. Thus, there is probably a narrow margin between the present typical United States intake and the "provisional tolerable intakes" (Fox, 1976).

The tentative upper limit set in the *WHO International Standards for Drinking Water* (World Health Organization, 1971) is 10 μg/liter. The amounts in drinking water for most industrialized countries are less; however, additional amounts may be dissolved from home plumbing, particularly from galvanized pipes. Thus, daily intake up to 10 μg from water appears to be a reasonable estimate (Fox, 1976).

There are very small amounts of cadmium in the air. It is estimated that approximately 0.02 μg may be inhaled daily by an adult man. Cigarette smoke can contribute significant amounts of cadmium to the total body burden. Menden *et al.* (1972) estimated that approximately 0.1 μg cadmium was inhaled from the mainstream smoke of each cigarette. The sidestream smoke contain a higher concentration of cadmium; however, the amount inhaled would be quite variable. It has been shown that the livers and kidneys of long-term smokers contain higher than average amounts of cadmium (Fox, 1976; Lewis *et al.,* 1972).

INTERRELATIONSHIP OF CADMIUM AND ZINC

The kidney is rich in zinc-dependent enzymes. The renal dysfunction caused by cadmium may be due to adverse effects of cadmium on zinc enzymes necessary for reabsorption and catabolism of proteins. Simultaneous administration of zinc to cadmium-exposed animals alleviates some of the renal symptoms caused by cadmium (Vigiliani, 1969). Cousins *et al.* (1973) found that the activity in the renal cortex of the zinc enzyme leucinaminopeptidase was decreased in swine exposed to high concentrations of cadmium in the diet. This decrease occurred at a cadmium concentration in the cortex of about 100 μg/g wet weight (Piscator, 1976).

In "normal" human subjects, the increase in cadmium concentration in renal cortex with age is accompanied by an equimolar increase in zinc concentrations (Piscator and Lind, 1972; Hammer *et al.,* 1973). This observation is valid for cadmium concentrations up to 75 μg/g wet weight. Human data are lacking, however, for the cadmium range of 75–200 μg/g. The relationship between cadmium and zinc in this range has been studied in normal horses, and it has been found that whereas at cadmium concentrations below 75 μg/g, there was an equimolar increase in zinc with increased cadmium, such a relationship could not be found in the higher range; i.e., zinc did not increase to the same extent as cadmium (Piscator, 1976). These observations indicate that there could be a progressive relative zinc deficiency in the renal cortex at cadmium concentrations between 100 and 200 μg/g, and that with increasing zinc deficiency, tubular dysfunction might appear. The retention of zinc in the liver and kidney caused by cadmium excess may also cause depletion of zinc in other organs. Thus, Petering *et al.* (1971) showed that when the intake of zinc in rats was marginal, exposure to cadmium caused a decrease in the zinc concentrations in the testes. Such an effect was not seen when the intake of zinc was increased. There is thus evidence for cadmium interference with metabolism and utilization of zinc, and it is obvious that in studies on effects of cadmium, the intake and organ levels of zinc must also be studied (Piscator, 1976).

CADMIUM TOXICITY

It has been known for several years that cadmium can markedly alter the metabolism and function of several essential elements, including zinc, iron, manganese, copper, selenium, and calcium. With individual deficiencies of zinc, iron, copper, calcium, vitamin D, or protein, the toxicity of cadmium and sometimes the tissue accumulation are markedly increased (Fox, 1976).

It has been shown that an excess intake of zinc, iron, copper, selenium, ascorbic acid, or protein over and above its daily requirement protects against various effects of cadmium. Fox *et al.* (1973) reported that the toxicity of cadmium was decreased when the dietary protein was supplied by dried eggwhite as compared with either isolated soybean protein or the combination of casein plus gelatin. The animals showed better growth response, were less anemic, and had higher tissue concentrations of zinc and iron when dietary protein was supply by dried eggwhite. On the other hand, Stowe *et al.* (1974) reported that high dietary pyridoxine levels increased the severity of the anemia produced by dietary cadmium (Fox, 1976).

Simultaneously supplementing a diet with amounts of zinc, copper, and manganese appreciably above the requirement level of each, with amounts of cadmium far in excess of the daily intake of man, resulted in decreased concentrations of cadmium in the kidneys of young Japanese quail (Fox, 1976). This effect was observed with dietary concentrations of 10, 20, and 40 mg cadmium/kg diet (Fox, 1976).

The need for protecting against unavoidable exposure to toxic elements may make it desirable for man to consume slightly more than the requirement levels of some nutrients. As more information is obtained, it is reasonable to expect that the quantities of essential nutrients that provide protection against toxic elements will be a consideration in establishing requirements for man (Fox, 1976).

CADMIUM AND HYPERTENSION

Hypertensive subjects have abnormally high concentrations of renal cadmium, and elevated blood pressures in animals following chronic cadmium administration orally have been observed (Perry, 1976). These observations provide support for early speculations relating cadmium to hypertension (Perry, 1976).

The evidence that cadmium can increase blood pressure in animals seems incontrovertible. Parenteral cadmium can induce acute transient hypertension in animals (Perry and Erlanger, 1971b; Schroeder *et al.,* 1966).

The induction of hypertension in animals by feeding cadmium was first reported by Schroeder and Vinton (1962). During tbe next 12 years, Schroeder extended his initial observations in numerous reports (Schroeder, 1964; Schroeder and Buckman, 1967; Schroeder *et al.,* 1968a, b, 1970; Kanisawa and Schroeder, 1969). Recently, it was confirmed that chronically fed cadmium could raise systolic pressure in animals (Perry and Erlanger, 1971a, 1974); however, some investigators have failed to induce hypertension by feeding cadmium to animals (Perry, 1976; Friberg *et al.,* 1971).

The mechanism of cadmium-induced hypertension in animals remains obscure. The most likely mechanism involves an effect of cadmium on salt and water metabolism. Several experiments indicate that cadmium may produce sodium retention. Vander (1962) observed that cadmium injected into one renal artery decreased sodium excretion on that side. Repeated subcutaneous injections of cadmium produced an early sodium loss followed by sodium retention (Perry *et al.,* 1971). Hyperreninemia was reported in cadmium-fed rats (Perry and Erlanger, 1973). Doyle and coworkers presented data to show that ingested cadmium induces significant retention of a single intravenous injection of radiosodium (Doyle *et al.,* 1974b; Perry, 1976).

Cadmium-induced hypertension in rats, although real, may be relatively small in magnitude. Most human hypertension is also mild. Of the 25 million Americans who are estimated to have hypertension, at least two thirds have diastolic pressures below 105 mm Hg. Nonetheless, in man at least, even such mild elevations in blood pressure can double the risk of heart attack or stroke, the major causes of disability and death. Moreover, like cadmium-induced hypertension in rats, mild human hypertension has no obvious associated findings. In rats, the small amounts of cadmium that induce hypertension produce none of the usual toxic manifestations of cadmium. In man, likewise, mild hypertension is not accompanied by any other clinical signs or symptoms (Perry, 1976).

Although at present there is no proof, pro or con, that cadmium is in any way involved in human hypertension, cadmium is an increasingly prevalent and serious environmental pollutant, and it thus becomes very pertinent to determine the maximum cadmium exposure that can be tolerated without affecting blood pressure. This level may be difficult to define. Obviously, the hypertensive effect of cadmium seems very likely to be conditioned by complex interactions with other substances, such as zinc, selenium, copper, and possibly many other things including hard water. Therefore, any such definition of permissible limits of cadmium exposure must take into account the rest of the environment (Perry, 1976).

TISSUE ACCUMULATION

The accumulation of cadmium in the whole body and in the liver, kidney, or duodenum of experimental animals can be determined very precisely in fairly short-term experiments by the use of radioisotopes. Cadmium-115m is suitable for whole-body counting, whereas either cadmium-109 or cadmium-115m is satisfactory for counting individual tissues following solubilization. Cadmium-109 is available in carrier-free form, so very small amounts of stable cadmium accompany the tracer. Thus, when foods are labeled with cadmium-109, it is possible to develop bioassays based on metabolism and tissue accumulation of cadmium at dietary levels similar to those of man (Fox, 1976).

CHRONIC CADMIUM TOXICITY

It has been known for more than a century that cadmium can cause acute poisoning in man. The occurrence of chronic cadmium poisoning was established only about 25 years ago (Friberg, 1948, 1950). Friberg made detailed examinations of cadmium-exposed workers and found that lung damage, mainly emphysema, and renal dysfunction were the major features. Since then, many similar investigations have been performed in several countries, and exposure to cadmium compounds is now recognized as a serious occupational hazard (Piscator, 1976).

OCCUPATIONAL POISONING

In a Swedish factory producing alkaline batteries with nickel and cadmium electrodes, a number of deaths had occurred in the 1930's and early 1940's, and the causative agent was not known. There were also complaints about such symptoms as shortness of breath and fatigue. Careful studies by Friberg, both clinical and experimental, revealed that cadmium oxide dust was responsible (Friberg, 1948, 1950). It caused emphysema of the lungs and renal damage, these two being the most prominent findings. Anemia, slight liver damage, anosmia, and a yellow coloring of the teeth were other significant findings. The exposure had been high, probably several milligrans per cubic meter of air for many years (Piscator, 1976).

Friberg's findings were confirmed by studies in West Germany and the United Kingdom (Baader, 1951; Hunter, 1954). Further reports from these countries and during later years also from Japan, France, and Belgium have shown that renal damage is the most common finding, whereas lung damage and anemia are uncommon. Improved working conditions and lower cadmium concentrations in air have resulted in less intense exposure. Most data are from studies on male workers. Already in 1942, however, osteomalacia was reported to have occurred in a French factory where there was exposure to cadmium (Nicaud *et al.,* 1942). Of six cases, four were women. In a study in the U.S.S.R., it was found that newborns from cadmium-exposed women had lower weights than children of nonexposed women. Since cadmium does not traverse the placenta to any significant extent, this effect might well be due to a zinc deficiency in the fetus induced by cadmium excess (Piscator, 1976).

CHRONIC POISONING VIA FOOD

The most severe form of chronic cadmium poisoning is itai-itai disease. It was first seen in women above 45 years of age in Fuchu, Toyama Prefecture, Japan. Exposure to cadmium had occured through the ingestion of rice grown on fields irrigated by water from a river that had been contaminated by a mine many miles upstream. The concentration of cadmium in the rice for many years had been around 1 μg/g, and the daily intake of cadmium must have been 300 μg or more, which is excessive in comparison with the average intake of 50 μg daily in some European countries and the United States. Itai-itai disease is characterized by osteomalacia and received its name from the severe pain caused by fractures of the softened bones. The renal dysfunction is severe, and there is an increase in the excretion of protein, glucose, amino acids, and phosphorus similar to that seen in Fanconi syndrome. Cadmium concentrations in the liver are high, of the same magnitude as found in exposed workers, but renal concentrations of cadmium are often very low due to losses of cadmium by the renal dysfunction (Friberg *et al.,* 1974). Predisposing factors are the low intakes of calcium and Vitamin D, and many pregnancies and lactation periods, which themselves cause depletion of calcium. Among the males in the area, proteinuria and glucosuria are common findings, but osteomalacia is uncommon, which may be explained by a better calcium balance. Itai-itai disease is an extreme manifestation of chronic cadmium poisoning, but in several other cadmium-polluted areas of Japan, only tubular proteinuria has been reported (Piscator, 1976).

EFFECTS OF CADMIUM ON THE HUMAN KIDNEY

Friberg reported that cadmium-exposed workers had a high prevalence of proteinuria in comparison with controls (Piscator, 1976). Further studies showed that this proteinuria was not of the classic type seen in chronic nephritis or nephrosis. The proteins had a different electrophoretic pattern and were of lower molecular weight than albumin. A decreased ability to concentrate the urine and a reduction in inulin clearance were other signs of renal dysfunction (Friberg, 1948, 1950; Piscator, 1976).

The tubular proteinuria due to cadmium toxicity was caused by a decrease in reabsorption of proteins from the glomerular filtrate (Piscator, 1966). The excretion of protein was related to cadmium exposure time. The low-molecular-weight proteinuria was regarded as the first sign of an effect of cadmium on renal function. By using immunological and electrophoretic methods for determination of specific proteins, it was possible to detect small increases in urinary excretion of such proteins, e.g., β_2-microglobulin. Glucosuria and aminoaciduria generally appear later than the protenuria. The excretion of cadmium is low as long as there is normal renal function, but when the excretion of protein increases, there is also an increase in the excretion of cadmium (Piscator, 1976).

In the Japanese study, the proteinuria was of the same type as seen in cadmium-exposed workers in Sweden, and the cadmium excretion was considerably higher in patients with itai-itai disease in comparison with that in people from the nonpolluted areas (Friberg *et al.,* 1974; Piscator, 1976).

The critical concentration of cadmium in the renal cortex, i.e., the concentration at which sensitive persons may get tubular dysfunction, has been estimated to be 200 μg/g wet weight (Friberg *et al.,* 1974; Piscator, 1976).

Experiments on animals verified that exposure to cadmium causes renal tubular dysfunction (Axelsson and Piscator, 1966; Nordberg, 1972). Autoradiographic studies by Berlin, *et al.* (1964) showed that cadmium accumulated mainly in the proximal part of the renal tubule, the part of the tubule in which protein reabsorption occurs. It has also been indicated that cadmium bound to metallothionein may be filtered through the glomeruli and reabsorbed (Nordberg, 1972). It is thus conceivable that cadmium will accumulate in the kidney mainly at a site in which there is reabsorption of protein. This also means that the first function to be disturbed when there is excessive accumulation of cadmium should be protein reabsorption, which fits well with the experience from investigations on humans (Piscator, 1976).

It was observed by Nordberg (1972) that in mice exposed to cadmium, the urinary excretion of cadmium was very low as long as the renal function was normal, but a sharp rise in cadmium excretion occurred when the tubular proteinuria appeared. The presence of cadmium in a low-molecular-weight urine protein fraction, conceivably metallothionein, was demonstrated. This finding may suggest that the decreased reabsorption of proteins also caused a decrease in the reabsorption of metallothionein. The continued increase in cadmium excretion may eventually lead to a depletion of renal cadmium as seen in itai-itai patients (Piscator, 1976). Although the critical level of cadmium in the renal cortex is around 200 μg/g wet weight in calcium-deficient rats, the excretion of ribonuclease was increased at a cadmium concentration in the renal cortex of about 90 μg/g wet weight, indicating that under certain circumstances, the critical level might be below 200 μg/g (Piscator, 1976).

EFFECTS OF CADMIUM ON BONE

Since osteomalacia has been found both in exposed workers and in Japanese women exposed to cadmium via rice, several studies have been carried out concerning mineral metabolism in cadmium toxicity. The concentrations of cadmium in bone tissue are low even at high body burdens, and there is little evidence for a direct action of cadmium on bone. In short-term experiments on calcium-deficient rats given cadmium in drinking water (25 μg/g for 2 months) and long-term experiments (7.5 μg/g for 13 months), calcium accretion in bone was not decreased in cadmium-exposed animals (Larsson and Piscator, 1971). It was observed, however, that cadmium accelerated the osteoporotic process caused by calcium deficiency alone.

It is possible that interference with intestinal absorption of calcium and endocrine disturbances due to cadmium excess were responsible for osteoporosis. In the short-term experiment, the increase in parathyroid volume, which is caused by calcium deficiency, was inhibited by cadmium. In the long-term experiment, there were signs of slight renal tubular damage already at a cadmium concentration in the renal cortex of about 90 μg/g wet weight, indicating that the kidneys of a calcium-deficient animals may be more sensitive to cadmium than those of normal animals (Piscator, 1976).

The bone changes in itai-itai disease occurred mainly in women with low intakes of calcium and greater losses of calcium due to multiple pregnancies. The exposure to cadmium caused renal tubular dysfunction, which caused further losses of minerals. In Swedish factory workers with renal tubular damage but high intakes of calcium, bone changes were not seen (Friberg, 1950; Piscator, 1976).

Since the most active form of vitamin D is produced in the kidney, it is also conceivable that the accumulation of cadmium may interfere with the synthesis of this form, which may further contribute to the disturbances in mineral metabolism (Piscator, 1976).

OTHER EFFECTS OF CADMIUM

Anemia has been seen in exposed workers and in animal experiments. This anemia may be due to interference with the absorption of iron and mild hemolysis (Friberg, *et al.*, 1974; Piscator, 1976).

The liver may contain large amounts of cadmium, but clinical tests for signs of liver damage are often negative. Animal experiments by Stowe *et al.* (1972) indicate, however, that clinical tests generally used for studies of liver function, e.g., glutamic oxalacetic transaminase (GOT) and glutamic pyruvic transaminase (GPT), may be negative even when morphological changes are manifest. Experiments by Sporn *et al.* (1970) on rats given small amounts of cadmium in drinking water for 1 year indicate that at liver levels of cadmium of the same magnitude as found in normal humans, some metabolic pathways in the liver may be affected (Piscator, 1976).

ACUTE CADMIUM POISONING

Acute cadmium poisoning is characterized by severe nausea, salivation, vomiting, diarrhea, abdominal pain, and neuralgia. Cadmium is soluble in an acid medium; therefore, storage of acid food or citrus juices in cadmium-plated containers has in the past caused poisoning. Sales of containers plated with cadmium are banned in many states to prevent chemical poisoning from this source. The lethal dose is unknown, but as little as 10 mg has caused serious symptoms that are mainly gastrointestinal.

Treatment

For acute poisoning due to ingestion, gastric lavage followed by demulcents is recommended. A chelating agent such as calcium-ethylenediaminetetraacetate (calcium-EDTA), 0.5 g every 6 hr for 1 or 2 weeks, has been found to be effective. In serious situations, it should be given intravenously. In inhalation exposure, the patient should be removed from further exposure and given supportive therapy for pulmonary edema, and calcium-EDTA should be started as described above.

REFERENCES

Anwar, R. A., Langham, R. F., Hoppert, C. A., Alfredson, B. V., and Byerrum, R. U. 1961. Chronic toxicity studies. III. Chronic toxicity of cadmium and chromium in dogs. *Arch. Environ. Health* **3,** 456–460.

Axelsson, B., and Piscator, M. 1966. Renal damage after prolonged exposure to cadmium. *Arch. Environ. Health* **12,** 360–373.

Baader, E. W. 1951. Die chronische Kadmiumvergiftung. *Dtsch. Med. Wochenschr.* **76,** 484–487.

Berlin, M., Hammarström, I., and Maunsbach, A. B. 1964. Microautoradiographic localization of water-soluble cadmium in mouse kidney. *Acta Radiol.* **2,** 345–352.

Chaube, S., Nishimura, H., and Swinyard, C. A. 1973. Zinc and cadmium in normal human embryos and fetuses. *Arch. Environ. Health* **26,** 237–240.

Cheften, H., Cotta-Ramusino, F., Egan, H., Kojima, K., Miettinen, J. K., Smith, D. M., Berglund, F., Blumenthal, H., Golberg, L., Kazantzis, G., Piscator, M., Truhaut, R., Tsubaki, T., and Zajcev, A. N. 1972. Evaluation of certain food additives and the contaminants mercury, lead, and cadmium. *W.H.O. Tech. Rep. Ser.* **505,** 1–32.

Cousins, R. J., Barber, A. K., and Trout, J. R. 1973. Cadmium toxicity in growing swine. *J. Nutr.* **103,** 964–972.

Decker, L. E., Byerrum, R. U., Decker, C. F., Hoppert, C. A., and Langham, R. F. 1958. Chronic toxicity studies. I. Cadmium administered in drinking water to rats. *AMA Arch. Ind. Health* **18,** 228–231.

Doyle, J. J., Pfander, W. H., Grebing, S. E., and Pierce, J. O., II. 1974a. Effect of dietary cadmium on absorption and cadmium tissue levels in growing lambs. *J. Nutr.* **104,** 160–166.

Doyle, J. J., Bernhoft, R. A., Vo-Khactu, K. P., and Sandstead, H. H. 1974b. The effects of a low level of dietary cadmium on some biochemical and physiological parameters in rats. VIII Annual Conference on Trace Substances in Environmental Health, University of Missouri, Columbia, pp. 403–409.

Evans, G. W., Majors, P. F., and Cornatzer, W. E. 1970. Mechanism for cadmium and zinc antagonism of copper metabolism. *Biochem. Biophys. Res. Commun.* **40,** 1142–1148.

Fox, M. R. S. 1976. Cadmium metabolism—A review of aspects pertinent to evaluating dietary cadmium intake by man. In: *Trace Elements in Human Health and Disease,* Vol. II (A. S. Prasad, ed.). Academic Press, New York, pp. 401–416.

Fox, M. R. S., Jacobs, R. M., Fry, B. E., Jr., and Harland, B. F. 1973. Effect of protein source on response to cadmium. *Fed. Proc. Fed. Amer. Soc. Exp. Biol.* **32,** 924.

Friberg, L. 1948. Proteinuria and emphysema among workers exposed to cadmium and nickel dust in a storage battery plant. *Proc. Int. Congr. Ind. Med.* **9,** 641–644.

Friberg, L. 1950. Health hazards in the manufacture of alkaline accumulators with special reference to chronic cadmium poisoning. *Acta Med. Scand.* **138**(Suppl. 240), 1–124.

Friberg, L., Piscator, M., and Nordberg, G. 1971. *Cadmium in the Environment,* 1st ed. CRC Press, Cleveland, Ohio, pp. 1–166.

Friberg, L., Piscator, M., Nordberg, G., and Kjellström, T. 1974. *Cadmium in the Environment,* 2nd ed. CRC Press, Cleveland, Ohio, pp. 1–248.

Hammer, D. I., Colucci, A. K., Hasselblad, V., Williams, M. E., and Pinkerton, C. 1973. Cadmium and lead in autopsy tissues. *J. Occup. Med.* **15,** 956–963.

Harland, B. F., Fry, B. E., Jr., Jacobs, R. M., and Fox, M. R. S. 1973. Response of young Japanese quail to graded levels of dietary cadmium. *Abstr. IX Int. Congr. Nutr.,* p. 53.

Henke, G., Sachs, H. W., and Bohn, G. 1970. Cadmiumbestimmungen in Leber und Nieren von Kindern und Jugendlichen durch Neutronenaktivierungsanalyse. *Arch. Toxikol.* **26,** 8–16.

Hunter, D. 1954. Cadmium poisoning. *Arch. Hig. Rada* **5,** 221–224.

Kägi, J. H. R., and Vallee, B. L. 1960. Metallothionein: A cadmium- and zinc-containing protein from equine renal cortex. *J. Biol. Chem.* **235,** 3460–3465.

Kanisawa, M., and Schroeder, H. A. 1969. Renal arteriolar changes in hypertensive rats given cadmium in drinking water. *Exp. Mol. Pathol.* **10,** 81–98.

Kirkpatrick, D. C., and Coffin, D. E. 1974. The trace metal content of representative Canadian diets in 1970 to 1971. *Canad. Inst. Food Sci. Technol. J.* **7,** 56–58.

Kjellström, T. 1971. A mathematical model for the accumulation of cadmium in human kidney cortex. *Nord. Hyg. Tidskr.* **53,** 111–119.

Larsson, S., and Piscator, M. 1971. Effect of cadmium on skeletal tissue in normal and calcium-deficient rats. *Isr. J. Med. Sci.* **7,** 495–497.

Lewis, G. P., Jusko, W. J., Coughlin, L. L., and Hartz, S. 1972. Contribution of cigarette smoking to cadmium accumulation in man. *Lancet* **1,** 291–292.

Lucis, O. J., Lucis, R., and Shaikh, Z. A. 1972. Cadmium and zinc in pregnancy and lactation. *Arch. Environ. Health* **25,** 14–22.

Menden, E. E., Elia, V. J., Michael, L. W., and Petering, H. G. 1972. Distribution of cadmium and nickel of tobacco during cigarette smoking. *Environ. Sci. Technol.* **6,** 830–832.

Murata, I., Hirono, T., Saeki, Y., and Nakagawa, S. 1970. Cadmium enteropathy, renal osteomalacia ("itai itai" disease in Japan). *Bull. Soc. Int. Chir.* **29,** 34–42.

Nicaud, P., Lafitte, A., and Gros, A. 1942. Les troubles de l'intoxication chronique par le cadmium. *Arch. Mal. Prof.* **4,** 192–202.

Nordberg, G. 1972. Cadmium metabolism and toxicity. *Environ. Physiol. Biochem.* **2,** 7–36.

Nordberg, G. F., Piscator, M., and Lind, B. 1971. Distribution of cadmium among protein fractions of mouse liver. *Acta Pharmacol. Toxicol.* **29,** 456–470.

Nordberg, G. F., Nordberg, M., Piscator, M., and Vesterberg, O. 1972. Separation of two forms of rabbit metallothionein by isoelectric focusing. *Biochem. J.* **126,** 491–498.

Perry, H. M., Jr. 1976. Review of hypertension induced in animals by chronic ingestion of cadmium. In: *Trace Elements in Human Health and Disease,* Vol. II (A. S. Prasad, ed.). Academic Press, New York, pp. 417–430.

Perry, H. M., Jr., and Erlanger, M. W. 1971a. Hypertension in rats induced by long-term low-level cadmium ingestion. *Circulation* **44**(Suppl. II), 130.

Perry, H. M., Jr., and Erlanger, M. 1971b. Hypertension and tissue metal levels after intraperitoneal cadmium, mercury, and zinc. *Amer. J. Physiol.* **220,** 808–811.

Perry, H. M., Jr., and Erlanger, M. 1973. Elevated circulating renin activity in rats following doses of cadmium known to induce hypertension. *J. Lab. Clin. Med.* **82,** 399–405.

Perry, H. M., Jr., and Erlanger, M. 1974. Metal-induced hypertension following chronic feeding of low doses of cadmium and mercury. *J. Lab. Clin. Med.* **83,** 541–547.

Perry, H. M., Jr., Perry E. F., and Purifoy, J. E. 1971. Antinatriuretic effect of intramuscular cadmium in rats. *Proc. Soc. Exp. Biol. Med.* **136,** 1240–1244.

Petering, H. G., Johnson, M. A., and Stemmer, K. L. 1971. Studies of zinc metabolism in the rat. I. Dose–response effects of cadmium. *Arch. Environ. Health* **23,** 93–101.

Piscator, M. 1966. *Proteinuria in Chronic Cadmium Poisoning.* Beckman's, Stockholm, p. 29.

Piscator, M. 1976. The chronic toxicity of cadmium. In: *Trace Elements in Human Health and Disease,* Vol. II (A. S. Prasad, ed.). Academic Press, New York, pp. 431–441.

Piscator, M., and Lind, B. 1972. Cadmium, zinc, copper and lead in human renal cortex. *Arch. Environ. Health* **24,** 426–431.

Pulido, P., Kägi, J. H. R., and Vallee, B. L. 1966. Isolation and some properties of human metallothionein. *Biochemistry* **5,** 1768–1777.

Richardson, M. E., Fox, M. R. S., and Fry, B. E., Jr. 1974. Pathological changes produced in Japanese quail by ingestion of cadmium. *J. Nutr.* **104,** 323–338.

Schroeder, H. A. 1964. Cadmium hypertension in rats. *Amer. J. Physiol.* **207,** 62–66.

Schroeder, H. A., and Buckman, J. B. 1967. Cadmium hypertension: Its reversal in rats by a zinc chelate. *Arch. Environ. Health* **14,** 693–697.

Schroeder, H. A., and Vinton, E. H., Jr. 1962. Hypertension induced in rats by small doses of cadmium. *Amer. J. Physiol.* **202,** 515–518.

Schroeder, H. A., Kroll, S. S., Little, J. W., Livingston, P. O., and Myers, M. A. G. 1966. Hypertension in rats from injection of cadmium. *Arch. Environ. Health* **13,** 788–789.

Schroeder, H. A., Nason, A. P., Prior, R. E., Reed, J. B., and Haessler, W. T. 1968a. Influence of cadmium on renal ischemic hypertension in rats. *Amer. J. Physiol.* **214,** 469–474.

Schroeder, H. A., Nason, A. P., and Mitchener, M. 1968b. Action of a chelate of zinc on trace metals in hypertensive rats. *Amer. J. Physiol.* **214,** 796–800.

Schroeder, H. A., Baker, J. T., Hansen, N. M., Size, J. G., and Wise, R. A. 1970. Vascular reactivity of rats altered by cadmium and a zinc chelate. *Arch. Environ. Health* **21,** 609–614.

Shaikh, Z. A., and Lucis, O. J. 1971. Isolation of cadmium-binding proteins. *Experientia* **27,** 1024–1025.

Shaikh, Z. A., and Lucis, O. J. 1972. Cadmium and zinc binding in mammalian liver and kidneys. *Arch. Environ. Health* **24,** 419–425.

Sporn, A., Dinu, I., and Stoenescu, L. 1970. Influence of cadmium administration on carbohydrate and cellular energetic metabolism in the rat liver. *Rev. Roum. Biochim.* **7,** 299–305.

Starcher, B. C. 1969. Studies on the mechanism of copper absorption in the chick. *J. Nutr.* **97,** 321–326.

Stowe, H. D., Wilson, M., and Goyer, R. A. 1972. Clinical and morphologic effects of oral cadmium toxicity in rabbits. *Arch. Pathol.* **94,** 389–405.

Stowe, H. D., Goyer, R. A., Medley, P., and Cates, M. 1974. Influence of dietary pyridoxine on cadmium toxicity in rats. *Arch. Environ. Health* **28,** 209–216.

Tsuchiya, K., and Sugita, M. 1971. A mathematical model for deriving the biological half-life of a chemical. *Nord. Hyg. Tidskr.* **53,** 105–110.

Vallee, B. L., and Ulmer, D. D. 1972. Biochemical effects of mercury, cadmium and lead. *Annu. Rev. Biochem.* **41,** 91–128.

Vander, A. J. 1962. Cadmium enhancement of proximal tubular sodium reabsorption. *Amer. J. Physiol.* **203,** 1005–1007.

Vigiliani, E. C. 1969. The biopathology of cadmium. *Amer. Ind. Hyg. Assoc. J.* **30,** 329–340.

Wilson, R. H., DeEds, F., and Cox, A. J., Jr. 1941. Effects of continued cadmium feeding. *J. Pharmacol. Exp. Ther.* **71,** 222–235.

Winge, D. R., and Rajagopalan, K. V. 1972. Purification and some properties of Cd-binding protein from rat liver. *Arch. Biochem. Biophys.* **153,** 755–762.

Wiśniewska-Knypl, J. M., and Jablońska, J. 1970. Selective binding of cadmium *in vivo* on metallothionein in rat's liver. *Bull. Acad. Pol. Sci. Ser. Sci. Biol.* **18,** 321–329.

World Health Organization. 1971 *International Standards for Drinking Water,* 3rd ed. World Health Organization, Geneva, p. 70.

Yoshikawa, H., Hara, N., and Kawai, K. 1960. Experimental studies on cadmium stearate poisoning. I. Dissociation curve and toxicity. *Bull. Natl. Inst. Ind. Health* **3,** 61–69.

CHAPTER 12

LEAD

INTRODUCTION

Lead is recognized as a highly toxic cumulative element in man and animals. During recent years in industrialized nations, long-time exposure to lead has been recognized as a health hazard. The effect of lead on heme synthesis is widespread and is of special interest to hematologists. Recent data indicate that the sources of lead are multiple, and that it affects biochemical and neuropsychological functions adversely.

BIOCHEMISTRY

Lead inhibits nearly all the enzymatic steps involved in heme synthesis. One of the primary effects of lead is on immature erythrocytes, the production of which appears to be increased by lead. Nearly all the blood lead is found in red cells. One clinical characteristic of plumbism is the appearance of basophilic stippled red cells in both bone marrow and peripheral circulation. These stippled cells contain mitochondria and therefore resemble reticulocytes. The stippling is due to the agglutination of ribosomes (Jensen *et al.,* 1965).

Lead inhibits the uptake of iron from transferrin by the reticulocyte. This inhibition is independent of the more direct adverse effect of lead on ferrochelatase that affects iron utilization (Morgan and Baker, 1969). There is also evidence that globin synthesis is inhibited in the presence of lead, but the mechanism is not known. An additional effect of lead is to decrease the life span of red cells by some unknown mechanism.

The initial reaction in heme synthesis (see Chapter 5, Fig. 6) is the combination of succinyl-CoA with glycine to form δ-aminolevulinic acid. This reaction is catalyzed by the enzyme δ-aminolevulinic acid synthetase (ALA-S), which is a mitochondrial enzyme. A major effect of lead is to inhibit this enzyme (Chisholm, 1964; Smith, 1976). The next step involves combination of the two ALA molecules into porphobilinogen. This reaction is catalyzed by the enzyme δ-aminolevulinic acid dehydrase (ALA-D) (a zinc-dependent enzyme) and is inhibited to an even greater extent by lead. This reaction occurs in the cytoplasm of the cell. The inhibition of this enzymatic step causes an increased urinary excretion and an increase in the blood level of ALA. This increase occurs even though ALA-S is also inhibited. The next step in the heme-synthesis pathway is a combination of four porphobilinogens to form coproporphyrinogen. These reactions occur extramitochondrially and are synthesized by the enzymes synthetase and cosynthetase. Although lead inhibits these steps as well, coproporphyrinogen excretion in the urine is increased. The next step is the conversion of coproporphyrinogen to protoporphyrin IX, which occurs intramitochondrially, catalyzed by an oxidase. The final step is the addition of ferrous iron to protoporphyrin to form heme, a reaction catalyzed by the enzyme ferrochelatase. Lead inhibits both ferrochelatase and ALA-D almost totally. Lead interferes with the incorporation of iron into the tetrapyrrole ring, resulting in its replacement by zinc. Consequently, increased levels of zinc protoporphyrin or its extraction product, free erythrocyte protoporphyrin, occur as a result of lead toxicity (Needleman, 1977). It is obvious that heme may not be synthesized either for the reason of an insufficient protoporphyrin due to lead toxicity or due to an inhibition in ferrochelatase.

Lead also affects other heme enzymes, notably cytochrome P_{450} in the liver (Alvares *et al.,* 1972). An adverse effect of lead on adenyl cyclase in brain and pancreas was recently observed (Nathanson and Bloom, 1975; Walton and Baldessarini, 1976; Needleman, 1977). A relatively low concentration of lead was demonstrated to affect collagen synthesis adversely (Vislica *et al.,* 1977). Lead inhibits certain ATPases and also inhibits lipoamide dehydrogenase, an enzyme crucial to cellular oxidation.

METABOLISM

Under normal conditions, 1–10% of the lead ingested is absorbed. The exact percentage depends on the chemical form of the lead, such as whether it is organically bound, tied up in insoluble oxides, or physically bound in a way that it is accessible only with difficulty, such as in large paint flakes. Obviously, more soluble forms are more readily absorbed than less soluble forms. Recent studies indicate, however, that a much higher rate of absorption might be present in children. Normal children may absorb as much as 50% of the ingested dose (Alexander, 1974).

The retention of inhaled lead is around 30–50%, and may be higher if the particle size is small. Lead has an adverse effect on iron deficiency, and iron deficiency increases the absorption of lead. These effects may be one of the causes for the apparent increase in lead burden in children with iron deficiency (Lin-Fu, 1973a,b; Mahaffey, 1974; Smith, 1976). This interaction of lead and iron, relating to absorption, is in addition to its effect on the iron uptake from transferrin by the reticulocytes and the inhibition of the enzyme ferrochelatase, which catalyzes the incorporation of iron into porphyrin. Another factor that can affect the absorption of lead is calcium. Recent studies indicate that more lead is absorbed in the presence of low calcium than in the presence of high calcium. This finding implies a competitive interaction between the two divalent cations lead and calcium. Increased lead absorption has been observed in the presence of low protein intake (Lin-Fu, 1973a,b; Mahaffey, 1974; Smith, 1976). Very high dietary levels of lead (0.5% lead as lead acetate) reduce plasma copper ceruloplasmin levels in rats, and decreased dietary copper levels have been associated with increased erythrocyte lead concentrations (Underwood, 1977).

Excess dietary zinc has been shown to be protective against lead toxicity in rats. This effect is mediated by an inhibition of lead absorption (Cerklewski and Forbes, 1976). A similar protective effect of excess zinc against lead toxicity was noted in young horses (Willoughby *et al.*, 1972).

Absorbed lead enters the blood and reaches the bones and soft tissues of the body. It is gradually excreted via the bile into the small intestine and eliminated in the feces. Approximately 97% of ingested lead is excreted in the feces and only 2% is excreted in the urine in calves (Underwood, 1977).

An increase in lead concentration occurs with age in human tissues under environmental conditions in the United States, indicating that excretion does not keep pace with total intake. In the rat, similar tissue accumulation of lead resulted in some loss of hair and body weight, although the life span was not affected.

The greatest subcellular accumulation of lead in the kidneys is found in the supernatant fraction, but lead also accumulates in the microsomal fraction and the mitochondria. Mitochondrial accumulation of lead in the kidneys is potentially harmful to normal renal function, because ADP-stimulated respiration in mitochondria is inhibited on incubation with lead.

The lead present in the soft tissues is readily mobilized by chelating agents, whereas the lead stored in bone is less easily released by such means. Increased levels of circulating corticosteroids and of parathormone enhance the mobilization of lead from bone. Release of lead from bone may also occur in pregnancy or due to trauma and infection. Lead can cross the placental barrier easily and thus affect the fetus.

LEAD TOXICITY

SOURCES OF EXPOSURE

Several investigators in the past believed that the only significant sources of increased lead ingestion were plaster, paint, or industrial exposure. This is probably true for acute poisoning with blood levels over 80 μg/

100 ml, in which symptoms of toxicity are seen. It is probably not true for subjects with signs of increased ingestion of lead who have lead levels between 40 and 80 μg/100 ml (Lin-Fu, 1973a,b; Smith, 1976).

Other potential sources of exposure include house dust, in which the lead content may vary between 65 and 1000 μg/g dust (Fairey and Gray, 1970; Haar and Aronow, 1974; Sayre *et al.,* 1974), and dirt. The lead content of dirt is usually higher in the inner city, near highways, around houses painted with lead paint, and in junkyards or other places where old batteries and other types of debris are found (Haar and Aronow, 1974). Airborne contamination with lead has been considered an important source, particularly in the vicinity of lead smelting, battery plants, or other industrial operations that involve lead (National Research Council, 1972). Although the importance of lead pollution arising from gasoline additives is under dispute, it has been decided that all new cars must use gasoline without lead-containing additivies, which would alleviate this problem within a few years. There is no question about the increased lead content of dirt and water near highways, which is most likely derived from tetraethyl lead from exhaust fumes (Smith, 1976).

Another source of lead is paper and newsprint (Lin-Fu, 1973a,b). This sourse could cause a problem in children who chew paper or make spitballs, or in other situations that might allow them to either ingest or have in their mouths newsprint or ink. Lead may also be available for ingestion from solder on cans (Mitchell and Aldous, 1974), particularly when acidic types of food are stored in the can at room temperature for a period of time after the can is opened. Tubes of toothpaste, which often contain lead, may contribute to lead ingestion by children, either by the direct chewing of the tube or from the lead being dissolved into the toothpaste (Berman and McKiel, 1972; Shapiro *et al.,* 1973).

None of these sources in itself, with the exception of the air around smelting and battery plants, is enough to cause acute toxic levels of lead, but all are likely to be involved in the cases in which evidence of increased lead burdens are found (Smith, 1976).

Mitchell and Aldous (1974) reported that canned baby foods may contain large amounts of lead. Canned evaporated milk may contain as much as 202 μg lead/liter, and canned fruit juices may average 100 μg lead/liter. The total daily intake of lead from dietary sources for an adult may range from 280 to 300 μg/day in the Western world.

CLINICAL FEATURES

The clinical symptoms of lead poisoning, when they develop, are similar whether it is so-called "acute" or "chronic" poisoning; chronic poisoning refers to prolonged exposure to lead. The symptomatology has been divided into alimentary, neuromuscular, and encephalopathic forms.

The symptoms that are common to all three are anemia, insomnia, headache, dizziness, irritability, and lead-line stippling of the gum. The alimentary form is also characterized by colicky pain. The neuromuscular form involves weakness of the muscle groups, with a characteristic wrist drop. In the encephalopathic form, which occurs primarily in children, the presenting manifestations include coma, convulsions, mania, or delirium. There is often a history of antecedent behavioral change, such as irritability, insomnia, restlessness, loss of memory, hallucinations, or confusion (Smith, 1976).

Damage to the central nervous system, causing lead encephalopathy and neuropathy, is a common feature of lead toxicity, particularly in children. Behavioral problems, intellectual impairment, and hyperactivity may be seen in children due to chronic lead poisoning (Needleman, 1977). The mechanism by which lead affects the central nervous system is obscure. Both impulse transmission and acetylcholine release are affected adversely due to lead toxicity. The DNA content of the cerebellum was found to be decreased in lead-intoxicated suckling rats (Underwood, 1977).

Anemia is a common feature of lead toxicity. The anemia is due to the adverse effect of lead on heme synthesis and also its adverse effect on copper and iron metabolism. Chronic lead toxicity is further manifested by renal tubular dysfunction with aminoaciduria and glycosuria. Lead exposure shortens the life span of rats and reduces their resistance to infections. Endocrine abnormalities such as decreased excretion of pituitary gonadotropic hormones, low thyroid uptake of radio iodine, and decreased response to exogenous ACTH were observed in a small number of lead-intoxicated patients due to drinking "moonshine" whiskey (Sandstead, 1973).

The effects of lead exposure during pregnancy include severe reproductive damage in occupationally exposed women, and lead has been found to be teratogenic in laboratory animals. Higher placental levels of lead were reported in malformed and stillborn fetuses in comparison with normal infants (Needleman, 1977).

DIAGNOSIS

The laboratory methods of detection most commonly used for screening populations for relatively high lead burdens involve the analysis of either blood or urine for certain precursor products of heme synthesis, or for lead itself.

A sensitive method is the measurement of ALA in either urine or serum (Chisholm, 1964; Haeger-Aronson, 1960; Robinson, 1974). Reports using this technique have demonstrated that there is a correlation between lead levels and ALA levels of lead workers (Haeger-Aronson, 1960; Robinson, 1974; Smith, 1976).

Analysis of free erythrocyte protoporphyrin is another very useful diagnostic procedure. Granick *et al.* (1972) and Piomelli *et al.* (1973) have developed micromethods that permit analysis of only 1–2 μl whole blood using a simple fluorometric procedure. Blood levels less than 80 μg/100 ml erythrocytes usually indicate very low lead exposure, whereas levels between 80 and 100 would be consistent with moderate lead exposure, and levels greater than 100 indicate more chronic lead exposure. The values can reach as high as 2000 μg/100 ml and correlate exponentially with lead levels (Smith, 1976).

A direct method for detecting lead toxicity is to assay whole blood for lead levels. There are several techniques available, but primarily the use of atomic absorption spectrometry has made this a very simple assay using small quantities of blood. It is normally considered that blood levels less than 40 μg/100 ml indicate a low lead burden, levels between 40 and 60 μg/100 ml indicate a moderate lead burden, and acute lead toxicity does not appear until 80–100 μg/100 ml whole blood (Smith, 1976).

TREATMENT

If the poison has been recently ingested, the stomach should be lavaged with warm water or 1% sodium sulfate solution. A saline cathartic, such as 30 g magnesium sulfate, should be given to flush the lead from the intestinal tract and reduce absorption. Eggwhite, milk, or other demulcents are also useful for this purpose (Arena, 1970).

To control colicky pain, calcium glutamate, 1 g, is given intravenously as a 10% solution. This may be repeated as necessary. Morphine sulfate, 15–30 mg, to control pain, may be given.

For chronic toxicity, versenate (calcium disodium edetate) should be administered. Calcium disodium versenate is the calcium chelate of ethylenediaminetetraacetic acid (EDTA). A 1-g ampule of "versenate" is diluted with 250–500 ml normal saline for intravenous administration. This is given as a drip for 1 hr, twice daily, for periods of up to 5 days. The treatment is interrupted for 2 days, following which another course is given for 5 days. For children, the dose is 0.5 g/30 lb body weight. The side effects of versenate include nephrotoxicity, hypokalemia, malaise, fatigue, thirst, numbness, tingling, fever, chills, headache, nausea, vomiting, sneezing, rhinorrhea, and thrombophlebitis (Arena, 1970).

A structural analogue of EDTA is diethylenetriamine pentaacetic acid (DPTA), which offers more promise than $CaNa_2EDTA$ in promoting excretion of Pb, Fe, Co, Zn, Cr, and Mn. It is given intramuscularly at intervals of 2 weeks with a dosage of 2–4 ml (0.5–1.0 g) of a 25% solution (Arena, 1970).

Other therapeutic agents include penicillamine (20–40 mg/kg per day), and BAL (British anti-lewisite) (4 mg/kg). A combination of BAL and EDTA may be more effective for the treatment of lead encephalitis. BAL is given alone initially and every 4 hr thereafter with EDTA (12.5 mg/kg) intramuscularly, at separate sites, for 5 days (Arena, 1970).

REFERENCES

Alexander, F.W. 1974. The uptake of lead by children in differing environments. *Environ. Health Perspect.* **7,** 155–159.

Alvares, A. P., Leigh, S., Cohn, J. and Kappas, A. 1972. Lead and methyl mercury: Effects of acute exposure on cytochrome P450 and the mixed function oxidase system in the liver. *J. Exp. Med.* **135,** 1406–1409.

Arena, J. M. 1970. *Poisoning: Toxicology—Symptoms—Treatments,* 2nd ed. Charles C Thomas, Springfield, Illinois, pp. 198–207.

Berman, E., and McKiel, K. 1972. Is that toothpaste safe? *Arch. Environ. Health* **25,** 64–65.

Cerklewski, F. L., and Forbes, R. M. 1976. Influence of dietary zinc on lead toxicity in the rat. *J. Nutr.* **106,** 689–696.

Chisholm, J. J., Jr. 1964. Disturbances in the biosynthesis of heme in lead intoxication. *J. Pediatr.* **64,** 174–187.

Fairey, F. S., and Gray, J W., III. 1970. Soil lead pediatric lead poisoning in Charleston, S. C. *J. S. C. Med. Assoc.* **66,** 79–82.

Granick, S., Sassa, S., Granick, J. L., Levere, R. D., and Kappas, A. 1972. Assays for porphyrins, delta-aminolevulinic acid dehydratase, and porphyrinogen synthetase in microliter samples of whole blood: Applications to metabolic defects involving the heme pathway. *Proc. Natl. Acad. Sci. U.S.A.* **69,** 2381–2385.

Haar, G. T., and Aronow, R. 1974. New information on lead in dirt and dust as related to the childhood lead problem. *Environ. Health Perspect.* **7,** 83–89.

Haeger-Aronson, B. 1960. Studies on urinary excretion of δ-aminolevulinic acid and other heme precursors in lead workers and lead-intoxicated rabbits. *Scand. J. Clin. Lab. Invest.* **12** (Suppl. 47), 1–128.

Jensen, W. N., Moreno, G. D., and Bessis, M. C. 1965. An electron microscopic description of basophilic stippling in red cells. *Blood* **25,** 933–943.

Lin-Fu, J. S. 1973a. Vulnerability of children to lead exposure and toxicity. Part I. *N. Engl. J. Med.* **289,** 1229–1233.

Lin-Fu, J. S. 1973b. Vulnerability of children to lead exposure and toxicity. Part II. *N. Engl. J. Med.* **289,** 1289–1293.

Mahaffey, K. 1974. Nutritional factors and susceptibility to lead toxicity. *Environ. Health Perspect.* **7,** 107–112.

Mitchell, D. G., and Aldous, K. M. 1974. Lead content of foodstuffs. *Environ. Health Perspect.* **7,** 59–64.

Morgan, E. H., and Baker, E. 1969. The effect of metabolic inhibitors on transferrin and iron uptake and transferrin release from reticulocytes. *Biochim. Biophys. Acta* **184,** 442–454.

Nathanson, J. A., and Bloom, F. E. 1975. Lead-induced inhibition of brain adenyl cyclase. *Nature (London)* **255,** 419–420.

National Research Council. 1972. *Biologic Effects of Atmospheric Pollutants: Lead. Airborne Lead in Perspective.* Committee on Biologic Effects of Atmospheric Pollutants, Division of Medical Sciences, National Research Council, National Academy of Sciences, Washington, D.C.

Needleman, H. L., 1977. Exposure to lead: Sources and effects. *N. Engl. J. Med.* **297,** 943–945.

Piomelli, S., Davidow, B., Guinee, V. P., Young, P., and Gay, G. 1973. The FEP (Free Erythrocyte Porphyrins) test: A screening micromethod for lead poisoning. *Pediatrics* **51,** 254–259.

Robinson, T. R. 1974. δ-Aminolevulinic acid and lead in urine of lead anti-knock workers. *Arch. Environ. Health* **28,** 133–138.

Sandstead, H. H. 1973. In: *Trace Substances and Environmental Health—6: Proceedings of the 6th University of Missouri Annual Conference,* p. 223.

Sayre, J. W., Charney, E., Bostal, J., and Pless, I.B. 1974. House and hand dust as a potential source of childhood lead exposure. *Amer. J. Dis. Child.* **127,** 167–170.

Shapiro, I. M., Cohen, G. H., and Needleman, H. L. 1973. The presence of lead in toothpaste. *J. Amer. Dent. Assoc.* **86,** 394–395.

Smith, J. L. 1976. Metabolism and toxicity of lead. In: *Trace Elements in Human Health and Disease,* Vol. II (A.S. Prasad, ed.). Academic Press, New York, pp. 443–452.

Underwood, E. J. 1977. *Trace Elements in Human and Animal Nutrition,* 4th ed. Academic Press, New York, pp. 410–423.

Vislica, D. T., Ahrens, F. A., and Ellison, W. R. 1977. The effect of lead on collagen synthesis and proline hydroxylation in the Swiss mouse 3 to 6 fibroblast. *Arch. Biochem. Biophys.* **179,** 15–23.

Walton, K. G., and Baldessarini, R. 1976. Effects of Mn^{++} and other divalent cations on adenylate cyclase activity in rat brain. *J. Neurochem.* **27,** 557–564.

Willoughy, R. A., MacDonald, E., McSherry, B. J., and Brown, G. 1972. Lead and zinc poisoning and the interaction between Pb and Zn poisoning in the food. *Canad. J. Comp. Med.* **36,** 348–359.

CHAPTER 13

MERCURY

INTRODUCTION

Mercury occurs widely in the biosphere. It is a toxic element that presents occupational hazards associated with both ingestion and inhalation. It is used extensively in industry and agriculture. The alkyl derivatives of mercury are more toxic than other chemical forms and can enter the food chain through the activity of microorganisms with the ability to methylate the mercury present in industrial wastes (Underwood, 1977).

The various forms of mercury can be classified as "inorganic" and "organic" (Table XXVI). Inorganic mercury consists of metallic mercury and of the dissociable salts of mercurous and mercuric mercury. Mercury present in molecules in which it is linked directly to a carbon atom is referred to as "organic" mercury. The short-chain alkyl mercurials and the aryl- and alkoxyalkyl mercurials belong in this category. The anion in Table XXVI is depicted as chloride. A large variety of anions may be found in combination with the mercury cation, but have little effect on its toxic properties (Clarkson, 1976).

The physicochemical classification of mercury does not correlate well with its toxic properties. For example, the toxicity of metallic mercury vapor differs distinctly from that of the mercurous and mercuric salts. The signs and symptoms of poisoning due to phenylmercury compounds differ from those due to exposure to the short-chain alkyl mercurials. Toxicologically speaking, the short-chain alkyl mercurials occupy a unique position. They cause irreversible damage to the central nervous system and are fetotoxic. Exposure to metallic mercury vapor may also cause damage to the nervous system, but usually these changes are reversible, especially at lower exposures. There is no evidence that metallic vapor is toxic to the fetus. Exposure to inorganic mercury as well as to the aryl- and alkoxyalkyl compounds leads to accumulation of mercury in the kidneys, the primary

Table XXVI. Organic and Inorganic Forms of Mercury[a]

Inorganic	
Metallic	Hg^0
Mercurous salts	Hg_2Cl_2
Mercuric salts	$HgCl_2$
Organic	
Alkylmercury compounds	CH_3HgCl
Arylmercury compounds	C_6H_5HgCl
Alkoxarylmercury compounds	CH_3OCH_2HgCl

[a]From Clarkson (1976).

target organs. Involvement of the central nervous system with these classes of compounds is minimal.

BIOCHEMISTRY AND METABOLISM

Inorganic mercury compounds are relatively poorly absorbed. Taguchi (1971) reported, 73, 45, and 6% absorption of mercury in rats after administration of methylmercury chloride, phenylmercuric acetate, and mercuric acetate, respectively. Following absorption, the inorganic, aryl-, and methoxyalkyl mercury compounds behave similarly, due to the rapid degradation of the two latter forms to inorganic mercury. Simple alkyl forms of mercury are not only better absorbed, but are also better retained, more firmly bound in the tissues, and induce higher brain mercury contents than aryl mercury compounds (Underwood, 1977).

Simple alkyl mercury compounds and other mercurials also differ in their excretory pattern. With methylmercury, much of the biliary mercury is present as a methyl mercury–cysteine complex, most of which is reabsorbed, whereas with other mercurials, mercury is excreted via the bile and the feces in inorganic or protein-bound form.

The placenta presents an effective barrier against the transfer of inorganic mercury in rats, but the transfer of methylmercury to the fetus greatly exceeds that of either mercuric chloride or phenylmercuric acetate in mice (Underwood, 1977). According to Taguchi (1971), over 20% of the methyl-mercury administered to the pregnant rat can be transferred to the fetus, with a tendency for this mercury to accumulate in the brain.

Methyl forms of mercury do not occur in animal cells and tissues in significant amounts, unless ingested or injected as such. In other words, the animal body has an extremely limited capacity to convert inorganic and various organic forms of mercury into the more toxic methyl forms. This ability to transform mercury is confined to microorganisms, and it is their activity that can introduce methylated mercury compounds into the food chain (Underwood, 1977).

The main mercury-binding protein in rat kidney cytosol is a stable metallothioneinlike protein. The mercury-binding capacity of the thioneins is extremely high, and zinc and cadmium have been completely displaced from metallothionein from rat liver *in vitro*. A nonhistone protein component into which mercury is rapidly incorporated was also isolated from rat kidney (Underwood, 1977).

A mutual antagonism between selenium and mercury is known to exist, and selenium is known to be protective against mercury toxicity in rats and Japanese quails (Ganther *et al.,* 1972). The biochemical mechanism responsible for this antagonism is not known. Selenium does not ameliorate or prevent methylmercury toxicity by increasing the rate of methylmercury breakdown. Selenium appears to effect a redistribution of mercury in the body.

Mercury appears to suppress the mitochondrial oxidative phosphorylation in the rat kidney. This inhibition may be directly correlated with the death of the animal due to mercury toxicity.

MERCURY TOXICITY

The toxicity of metallic mercury vapor and of methylmercury compounds shows remarkable species differences. For example, the pigeon is able to withstand an atmosphere of mercury vapor approximately 100 times greater than that which produces adverse effects in humans (Armstrong *et al.,* 1963). Species differences in sensitivity to methylmercury are of the order of 10- to 100-fold (Berglund *et al.,* 1971). Data on human exposure to both methyl and metallic mercury are now available, since large numbers of people have been exposed to these forms of mercury in the past, resulting in many cases of poisoning. Such studies are of considerable importance from the public health point of view, since it is likely that occupational exposure to metallic mercury vapor and exposure to methylmercury compounds in food (particularly food containing fish and fish products) will continue (Clarkson, 1976).

In man at low exposures to metallic mercury vapor, there was a significant (10–50 $\mu g/m^3$) increase in complaints of loss of appetite (Smith *et al.,* 1970). It was not until the exposure rose to 240 $\mu g/m^3$, however, that the frequency of objective tremors showed a sharp increase. Indeed, the classic triad of symptoms of mercurialism—tremor, erethism, and gingivitis—appears only at exposures higher than 240 $\mu g/m^3$. In the study by

Smith *et al.* (1970), the symptoms of loss of appetite and the complaint of loss of weight were the first to appear.

There is no general agreement as to the lowest air level of mercury that produces detectable adverse effects. Russian workers (Friberg and Nordberg, 1973) claimed to see effects at very low concentrations of mercury vapor in air (on the order of 10 $\mu g/m^3$). This claim is based primarily on subjective symptoms in workers, with all the attendant difficulties of quantifying these effects. On the other hand, the objective signs associated with mercurialism do not occur until air levels are substantially above 100 $\mu g/m^3$. It is the concentration range from 10 to 100 $\mu g/m^3$ about which there is so much controversy at this time over possible adverse health effects (Clarkson, 1976).

Quantitative studies on the toxicity of methylmercury were reported recently from an outbreak of methylmercury poisoning in Iraq (Bakir *et al.*, 1973). This outbreak, which involved over 6000 cases admitted to hospital, was due to the ingestion of homemade bread prepared from wheat that had been treated with a methylmercury fungicide. People ingested contaminated bread for a period of about 2 months, after which signs and symptoms of methylmercury poisoning developed. The signs and symptoms were essentially similar to those described in previous cases of methylmercury poisoning (Berglund *et al.*, 1971), and included paresthesia, ataxia, constriction of the visual fields, slurred speech, and hearing difficulties. At body burdens of approximately 0.5–1.0 mg Hg/kg body weight, all the signs and symptoms of poisoning were evident, while at lower body burdens, only a few of these signs and symptoms were exhibited (Clarkson, 1976). The effects of methylmercury were first evident with the symptoms rather than the objective signs. For example, paresthesia, which was a complaint of loss of sensation or tingling in the extremities of the hands and feet or around the mouth, was the first effect due to methylmercury. Paresthesia is a nonspecific symptom with respect to methylmercury, and might be caused by a variety of other agents or disease states. According to Clarkson (1976), the true threshold point at which the effects of methylmercury become detectable could lie anywhere between 0.5 mg and 0.8 mg Hg/kg body weight.

Studies of the distribution of tracer doses of radioactive methylmercury in man allow a rough calculation of the chronic daily intake of methylmercury from food necessary to produce a body burden on the order of 0.5 mg/kg. A steady daily intake of between 280 and 420 μg/day might be expected to yield a body burden in the range of about 25 mg in a 70-kg adult. These figures would compare with an average daily intake in the general population of less than 20 μg/day (Berglund *et al.*, 1971; Clarkson, 1976).

FACTORS THAT AFFECT THE TOXICITY OF MERCURY IN MAN

Many factors can influence the toxicity of mercury. Studies on animals have indicated that the length of exposure to methylmercury plays an important role in determining the outcome of adverse effects. Berglund *et al.* (1971) point out that most studies on the toxicity of methylmercury in animals have not been carried out long enough to determine the lowest toxic dose. Chronic daily exposures continuing for weeks or months are necessary in most species, followed by an extensive latent period, before the first signs of poisoning appear. The stage of the life cycle at which exposure occurs can also be a decisive factor in determining the lowest toxic dose. Animal studies suggest that the prenatal stage of life may be most sensitive to insult from methylmercury (Clegg, 1971). The administration of mercury-binding compounds can result in a reduction in the toxicity of mercury. In the case of methylmercury, the administration must take place before irreversible damage to the nervous system has occurred. In effect, these mercury-binding agents modify the toxicity of mercury by effectively reducing the dose. More recent work indicates, however, that other types of interactions with chemicals are possible that result in a modification of the toxicity of mercury (Clarkson, 1976).

The period of exposure to methylmercury in the outbreak in Iraq was about 2–3 months (Bakir *et al.,* 1973). Assuming a 70-day clearance half-time from the body, the body burden would remain elevated for a period of about 1 year after the end of exposure. Thus, the victims of mercury poisoning in Iraq experienced an exposure period of not more than 15–18 months (Clarkson, 1976).

Blood levels of mercury in fishermen and shore workers in American Samoa employed in a fish canning factory were recently reported (Clarkson, 1976). Most of the fishermen had blood levels less than 100 ng/ml, but some had blood levels in the range of 100–200, and one fisherman had a blood level of 218 ng Hg/ml. The shore workers had blood levels that were substantially lower, though still considerably higher than the normal level found on the North American continent. The shore workers had a median blood level in the range of 20–40 ng/ml, with most of the workers being substantially below 100 ng/ml. The highest recorded blood level was 140 ng/ml.

The distribution in hair generally followed that observed in blood, except that the absolute level in hair was about 300 times higher. Most of the fishermen had hair levels below 30 μg/g, although some had levels as high as 55 μg/g. The shore workers had levels substantially lower than those seen in the fishermen, with most falling below 10 μg/g, and all below 25 μg/g (Clarkson, 1976). The clinical data in these studies indicated that no signs or symptoms were attributable to methylmercury exposure in the fishermen. Only one of the fishermen complained of a mild aching in his limbs, but this was attributed to a brain stem lesion of an undetermined type.

These results suggest that length of exposure is not an important factor in determining response to methylmercury in humans. It must also be admitted, however, that these data on the Samoan fishermen suffer from the weakness that only a few fishermen had blood levels in the range associated with signs and symptoms in the Iraq study. The majority of the fishermen and all the shore workers except one had blood levels lower than 100 ng/ml. This is more than a factor of 2 below the minimum threshold effect noted in Iraq (Clarkson, 1976).

The relationship between length of exposure and toxicity of metallic mercury vapor is not known. Occupational exposures can vary from days or weeks to periods of 10–20 years or more. Information is also lacking on the kinetics of elimination of mercury from man following exposure to metallic mercury vapor. The rate of elimination cannot be the same immediately following a single dose as that seen after long-term chronic exposure (Clarkson, 1976).

EFFECTS OF PRENATAL AND EARLY POSTNATAL EXPOSURE TO METHYLMERCURY

The effects of prenatal exposure to methylmercury and early postnatal exposure to ingestion of methylmercury by breast-fed infants were observed in the Iraq study (Clarkson, 1976). Iraqi infants are usually breast-fed for the first 2 years of life. They usually begin to consume some solid foods at about the age of 1 year. Thus, infants born in the 6 months just prior to the consumption of the contaminated bread by the mother had exposure to methylmercury only in breast milk. Infants older than this would receive mercury not only from breast milk, but possibly also by eating some contaminated bread.

The concentration of mercury in one infant blood was noted to decline at a slower rate than that of the mother. At first, the infant's blood was lower than that of the mother, but later, infant blood mercury levels were usually higher than those seen in the mother. The primary reason for this lower rate of decline in infant blood level was the continued ingestion of methylmercury from mother's milk. Although the milk levels were significantly lower than the blood level, the daily intake of methylmercury from milk could make a substantial difference in the overall methylmercury balance in the infant. Methylmercury was excreted only slowly from the body (in adults, 1% of the body burden was excreted per day); thus, a small intake could significantly affect blood levels of methylmercury (Clarkson, 1976).

Despite the slower decline in methylmercury levels in the infant than in the mother, no signs of methylmercury poisoning were seen in infants who had received only postnatal exposure to methylmercury. Most infants received methylmercury only from milk, but some infants may have received additional mercury from contaminated bread. Despite blood levels as high as 1000 ng/ml, no signs of poisoning were evident at this early stage after exposure. It is possible that signs of methylmercury poisoning may manifest themselves as the infants get older (Clarkson, 1976).

A group of 15 infant–mother pairs in which prenatal exposure had occurred was the subject of a report by Amin-Zaki *et al.* (1974b). Clinical evidence of methylmercury poisoning was evident in 6 of the 15 mothers and in at least 6 of the 15 infants. Of the 6 infants, 5 were severely affected, suffering from gross impairment of motor and mental development. There was only one case in which the infant had signs of methylmercury poisoning and the mother was free of signs and symptoms herself. This is in marked contrast to the report from Minamata (Harada, 1966), in which evidence was presented that 21 infants were born suffering from severe cerebral palsy, whereas the mothers were free from or exhibited only minimal signs and symptoms of methylmercury poisoning. The reason for this difference is not known, but the Japanese infants were examined several years after birth, while the preliminary report on Iraq was based on studies within approximately 6 months of the outbreak. Mercury levels in the blood of infants and mothers were not reported in the cases of prenatal poisoning in Japan (Clarkson, 1976).

The ultimate question on the relative sensitivity of prenatal vs. adult life has not been settled by the Iraq data. The possibiity that the infants prenatally exposed and those postnatally exposed from milk may develop problems in mental and physical development at a later stage in life cannot be excluded at present (Clarkson, 1976). Careful long-term follow-up studies on the infants exposed to methylmercury in Iraq are needed.

There are no reports in the literature of prenatal poisoning due to exposure to metallic mercury vapor. Substantial numbers of females of childbearing age have been and still are employed in industries in which occupational exposure occurs. The absence of reports of prenatal poisoning therefore suggests that metallic mercury vapor may not present a significant hazard to prenatal life. Nevertheless, we do not know how carefully such effects have been looked for in exposed populations (Clarkson, 1976).

Studies on animals reported by Clarkson *et al.* (1972) indicate that metallic mercury vapor may cross into the fetus much more rapidly than ionic mercury. The mercury content of the fetus is 10 times higher following exposure to metallic mercury than after a similar dose of mercury chloride. In contrast, the accumulation of ionic mercury in the placenta is much higher than that after exposure to metallic mercury vapor. When the mercury level in the fetus is compared to that in maternal blood, the distinction between the two forms of mercury is even more dramatic. The fetal tissue/maternal blood ratio is about 60 times higher after exposure to metallic vapor than after an equivalent dose of mercury chloride (Clarkson, 1976).

The preferential transport of metallic vapor vs. ionic mercury across the placenta parallels the same type of selectivity in the case of the blood–brain barrier. Metallic mercury vapor produces adverse effects primarily on the central nervous system, whereas ionic inorganic mercury affects primarily the kidneys and gastrointestinal tract. The preferential transport of metallic vapor into the fetus warrants further studies on possible fetotoxic effects (Clarkson, 1976).

INTERACTION OF MERCURY WITH OTHER CHEMICALS

Except for reports of patients given mercury-complexing agents, no information is available in man on the interaction of other chemicals with mercury compounds. Studies by Ganther *et al.* (1972) on rats and Japanese quails suggest that the presence of selenium in the diet can diminish or at least delay the toxic effects of methylmercury compounds. The mechanism of this interaction is unknown. If it could be demonstrated that selenium is also protective in man, the significance would be considerable. Certain species of oceanic fish, such as tuna, which are a source of methylmercury in the diet, also contain quantities of selenium that could diminish the hazard from methylmercury (Clarkson, 1976).

On contact with blood and tissues, metallic mercury vapor is oxidized to ionic mercury (Clarkson, 1972, 1976). On entering the alveolar spaces of the lung, metallic mercury vapor rapidly crosses the pulmonary membranes and dissolves in blood. The dissolved vapor rapidly crosses into the red cell, where it is oxidized to ionic mercury. The process of oxidation is believed to be enzyme-mediated, and Kudsk (1972) speculated that catalase might be the enzyme involved. Despite transport into and oxidation within red blood cells, sufficient metallic mercury remains dissolved within the bloodstream so that appreciable amounts are present when the blood passes by the blood–brain barrier, allowing diffusion of metallic vapor into the brain. In this tissue, it is believed to be oxidized to ionic mercury. Once transformed into the ionic form, mercury rapidly reacts with protein SH groups and is retained in the tissue (Clarkson, 1976).

The retention and deposition of metallic mercury vapor can be influenced by other chemicals, probably through inhibition of the oxidation process. Ethanol and the herbicide 3-amino-1,2,4- triazole, chemicals that have no obvious structural similarities, both produce similar and dramatic effects on the retention and distribution of mercury following exposure to metallic mercury vapor. Kudsk (1965) observed that the retention of mercury was dramatically diminished in workers ingesting moderate amounts of alcohol under conditions of occupational exposure to metallic mercury vapor (Clarkson, 1976).

In experimental animals, although the retention of methylmercury in lungs and liver was reduced due to alcohol ingestion, the opposite effect was seen in the brain. Thus, it would appear that blood levels of mercury may give misleading information in people who have ingested alcohol.

Aminotriazole produces effects essentially similar to alcohol except that the levels in blood are not influenced to the same extent. This herbicide is an inhibitor of the enzyme catalase, and it may be that both alcohol and amino-triazole inhibit this enzyme, which may be responsible for the oxidation of elemental mercury vapor. These changes in the retention and deposition of mercury following exposure to alcohol or aminotriazole indicate the potential for modifying the toxic effects of this form of mercury. However, no studies have yet been reported measuring the effects of these chemicals on the toxicity of inhaled vapor (Clarkson, 1976).

TREATMENT OF MERCURY POISONING

Acute Poisoning with Inorganic Mercury

Serious illness results from ingestion of 0.5 g mercuric chloride, but the illness is not fatal. Ingestion of 1.0 g is fatal in 50% of cases; of 1.5 g in all cases.

In cases of acute ingestion, the stomach should be washed with a 5–10% solution of sodium formaldehyde sulphoxylate, and treatment of shock or loss of electrolytes should be instituted as the need arises in individual patients (Arenas, 1970; Bidstrup, 1964).

BAL (British anti-lewisite; 2,3-dimercaptopropanol) should be administered as follows: initial dose of 300 mg i.m., followed by 150 mg in 2 hr, 150 mg in 4–6 hr, 1 or 2 doses of 150 mg in the next 12 hr, and thereafter 150 mg twice daily for 1 or 2 days (Arenas, 1970; Bidstrup, 1964).

Chronic Poisoning with Inorganic Mercury

The symptoms of chronic toxicity include lassitude, anorexia, weight loss, metallic taste, and nephrotic syndrome. The treatment consists of the administration of $CaNa_2$-EDTA, 3 g daily i.v., for 5 days. This course is repeated as necessary. The other drug of choice is *N*-acetyl-DL-penicillamine, which is given in a dosage of 250 mg four times daily for 10 days. This course may be repeated after an interval of 2–3 weeks, as indicated by the patient's condition (Arenas, 1970; Bidstrup, 1964).

Poisoning with Organic Mercury Compounds

Symptomatic treatment should be given. BAL is of no value in acute poisoning; it may have some beneficial effect in chronic cases, since there may be some inorganic mercury remaining in tissues that may be removed and excreted. The patient must be removed from further exposure. Physiotherapy, exercise, and speech therapy may have to be instituted for rehabilitative purposes (Arenas, 1970; Bidstrup, 1964).

REFERENCES

Amin-Zaki, L., Elhassani, S., Majeed, M. A., Clarkson, T. W., Doherty, R. A., and Greenwood, M. R. 1974a. Studies of infants postnatally exposed to methylmercury. *J. Pediatr.* **85,** 81–84.

Amin-Zaki, L., Elhassani, S., Majeed, M. A., Clarkson, T. W., Doherty, R. A., and Greenwood, M. R. 1974b. Intrauterine methylmercury poisoning in Iraq. *Pediatrics* **54,** 587–595.

Arenas, J. M. 1970. *Poisoning: Toxicology—Symptoms—Treatments,* 2nd ed. Charles C Thomas, Springfield, Illinois, pp. 105–109.

Armstrong, R. D., Leach, L. J., Belluscio, P. R., Maynard, E. A., Hodge, H. C., and Scott, J. K. 1963. Behavioral changes in the pigeon following inhalation of mercury vapor. *Amer. Ind. Hyg. Assoc. J.* **24,** 366–375.

Bakir, F., Damluji, S. F., Amin-Zaki, L., Murtadha, M., Khalidi, A., Al-Rawi, N. Y., Tikriti, S., Dhahir, H. I., Clarkson, T. W., Smith, J. C., and Doherty, R. A. 1973. Methylmercury poisoning in Iraq. *Science* **181,** 230–241.

Berglund, F., Berlin, M., Birke, G., Cederlöf, R., von Euler, U., Friberg, L., Holmstedt, B., Jonsson, E., Lüning, K. G., Ramel, C., Kerfving, S., Swensson, A., and Tejning, S. 1971. Methyl mercury in fish: A toxicologic–epidemiologic evaluation of risks: Report from an expert group. *Nord. Hyg. Tidskr.* (Suppl.) **4,** 1–364.

Bidstrup, P. L. 1964. *Toxicity of Mercury and Its Compounds.* Elsevier, London, pp. 1–112.

Clarkson, T. W. 1972. Recent advances in the toxicology of mercury with emphasis on the alkylmercurials. *CRC Crit. Rev. Toxicol.* **1,** 203–234.

Clarkson, T. W. 1976. Quantitative measures of the toxicity of mercury in man. In: *Trace Elements in Human Health and Disease,* Vol. II (A.S. Prasad, ed.). Academic Press, New York, pp. 453–475.

Clarkson, T. W., Magos, L., and Greenwood, M. R. 1972. Transport of elemental mercury into fetal tissues. *Biol. Neonate* **21,** 239–244.

Clegg, D. J. 1971. Embryotoxicity of mercury compounds. In: *Mercury in Man's Environment* (Royal Society of Canada, ed.). Royal Society of Canada, Ottawa, pp. 141–148.

Friberg, L., and Nordberg, G. 1973. Inorganic mercury—a toxicological and epidemiological appraisal. In: *Mercury, Mercurials, and Mercaptans* (M. W. Miller and T. W. Clarkson, eds.). Charles C Thomas, Springfield, Illinois, pp. 5–23.

Ganther, H. E., Goudie, C., Sunde, M. L., Kopecky, M. J., Wagner, P., Oh, S. H., and Hoekstra, W. G. 1972. Selenium: Relation to decreased toxicity of methylmercury added to diets containing tuna. *Science* **175,** 1122–1124.

Harada, Y. 1966. Study on Minamata disease. In: *Minamata Disease* (M. Katsuma, ed.). Kumamoto University, Japan, pp. 93–117.

Kudsk, F. N. 1965. Absorption of mercury vapor in the respiratory tract in man. *Acta Pharmacol. Toxicol.* **23,** 250–262.

Kudsk, F. N. 1972. Biological oxidation of elemental mercury. In: *Mercury, Mercurials and Mercaptans* (M. W. Miller and T. W. Clarkson, eds.). Charles C Thomas, Springfield, Illinois, pp. 350–371.

Smith, R. G., Vorwald, A. J., Patil, C. S., and Mooney, T. F., Jr. 1970. Effects of exposure to mercury in the manufacture of chlorine. *Amer. Ind. Hyg. Assoc. J.* **31,** 687–701.

Taguchi, Y. 1971. Studies on microdetermination of total mercury and the dynamic aspects of methyl mercury compound *in vivo*. II. Behavior of low concentrated methyl mercury compound *in vivo*. *Nippon Eiseigaku Zasshi (Jpn. J. Hyg.)* **25,** 563–573.

Underwood, E. J. 1977. *Trace Elements in Human Health and Nutrition,* 4th ed. Academic Press, New York, pp. 375–387.

INDEX

BILL & MIEKO ANDRESS
1757 ~~25421~~ HARDT STREET
LOMA LINDA, CA 92354
714-796-9450